ANESTHETIC MANAGEMENT OF DIFFICULT AND ROUTINE PEDIATRIC PATIENTS

SECOND EDITION

ANESTHETIC MANAGEMENT OF DIFFICULT AND ROUTINE PEDIATRIC PATIENTS

SECOND EDITION

Edited by

FREDERIC A. BERRY, M.D.

Professor
Departments of Anesthesiology and Pediatrics
University of Virginia School of Medicine
University of Virginia Health Sciences Center
Charlottesville, Virginia

CHURCHILL LIVINGSTONE
New York, Edinburgh, London, Melbourne

Library of Congress Cataloging-in-Publication Data

Anesthetic management of difficult and routine pediatric patients /
  edited by Frederic A. Berry. — 2nd ed.
    p.   cm.
    Includes bibliographical references.
    Includes index.
    ISBN 0-443-08678-8
    1. Pediatric anesthesia.   I. Berry, Frederic A., date
    [DNLM: 1. Anesthesia—in infancy & childhood.   WO 440 A5796]
RD139.A56   1990
617.9'6798—dc20
DNLM/DLC
for Library of Congress   90-2312
                                                       CIP

Second Edition © Churchill Livingstone Inc. 1990
First Edition © Churchill Livingstone Inc. 1986

Distributed in the United Kingdom by Churchill Livingstone, Robert Stevenson House, 1–3 Baxter's Place, Leith Walk, Edinburgh EH1 3AF, and by associated companies, branches, and representatives throughout the world.

Accurate indications, adverse reactions, and dosage schedules for drugs are provided in this book, but it is possible that they may change. The reader is urged to review the package information data of the manufacturers of the medications mentioned.

The Publishers have made every effort to trace the copyright holders for borrowed material. If they have inadvertently overlooked any, they will be pleased to make the necessary arrangements at the first opportunity.

Copy Editor: *Ann Ruzycka*
Production Designer: *Gloria Brown*
Production Supervisor: *Sharon Tuder*

Printed in the United States of America

First published in 1990

TO MY FAMILY

Suzanne, Fritz, Hayden, and Alex,
and all the other families of health-care providers
who unselfishly support us

CONTRIBUTORS

Frederic A. Berry, M.D.
Professor, Departments of Anesthesiology and Pediatrics, University of Virginia School of Medicine, University of Virginia Health Sciences Center, Charlottesville, Virginia

Raeford E. Brown, Jr., M.D.
Assistant Professor and Head, Section of Pediatric Anesthesia, Department of Anesthesiology, and Assistant Professor, Department of Pediatrics, The Bowman Gray School of Medicine of Wake Forest University, Winston-Salem, North Carolina

Roderick K. Calverley, M.D.
Clinical Professor, Department of Anesthesiology, University of California, San Diego, School of Medicine, San Diego, California

Charles G. Durbin, Jr., M.D.
Associate Professor, Departments of Anesthesiology and Surgery, University of Virginia School of Medicine, University of Virginia Health Sciences Center, Charlottesville, Virginia

Mark M. Harris, M.D.
Assistant Professor, Departments of Anesthesiology and Neurosurgery, University of Virginia School of Medicine, University of Virginia Health Sciences Center, Charlottesville, Virginia

Madelyn D. Kahana, M.D.
Assistant Professor, Departments of Anesthesiology and Pediatrics, University of Cincinnati College of Medicine, Children's Hospital Medical Center, Cincinnati, Ohio

Fred Koch, M.D.
Assistant Professor, Department of Anesthesiology, University of Virginia School of Medicine, University of Virginia Health Sciences Center, Charlottesville, Virginia

David J. Steward, M.D., F.R.C.P. (C)
Professor, Department of Anaesthesiology, University of British Columbia Faculty of Medicine; Anaesthetist-in-Chief, British Columbia's Children's Hospital, Vancouver, British Columbia, Canada

Douglas F. Willson, M.D.
Assistant Professor, Departments of Anesthesiology and Pediatrics, University of Cincinnati College of Medicine, Children's Hospital Medical Center, Cincinnati, Ohio

Andrew M. Woods, M.D.
Associate Professor, Department of Anesthesiology, University of Virginia School of Medicine, University of Virginia Health Sciences Center, Charlottesville, Virginia

PREFACE

This book was written for the purpose of sharing the clinical experiences and practices of a group of anesthesiologists in the management of the everyday problems of pediatric patients and some of the more difficult problems of a referral center.

A second purpose is to convey three important goals and how they may be met. The first goal is the peaceful separation of the patient and parents. It is said that the surgical experience affects not only the child, but the entire family. There is no such thing as "stress-free" surgery for the family. This is why we encourage the presence of the parents during the induction of anesthesia. In addition, the parents are thus given the opportunity to meet with the anesthesiologist. Another technique for the peaceful separation of parent and child is the use of premedication. The second goal is to provide postoperative comfort. Use of narcotics and regional anesthetic techniques are, of course, the first steps in controlling postoperative discomfort. However, it must be recognized that the presence of the parents in the recovery room is effective adjunctive therapy, as they can help to make the transition to consciousness smoother by their comforting familiarity. The recovery room also presents another opportunity for the anesthesiologist to meet with the parents. The third goal is to create and maintain a safe anesthesiology practice.

This book is not meant to be as basic and encompassing as Gregory's *Pediatric Anesthesia* or a handbook such as Steward's *Manual of Pediatric Anesthesia,* but somewhere in between. Controversial areas are discussed and our preferences given. This book is intended for the anesthesiology resident and student CRNA and the practicing anesthesiologist and CRNA.

We present here an extensive revision of the material in the first edition. In particular, the area of pain management and regional anesthesia has been expanded in keeping with the interests and needs of the pediatric patient.

Frederic A. Berry

CONTENTS

1

A MAGNIFICENT HERITAGE: THE HISTORY OF PEDIATRIC ANESTHESIA

Roderick K. Calverley
David J. Steward

Pediatric anesthesia has passed through two important periods in its history: a century of gradual change followed by four decades of almost explosive growth. There are anesthesiologists still in practice who have seen pediatric anesthesia evolve from the simple but hazardous routines of "rag and bottle" to the complexities of modern practice. The recent advances reviewed in the chapters that follow are all based on the achievements of earlier American, British, Canadian, and European pioneers whose contributions deserve our attention.

I became interested in the history of pediatric anesthesia during my residency, when I began to appreciate the rapid evolution of anesthetic practice. The anesthetics I was being taught to deliver were strikingly different from those I had received as a child, observed as a medical student, or provided as a general practitioner. My first experience of anesthesia came when I was 12. My anesthetist was a nun whose kind eyes captured my attention as she covered my mouth and nose with a gauze-covered metal mask. I smelled a strange odor. After my eyes closed I was still aware of her soft voice and the gentle caress of her fingers on my cheek. While some older patients have distasteful memories of their first anesthetic, the scent of ether still arouses in me a memory of her kind attention.

As a medical student in 1958 I followed the hospital course of a child distressed with acute otitis media and watched his myringotomy. The anesthesiologist began by proposing an imaginary journey to outer space as he positioned a metal mask a few inches over the boy's face. Within 5 minutes the administration of vinethane was completed. The child awoke in a moment to call out happily, "I've been to the moon!" I was captivated by the mystery of that anesthetic.

Later I learned firsthand of some of the hazards that the pioneers of anesthesia had overcome, and came to respect their mastery of clinical skills. As interns we had been instructed in the use of halothane by mask, but when I worked for a medical charity in a small, isolated hospital in southern Afghanistan in 1965, no anesthetists or modern anesthetics were available. Through my ignorance of an exceptionally potent drug, my first induction with ethyl chloride suffered from an overly enthusiastic rate of administration. My young patient became apneic and pulseless within 2 minutes but, to my profound relief, recovered promptly.

These experiences helped me appreciate the skills of the pioneers of pediatric anesthesia. They had mastered inhalation anesthesia without access to the devices that are now available to protect our patients from harm. Modern pediatric anesthesia was shaped by men and women who challenged adversity, overcame severe problems, and left us a great heritage. It has been a pleasure to explore this history by studying early accounts as well as by corresponding with and interviewing some of our forerunners and their students.

NINETEENTH CENTURY

No comprehensive accounts of pediatric anesthesia appeared in the nineteenth century. One finds only fragmentary comments by anesthetists and other physicians that show their reactions to newly discovered anesthetic drugs and, in time, an increasing knowledge of their action. Modern readers, however, can never learn every important detail of any one case from induction to recovery. While many intriguing questions remain unanswered, the reports of early anesthetists give us respect for their skills.

Diethyl Ether

Pediatric anesthesia ended a grotesque ordeal for children and parents. While many patients came to operations already in pain, elective pediatric surgery antedated the discovery of surgical anesthesia. Attempts to repair clubfoot, cleft lip, and cleft palate without anesthesia were recorded by Indian, European, and North American surgeons. By 1842 some writers partially corrected strabismus by tenotomy, as it had been realized that early surgery could preserve vision by the affected eye.

A child was among the first patients to experience an inhalation anesthetic. On July 3, 1842, Crawford W. Long's second subject was Jack, an 8-year-old boy, whom he anesthetized with ether dropped onto a towel for the amputation of a toe. Long reported that "the operation was performed without the boy evincing the least sign of pain."[1]

Other early accounts of pediatric anesthesia appeared in 1847. The first of these was James Robinson's book, *A Treatise on the Inhalation of the Vapour of Ether*. His youngest dental patient, an 8-year-old boy, gave an enthusiastic opinion of his anesthetic. "When he recovered he said... that he had been in heaven or somewhere else, for he had been exceedingly comfortable and happy."[2] While this patient might have complained of a painful tooth, Robinson's book also featured five descriptions of strabismus corrections performed under anesthesia. In the same year John Snow observed, "Children are, indeed, amongst the most favourable subjects for ether, recovering from its effects as promptly as they are brought under its influence, and it possesses more than the usual advantages in their cases, as, without it, their struggles would often interfere with the performance of the operation."[3]

Chloroform

John Snow's last book, *On Chloroform and Other Anaesthetics*, contained an important pharmocokinetic observation and reports of anesthesia for infants:

> The effects of chloroform are more quickly produced and also subside more quickly in children than in adults, owing no doubt to the quicker breathing and circulation. . . . I have given chloroform in a few cases as early as the ages of eight and ten days, and in a considerable number before the age of two months; and I have at this time, June 30th, 1857, memoranda of the cases of 186 infants under a year old to whom I have administered this agent. There have been no ill effects from it either in these cases, or in those of children more advanced in life; and it is worthy of remark that none of the accidents from chloroform which have been recorded, have occurred to young children.[4]

Despite his unqualified endorsement, John Snow was aware of the hazards of chloroform overdosage, which would come to be more widely appreciated many years later. He described a near-fatality from his own experience in which a surgeon accidentally pressed a chloroform-soaked sponge to the nostrils of a 6-year-old child. Although the child recovered, Snow noted that there was "no doubt that in this case the heart was paralyzed, or nearly so, by the chloroform. . . ."[4]

The safety of chloroform for children continued to be debated for decades. In 1867 Giraldes, a French surgeon, wrote: "I wish to protest against the immunity [from accidents due to chloroform] which people are disposed to attribute to childhood. That immunity does not exist."[5] A decade later a fanciful rebuttal was presented by Bergeron of Paris: "Chloroform is perfectly safe for children and infants and may be used from the day of birth. It owes its safety in part to the absence of all moral influences."[6] A century later it is difficult to recognize the relationship which Bergeron perceived between toxicity and morality, but his opinion was accepted by some colleagues.

In 1901 Frederic Hewitt, the first person to be knighted for services to anesthesia (which included a chloroform anesthetic for King Edward VII), wrote a more balanced assessment:

> Chloroform . . . is certainly inhaled with comparative ease by children. . . . It is a mistake, however, to suppose that children are not so susceptible as adults to the toxic effects of this agent and that with them fatalities are practically unknown. . . . Children may be rescued from conditions of respiratory and circulatory depression which in adults would be attended by a more immediate risk to life . . . [however] more fatalities . . . have been recorded than might be imagined.[7]

In 1894 James Guthrie, an astute British pediatrician, proved that children were susceptible to the hepatic toxicity of chloroform.[8] He presented case reports of postchloroform jaundice causing nine deaths in young children. As the hepatic and cardiovascular complications of chloroform became more widely appreciated, the drug gradually fell from use.

Ethyl Chloride

When anesthetists experimented with ethyl chloride during the last years of the nineteenth century, they were surprised by the rapid inductions that could be achieved. After anesthetizing a child George Lotheissen wrote: "We were astonished when after one minute, without any trace of preceding excitement, complete anaesthesia was established and the operation could be begun immediately. Scarcely was the mask removed than the patient opened her eyes and after a few seconds was completely herself and would not believe that the operation could be over so soon."[5]

The success of ethyl chloride anesthesia prompted the creation of a variety of masks for its administration. While some devices were of complex construction, others consisted of only a paper cone. Aristide Malherbe of Paris recommended a technique employing a handkerchief that was both simple and yet safer than a large mask. He folded a handkerchief into his hand, which was held "deeply hollowed to avoid too great an evaporating surface."[5] Malherbe's appreciation of the hazard of overdosage demonstrated excellent clinical judgment. With only chest or abdominal compression as methods of artificial respiration, carelessness during induction was sometimes fatal. Ethyl chloride continued to be used, most commonly as an induction agent for children, until halothane was marketed.

The Child Anesthestist of 1877

While many nineteenth-century anesthetists attended children, none became a pediatric anesthetist exclusively. In 1877 a child of 12 became his surgeon-father's anesthetist, and could be considered the first "pediatric anesthetist." The younger of the famous Mayo brothers, Charles Mayo gave his first anesthetic while his father, William Worrall Mayo, operated in a patient's home near Rochester, Minnesota. His older brother reported: "In the midst of the operation, the doctor who was giving the anesthetic fainted. Charlie climbed up onto a cracker box and gave the anesthetic, and he did it so well that from that time on he was the family anesthetist."[9]

TWENTIETH CENTURY
The First Decades

The first American text in the speciality, James T. Gwathmey's *Anesthesia*, was published in 1914. This encyclopedic study contains many valuable accounts of the pediatric techniques of that period. Unfortunately, most of this information was left scattered throughout several chapters and was not collected into a single discussion. This deficiency persisted for more than 30 years as other American authors neglected to prepare a separate chapter describing anesthesia for children. This oversight would frustrate the studies of residents and medical students for decades.

Inductions: "Steal the Child" With "a Sleepy Wind"

With the exception of rectal ether, almost every induction of that time required a mask technique that might be vigorously resisted by the child. To achieve a calm induction, Gwathmey counseled a gentle approach. "Infants should preferably be anesthetized in the mother's or nurse's arms. Care should be taken in anesthetizing children to make the operation as informal as possible. . . . Mental suggestion here plays a great part, as well as gentleness in voice and movement. . . . Immediately calling the child by the first name, puts them at their ease at once."[10]

A child's rejection of the unpleasant odor of some anesthetics could be avoided by disguising the smell. British anesthetists often added an inexpensive perfume to ethyl chloride. Although this might improve the patient's acceptance of the drug, the persistence of the scent exposed the anesthetist to an unexpected postanesthetic risk: anesthetists sometimes returned to their homes unaware that they still reeked of cheap perfume. Occasionally this aroused a wife's suspicions, which brought accusations that the anesthetist had spent his day in loose company. In America James Gwathmey encouraged another approach to achieve the same purpose. He added a few drops of the essence of bitter orange to mask the anesthetic without risking unwanted domestic repercussions. Some specialists have recently rediscovered Gwathmey's approach and camouflage anesthetic odors with fruit flavors.

Arthur Guedel advocated a clever induction technique in 1921. He counseled, "Steal the child."[11] This inventive specialist began with the mask concealed in his hand, which was held several inches over the child's face before it was lowered slowly to increase the inspired concentration without stress or struggle.

Another considerate approach was practiced by a British contemporary, Dr. Steven Coffin of London (Coffin S, personal communication). When Dr. Coffin entered practice in 1919, nitrous oxide inductions were popular. He realized that, although children welcomed soothing phrases, he must be careful to select an expression that could not be misinterpreted. He was concerned that a child might equate the instruction "to go to sleep" with the demise of a pet or the gloomy possibilities suggested in a line of a children's prayer, "If I should die before I wake." Dr. Coffin learned to offer nitrous oxide as "a sleepy wind," with much greater comfort to his young patients. His phrase "a sleepy wind" is still used by some English anesthetists. One of Dr. Coffin's warmest memories was of receiving a brief note from a young girl that thanked him for "a lovely wind."

Status Lymphaticus

Not every anesthetic ended happily. If a death occurred during surgery, the diagnosis of "status lymphaticus" was sometimes invoked to explain unexpected cardiorespiratory collapse. Some physicians assumed that this was due to hyperplasia of the thymus and other lymphatic structures. While a causal relationship was never proven, the postmortem diagnosis of "status lymphaticus" was widely accepted for many years.

James Gwathmey, who published an extensive review in 1914, wrote: "The majority of writers are agreed that a positive diagnosis of this condition during life is very difficult Most patients dying during or immediately after anesthesia have been young people or children, of flabby type, with enlarged adenoids, tonsils, thyroid (usually), high-arched palate, small mouth and throat, and weak heart sounds. During anesthesia a grayness of complexion or pallor is witnessed, with weak heart action and shallow breathing."[10] His suggestions for treatment stressed cardiac massage and artificial respiration. Gwathmey was not convinced of the existence of "status lymphaticus," for he concluded his discussion by supporting Yandell Henderson's belief that a poorly administered anesthetic was more often the cause of death than was status lymphaticus or heart disease.

The unfortunate cost of this erroneous belief was that the responsibility for death was placed on the patient rather than on the person who administered the anesthetic. While some clinicians were relieved of liability by this diagnosis of convenience, others questioned its existence. In 1939 Arthur Guedel wrote: "This may or may not be. Some investigators claim there is something to the condition, but just as many claim there is not. . . . Certainly status lymphaticus is at times a great help to the anesthetist. When he has a fatality under anesthesia with no other cleansing explanation he is glad to recognize the condition as an entity."[12]

As anesthetic care improved, status lymphaticus gradually disappeared from consideration. In 1948 Digby Leigh and Kathleen Belton stated, "If this calamity was not seen once in 18,000 anesthetics given to infants and children, then it is difficult to draw any other conclusion than that status lymphaticus is a diagnosis which covers a multitude of anesthetic or surgical sins."[13]

The history of this persisting myth demonstrates a recurrent danger—the power of an erroneous belief to prevent the admission of ignorance. If status lymphaticus had not provided a ready excuse for failure, a more forthright examination of deaths during surgery might have prompted better anesthetic care. We look back to "status lymphaticus" with bemusement but recognize that we may still be prisoners of other misconceptions.

Regional Anesthesia

The development of procaine and other synthetic local anesthetics increased the popularity of regional anesthesia. Although local anesthetics were often reserved for adults, who might be expected to be more cooperative, a few American surgeons used regional or infiltration anesthesia routinely for small children.

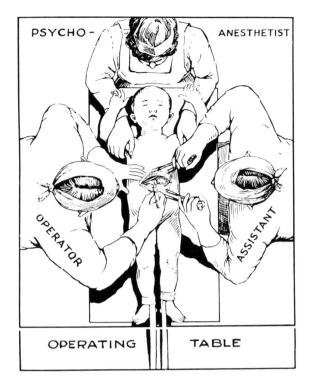

Fig. 1-1. Abdominal surgery in children: anesthetic technique and comfort with restraint. The child rests upon the arm-table, with pillow and sterile cotton pad. Gauze bandages are anchored to the cotton-padded ankles and to the operating table. The psychoanesthetist grasps the child's arms, controlling the child. The surgeon and his assistant sit on opposite sides. The operating table converts into an instrument table. (Modified from Farr,[14] with permission.)

The greatest enthusiast of this practice was the Minneapolis surgeon Robert Emmett Farr, whose 1923 text, *Practical Local Anesthesia*, contains fascinating photographs taken from his now-lost movies of surgical procedures on awake patients under local anesthesia. Much of Farr's work employed a high-volume, continuous-infiltration technique for both abdominal and extremity surgery in patients of all ages. In contrast with the authors of other regional anesthesia texts, Farr stressed his dependence on the support of an anesthetist by giving her a unique title. Even when supplemental inhalation anesthesia was not required, his "psycho-anesthetist" comforted and diverted his younger patients (Fig. 1-1).[14] "Upon opening the abdomen a condition of negative pressure is most desirable and the psychoanesthetist can be of great aid in bringing this about. Provided the child struggles or strains between the moment at which the peritoneum is incised and the stage when the incision is securely blocked by the dislocated pylorus, the small intestine may be extruded, complicating the procedure, embarrassing the surgeon and necessitating the introduction of long, narrow salt packs."[14]

Pediatric Anesthetic Literature

After 1920 students of pediatric anesthesia could find occasional articles to guide their practice. A well-constructed discussion was provided in 1925 by Charles Robson, the first Anesthetist in Chief of The Hospital for Sick Children,

Toronto. Robson described techniques to meet the challenges of pyloric obstruction, bronchoscopy, and the induction of anesthesia for a trauma patient with a full stomach. He emphasized the need for control of the airway and advocated that "every anesthetist should be able to pass an endotracheal catheter, by the sense of touch in any patient under anesthesia."[15] Since pediatric laryngoscopes had not been invented, Robson intubated by palpation.

In 1923 control of the airway had been encouraged in the first pediatric anesthesia text, *Anaesthesia in Children*, by C. Langton Hewer of St. Bartholomew's Hospital, London. Hewer stated, "The endo-tracheal method is probably the safest possible way of administering a general anesthetic, as a perfect airway is assured, and in the event of any untoward occurrence the lungs can be instantly inflated with pure oxygen."[16] This technique could not be applied routinely, however, for Magill's pediatric tubes had not yet been marketed.

While Hewer's book deserves admiration for his astute clinical observations, the 31 illustrations of his text reveal a major failing in pediatric practice of that time. Each picture shows equipment in sizes appropriate only for adults. Except for some small metal masks, pediatric equipment was not available commercially.

The Development of Pediatric Equipment

Ayre's T-Piece

The frustrations produced by inadequate apparatus persisted but eventually were to prompt an important advance in 1937. Before that time pediatric anesthesia had been what Philip Ayre of Newcastle-upon-Tyne described as "a protracted and sanguine battle between surgeon and anaesthetist with the poor unfortunate baby as the battlefield."[17] Ayre introduced his T-piece by saying: "In an endeavour to remedy the above distressing state of affairs (and spurred on by the caustic criticism of a candid surgeon!), the writer sought to devise a method by which the endotracheal technique could still be utilized without . . . drawbacks. . . . The following method is simple in the extreme, and has proved highly satisfactory."[18] Ayre's T-piece was an ingenious, lightweight, valveless non-rebreathing method for intubated patients. He first prepared the T-piece for use in neurosurgery, but it found its widest early application in cleft palate repairs. Philip Ayre's own speech was distorted by a cleft palate, which limited this great teacher's ability to address a large audience. He found pleasure, however, in recording the great number of variations that extended the applications of his original simple design.

Jackson Rees's Modification of the Ayre's T-Piece

After the Second World War the pace of development accelerated. A significant alteration was Gordon Jackson Rees's modification of the Ayre's T-piece to permit better control of ventilation.[19] Rees had conducted early studies of the use of muscle relaxants for pediatric anesthesia at the Alder Hey Hospital near Liverpool and had become dissatisfied with the pattern of controlled ventilation provided by the periodic obstruction of the outflow tube of the T-piece. In 1950 Rees extended the outflow limb and added an open-ended breathing bag, which could be used to monitor spontaneous ventilation or to control ventilation manually. This circuit maintains a wide popularity.

American and Canadian Anesthesia Circuits

At that time many American anesthetists favored rebreathing circuits employing soda-lime for carbon dioxide absorption. Waters' to-and-fro cannister, an early American innovation, proved to be awkward to use for infants. Within two decades of Brian Sword's successful reintroduction of the adult circle system in 1930, several American pediatric circle systems were developed.

After the Second World War anesthetists could choose from among the Adriani, Ohio, Mayo Clinic, Leigh, and Bloomquist circle systems. One of the limitations of the circle system was the effort demanded of the infant to overcome the valves. This could be corrected by the Revell circulator, which created a functionally valveless circuit with reduced resistance.[20]

Other North American innovations were non-rebreathing circuits employing unidirectional valves. Two early models came from the Montreal Children's Hospital and were designed for spontaneously breathing patients. The metal Leigh valve was improved by the substitution of lightweight rubber discs, thus creating the Stephen-Slater valve. Since these devices obliged the anesthetist to use both hands when controlling ventilation, they were eventually superseded by the Fink, Frumin, and Lewis-Leigh valves. While now rarely employed, these valves led to the development of the Rueben, Ambu, and Laerdal valves, which are now standard features of resuscitation devices.

Precordial and Esophageal Stethoscopes

Precordial monitoring had been developed by Harvey Cushing and his anesthetist, Griffith Davis, at the Johns Hopkins Hospital in 1907. The device had been almost forgotten for many years until its routine use in pediatrics was advocated by Robert M. Smith of Boston. Albert Codesmith, a Canadian contemporary at The Hospital for Sick Children, Toronto, launched an important new departure in 1954 by creating an esophageal stethoscope. He had become frustrated by the repeated dislodging of the chest piece under the surgical drapes and set about fabricating his first esophageal stethoscope from urethral catheters and soft rubber drains. His brief report not only reviewed the technique of its production but also heralded its clinical role as a monitor of both normal and adventitious respiratory and cardiac sounds.[21]

Pediatric Laryngoscopes

Many laryngoscopes used for children are miniature forms of adult blades, but the Seward laryngoscope, with its flat blade, was designed specifically for infants. Edgar Seward's motivation came when he was an obstetrical house officer in England and was called upon to resuscitate infants. "I can remember on occasion intubating a baby with pen torch (flashlight) in my mouth and a teaspoon handle acting as the tongue spatula. So I saw a need for a special laryngoscope...and created the blade." His account reminds us of a common theme: inventiveness often arises from frustation. As Dr. Seward observed, "The way to improve things is to give the task to a lazy chap, overwork him, and don't give him the tools to do the job." (Seward EH, personal communication.)

Mechanical Ventilators

Mechanical ventilators were used only rarely in the operating room before 1960. A major impetus to their development arose in 1952 during an international epidemic of poliomyelitis, when large numbers of patients required controlled ventilation. Since the need exceeded the limited supply of "iron lungs," teams of medical students and other volunteers provided continuous manual ventilation. British, Scandinavian, and American engineers, responding to the need, developed mechanical ventilators.

At first these machines were built only for adults, but several innovators, including Codesmith of Toronto, adapted these machines for pediatric use. One of the first British machines designed for infants was Jackson Rees' modification of a Starling pump. Doreen Vermuelen Cranch, an early pioneer of anesthesia in the Netherlands, encouraged the development of a miniature ventilator. Another early machine was created in South Africa as investigators provided long-term ventilation for infants with neonatal tetanus.

Anesthesia Masks

In 1960 Leslie Rendell-Baker recognized that pediatric masks needed improvement, for they contained a large dead space and often did not fit well (Rendell-Baker L, personal communication). He and a dental associate, Donald Soucek, created casts of the faces of intubated infants and young children. They used the casts to create masks that closely approximated the facial contours of their models. These masks were also modified to situate the orifice for the adapter directly over the patient's nose, which improved ventilatory exchange.

Their introduction of the Rendell-Baker masks marked an important advance in the standardization of pediatric anesthesia equipment. On the insistence of Ralph Tovell the diameter of the mask orifice was set at 22 mm so that the mask would fit standard adult breathing systems. Rendell-Baker and his associates of the American National Standards Institute designed the mask adapter so that it could be used for both the mask and the endotracheal tube.

Endotracheal Tubes

Sir Ivan Magill created some of the first endotracheal tubes for children and infants. Red-rubber Magill tubes of uniform internal diameter were the standard from 1930 until they were replaced by plastics.

Other endotracheal tubes had been designed for specialized purposes prior to the era of plastics. Philip Woodbridge and Ralph Tovell developed armored tubes that featured an internal coiled wire to prevent kinking when the patient's neck was flexed. In 1945 Frank Cole created tapered tubes to reduce the high airway resistance of long, narrow tubes in infants. His first tube was formed by cementing the tracheal segment of a 3.5-mm tube to the broader shaft of a 5.5-mm tube.[22] Cole tubes were routinely used in infant resuscitation and surgery. Some years later it was argued that the shoulder of the Cole tube prevented accidental endobronchial intubation, but errors in placement still occurred.

The introduction of plastic endotracheal tubes in 1959 came through the work of Mr. David Sheridan and other engineers (Sheridan D, personal communication). Pediatric anesthetists are also indebted to Mr. Sheridan for his development of the centimeter markings along the length of plastic tubes, which allow accurate placement of the tube within the trachea. Many clinicians believe that this has reduced the frequency of both accidental extubation and unintentional endobronchial intubation.

Pediatric Specialists

The growth of pediatric anesthesia was not confined to the development of apparatus. Anesthesiologists crossed several physiologic frontiers. Merel Harmel, Austin Lamont, and William McQuiston pioneered anesthesia for congenital heart surgery. Controlled hypotension, elective hypothermia, and cardiopulmonary bypass allowed surgeons to mend complex lesions that had previously been beyond repair. Research studies by James Eckenhoff, Virginia Apgar, Stanley James, Ernest Salanitre, Herman Rackow, and others gave all clinicians a better understanding of the special anesthetic needs of infants and children.

This great collection of information was transmitted to residents by dedicated teachers. While some clinician-instructors are remembered only by their students, a few wrote superb books that gained wide attention. The first widely popular text appeared in 1948. *Pediatric Anesthesia*, by Digby Leigh and Kathleen Belton, became an international classic.

The history of modern pediatric anesthesia can be discovered by anyone who reviews Leigh and Belton's books and those written by other early specialists, including Robert Smith, Ronald Stephen, and Harold Davenport. They deserve study by every student of pediatric anesthesia for they record a magnificent heritage: the coming of age of pediatric anesthesia.

EPILOGUE

For many years pediatric anesthesia was practiced using techniques that evolved "because they worked." Early texts on pediatric anesthesia recommended practices that to the author were found to be satisfactory in use or seemed to be the most approppriate in light of available general medical knowledge. It was not until the 1960s that any systematic approach to clinical investigation in pediatric patients came into use. Since that time we have increasingly been able to base our anesthesia practice on scientifically validated facts.

One of the joys of the historian is to be able to look back at the writings of the pioneers and relate their practical wisdon to current thoughts and practice. The first book on pediatric anesthesia published in North America, that authored by Digby Leigh and Kathleen Belton in 1948,[13] is a magnificent storehouse of such wisdom. On page 6, in the section dealing with preoperative preparation, the following passage can be seen: "In older children, breakfast is omitted if the operation is in the morning. For afternoon operations, a light breakfast is allowed but lunch is forbidden. . . . All patients are given clear fluids freely up to one hour before their journey to the operating room." Since that time, how many children have been needlessly subjected to prolonged periods of preoperative oral fluid restriction? Now, over 40 years later, we are just beginning once again to appreciate that oral fluids can indeed be safely given to children in the later preoperative period. A recent study has shown that the volume and acidity of the stomach contents of healthy children are not significantly different following 6, 4, or 2 hours of preoperative fasting.[23] Another recent study has demonstrated that adminstered fluids are rapidly cleared from the child's stomach.[24] On the basis of these and similar studies the trend in many pediatric centers is now to return to a more liberal approach to oral fluid administration—in fact to return to a routine that was suggested in 1948!

Leigh also anticipated by more than two decades some recent thoughts on the management of the preterm infant. Writing in the "Question the Experts" section of the journal, *Anesthesia and Analgesia*, in 1961 on the subject of intubation of the premature infant he stated: "First they should be anesthetized with cyclopropane, then they should be given succinylcholine 0.5–1 mg intramuscularly, then they should be intubated."[99] He evidently appreciated the need to provide anesthesia and analgesia to even the smallest infants for any potentially distressing procedure, a need that has only recently been generally accepted by all anesthesiologists.[25]

Robert Smith, in his book, *Anesthesia for Infants and Children*, first published in 1959,[26] laid the foundations for many of our routines of safe patient care. He was most concerned that patients should be carefully monitored: he stressed the need for the regular use of simple devices, such as the precordial stethoscope, but also envisioned the eventual everyday application of "oximeters, carbon dioxide analysers and electroencephalographs." Smith was also most concerned that the psychological considerations of pediatric anesthesia must be observed. He wrote: "In children old enough to have fear or apprehension the emotional factor may be an even greater source of concern than the child's physical condition. . . . Psychic preparation is considered first because when possible this is started before the child enters the hospital." Over the years since this has been written many studies of the hospitalized child have confirmed the wisdom of the approaches that were suggested by Smith.

Now that we can base much of our practice on the results of recent reputable clinical studies we might tend to ignore the writings of our predecessors. It will be a pity if we do this. History is fascinating, and may provide us with many a new idea.

REFERENCES

1. Long CW: An account of the first use of sulphuric ether by inhalation as an anaesthetic in surgical operations. South Med Surg J 5:705, 1849
2. Robinson J: A Treatise on the Inhalation of the Vapour of Ether for the Prevention of Pain in Surgical Operations. Webster & Co., London, 1847, p. 16 (reprinted by Bailliere Tindall, Eastbourne, 1983)
3. Snow J: On the Inhalation of the Vapour of Ether. Churchill, London, 1847, p. 28 (reprinted by Lea & Febiger, Philadelphia, 1959)
4. Snow J: On Chloroform and Other Anaesthetics. Churchill, London, 1858, pp. 49, 258–259
5. Duncum B: The Development of Inhalation Anaesthesia. Oxford University Press, London, 1947, pp. 341, 502, 512
6. Bergeron A: Chloroform in children (summary). Pac Med Surg J 18:440, 1876
7. Hewitt F: Anaesthetics and Their Administration. Macmillan, London, 1901, p. 116
8. Ellis RH (ed): W. Stanley Sykes Essays on the First Hundred Years of Anaesthesia, Vol. III. Churchill Livingstone, Edinburgh, 1982, pp. 136–149
9. Keys TE, Key JD: An overlooked tribute for Dr. William Worrall Mayo. Minn Med 67:375, 1984
10. Gwathmey JT: Anesthesia. Appleton, New York, 1914, pp. 327, 332
11. Guedel AE: Unpublished Personal Papers. Guedel Anesthesia Center, San Francisco
12. Guedel AE: Inhalation Anesthesia: A Fundamental Guide. MacMillan, New York, 1937, p. 129
13. Leigh MD, Belton MK: Pediatric Anesthesia. MacMillan, New York, 1948, p. 206
14. Farr RE: Practical Local Anesthesia. Lea & Febiger, Philadelphia, 1923, p. 492
15. Robson CH: Anesthesia in children. Curr Res Anesth Analg 4:240, 1925
16. Hewer CL: Anesthesia in Children. Paul B. Hoeber, New York, 1923, p. 70
17. Obituary of T. Philip Ayre. Br Med J 280:125, 1980
18. Ayre TP: Anaesthesia for hare-lip and cleft palate operations on babies. Br J Surg 25:131, 1937
19. Rees GJ: Anaesthesia in the newborn. Br Med J ii:1419, 1950
20. Revell DG: A circulator to eliminate mechanical dead space in circle absorption systems. Can Anaesth Soc J 6:98, 1959
21. Codesmith A: An endo-oesophageal stethoscope. Anesthesiology 15:566, 1954
22. Cole F: A new endotracheal tube for infants. Anesthesiology 6:87, 1945
23. Farrow-Gillespie A, Christensen S, Lerman J: Effects of fasting interval on gastric pH and volume in children. Anesth Analg 67:S59, 1988
24. Sandhar BK, Goresky GV, Shaffer EA, Strunin L: Preoperative fasting in children: How long is enough? Can J Anaesth 35:S141, 1988
25. Berry FA, Gregory GA: Do premature infants require anesthesia for surgery? Anesthesiology 67:291, 1987
26. Smith RM: Anesthesia for Infants and Children. CV Mosby, St. Louis, 1959

2

GENERAL PHILOSOPHY OF PATIENT PREPARATION, PREMEDICATION, AND INDUCTION OF ANESTHESIA

Frederic A. Berry

Physicians often ask what is the best premedication or what is the best induction technique. It is difficult to separate and isolate these issues without considering the place each holds in the anesthetic continuum. The anesthetic continuum includes the psychological preparation of the child and the family, the option of premedication, the induction technique, and postoperative analgesia. All of these factors need to be considered when planning an anesthetic. Although each must be addressed on an individual basis, there should be an overall plan for maintaining continuity within the anesthetic continuum.

THE PSYCHOLOGICAL PREPARATION OF THE CHILD AND THE FAMILY

To help prepare the child and the family psychologically for surgery, the anesthesiologist must recognize that the entire family is undergoing the mental stress of the surgery, even though the infant or child alone will undergo the operation. There is no such thing as "stress-free" surgery for the family. One of the signs of our times is our reliance on the concept of cause and effect: if an infant or child has a problem, there must be a cause. That thought is followed by another one: since there is a cause, it must be the "fault" of the parents. There are two major types of surgical problems in infants and children: congenital defects and acquired defects. Regardless of the type of surgical problem, the parents are made to feel guilty, and the mother often takes the larger share of the blame. "She" caused the problem through smoking, dietary indiscretion, medications, alcohol, or even some evil thought. In the case of acquired defects (accidents, infections, malignancies, and the like) the same sort of cause-and-effect thinking is brought to bear on the parents, and they are sometimes made to feel guilty about a situation that might or might not have been avoidable.

Regardless of the part the parents may have played in the problem, the time of surgery is not the time to heap guilt feelings upon the parents. There is a need during the surgical period to discuss with parents their emotions, because they feel guilty whether or not they had a direct or preventable part in causing the problem. If the parents did contribute to the cause, for example, by failing to put their child in a safety belt, then their guilt feelings need to be addressed in a compassionate manner so that they can begin to psychologically adjust— not only to the immediate care of their child but also to the long-term implications for the family. The ability of the anesthesiologist to communicate empathy and understanding is part of the art of medicine, and its practice is not limited to nurses, surgeons, and pediatricians. A simple statement to the parents such as "I know this must be tough for you" will often transmit our understanding and feelings, and open the avenues of communication.

Anesthesia and surgery represent a time of enormous stress for the child. The reasons for the stress are many but include:

1. Separation from parents
2. Strange surroundings
3. Painful procedures
4. Frightening procedures
5. Fear of dying

Examples of frightening procedures are computed tomography (CT) and magnetic resonance imaging (MRI). A plain CT scan without the injection of contrast material or MRI is a nonpainful procedure, but it certainly is frightening. This is particularly true for children under 5 years of age who have watched Saturday morning cartoons. They may see great similarities between being strapped on a scan table and slowly propelled through a small hole into a loud machine and Minnie Mouse being tied to the railroad tracks while an oncoming train thunders toward her.

Coping with the stresses and pain of the medical experience requires honest communication. This communication needs to be established between all members of the surgical and medical team, the parents, and the child. The younger the child, the more the communication is directed toward the parents. The older the child, the more the communication is directed toward the child. The methods of communication are "multifocal." Through our language, attitude, and touch we let the family and child know we care. The current practice of insurance companies of not allowing patients to be admitted the day before surgery except in exceptional circumstances has greatly interfered with establishing these lines of communication. There is no question but that insurance companies have limited their priorities to cost while the concept of the emotional well-being has been relegated to ancient history.

The experience of surgery and hospitalization may be a growing experience for children because they may learn how to deal with a stressful or painful experience. However, for a young child who is unable to communicate and unable to understand, the situation may be completely negative. It can also be negative for an older child who is able to understand, but the situation is not adequately explained, or much worse, not explained truthfully. This latter problem occurs in either of two ways: (1) the parents do not understand the situation and consequently are unable to communicate the true picture to the child, or (2) the physician or parents attempt to avoid upsetting the child because they are afraid the child cannot cope. Accordingly, they tell a little white lie: "It won't hurt." It doesn't take the child long to find out the truth. The child feels betrayed, and this damages the credibility of the parents and the entire medical team.

Some trauma is avoidable, such as unnecessary tests and unnecessary separation from the parents. Some trauma is unavoidable, however, but with care and concern it can be made less painful. An example of this is the use of local anesthesia whenever a painful procedure, such as a spinal tap, bone marrow biopsy, IV placement, or arterial sampling, has to be done. A reason often given for not using local anesthesia is that "the local hurts as much as the procedure." This is an erroneous line of thinking that admits a lack of clinical skill with local anesthetics and a failure to understand the pain and discomfort of these procedures. Administered slowly with a small needle, a local anesthetic will cause only very slight burning. The child is told what to expect and then distracted by the parent or the nurse. Some well-meaning physicians tell children that it is like a "bee sting." Bee stings are quite painful, much more so than the injection of local anesthesia, and children may become upset at the thought of a bee sting. I tell them it is like a "pinch," and then gently pinch them on the back of the hand to demonstrate the discomfort. Then I tell them to take a deep, deep breath and hold it as the local anesthetic is slowly injected. A recent addition to the bag of tricks for the anesthesiologist is EMLA cream. This cream is a eutectic mixture of lidocaine and prilocaine that can penetrate intact skin.[1] A eutectic mixture is a compound that has a lower melting point than any of its ingredients. EMLA cream has to be applied under an occlusive dressing 1 hour before venipuncture.

Children have a host of fears when they approach surgery. The appreciation and understanding of the fears are based on age. Young children are most concerned about the separation from their parents. With the development of memory comes the fear of pain in the form of needles or procedures. As children grow older, fear of the unknown becomes prominent as well. They are uncertain about what to expect. Older adolescents fear loss of self-determination and loss of dignity. A group of factors help us identify the child who is most at risk for problems with their surgical experience:

1. Age
2. Duration of hospitalization
3. Previous hospital experiences
4. Home and parental support

5. Type of surgery
6. Type of medical problem

Of all these factors, age is probably the most important.

Approach to the Patient Based on Age

Steward has developed a categorization of age that is very useful in identifying the various problems for anesthesia and surgery[2]:

1. 0 to 6 months
2. 7 months to 4 years
3. 4 to 6 years
4. 6 years to adolescence
5. Adolescence

0 to 6 Months

From 0 to 6 months is the age of maximum stress for the parents and least stress for the patient because the infant is not old enough to understand or remember. Called "the Golden Age of blissful ignorance," it is a period when the infant trusts almost everyone. There is no particular need for sedative premedication. The major premedication need at this age is an anticholinergic in the form of oral or intravenous glycopyrrolate. The induction technique for these infants is the choice of the anesthesiologist. If the infant has an IV, then an intravenous induction is used; if the infant does not have an IV, then an inhalation induction is used.

7 Months to 4 Years

Seven months to four years is the most vulnerable age for the child emotionally because the child's separation anxiety is at its maximum. There are certainly great differences among children and their ability to separate from their parents but as an age group this is the most difficult age. Another problem with this age group is that the child is becoming or already is old enough to remember, particularly if there have been negative experiences, but not old enough to understand the need for surgery.

One may wonder why most of the surgery for congenital defects is done at this time, but there are many positive reasons why this is necessary. Most major and minor surgery is done at this age because physiologically, the organ systems are mature and the child is now large enough to operate on. For procedures such as reconstructive craniofacial surgery, it is important to initiate the beginning of what may be multiple surgeries before the child develops a negative self-image and before peer groups and other parents have begun to have negative feelings and make negative remarks about the child. Also parents are anxious to get on with the repair of congenital defects since surgical defects are much more accepted by society than congenital defects. The guilt feelings of parents are greatly reduced as they feel they have done everything in their power to help their child. In addition to the feelings of guilt, parents experience feelings of grief. While this child was in utero the parents certainly had dreams about how wonderful this child would be. When the child is born with a congenital defect there is the development of grief as the parent realizes that this child will never be what they dreamed and that the child and family may be faced with a lifetime of adjustment.

This is the age where communication with the child should be attempted according to the age and response of the child. These children should be handled as outpatients whenever possible, since this minimizes the time of separation from their family and encourages a rapid reunion with the family. This is a particularly difficult age for infants and children who require hospitalization. Korsch describes the situation beautifully: "These young children have no assurance that painful experiences will ever stop, that assaults by caretakers have any reliable limit or that the dreary lonely nights in the hospital will definitely come to an end."[3]

4 to 6 Years

The age of 4 to 6 years is when most children understand the major implications of the surgical experience and may be able to tolerate separation from their parents without a great deal of negative feelings. This is the age when the child needs to be the primary focus of communication, with the parents being second. The child should be asked whether or not he would like premedication and should be given an explanation of what the options are. The various induction options should also be discussed. Even though children at this age may not fully understand the facts, they do understand the feelings.

6 Years to Adolescence

The age of 6 years to adolescence has been called "the true Golden Age." With few exceptions, these children are able to understand, with a reasonable explanation, what is going to happen to them. They still think their parents are relatively intelligent and believable. This will soon fade in the teenage years. They are aware of their body and they are aware of surgery. They often have fears that they are able to communicate. The major immediate fear they have is that they may awaken during the surgery. We must carefully inform them that the anesthetic will last the entire period of surgery and that we have special techniques and medications that will be used so that they will be comfortable when they do awaken from their surgery. The final question I ask a child of this age is "What worries you most?" Like children of 4 to 6 years, children from 6 years to adolescence should be the primary focus of communication, and all discussion about premedication, induction, and other treatment options should be directed toward them.

Adolescence

Adolescents can be very enjoyable patients for the medical team. They are in the age of Superman and Wonder Woman. They certainly understand what is happening in their world and what is going on with their body, and if appropriately informed, will understand what to expect with anesthesia and surgery. They are also developing their sexuality. They have major concerns about dignity, which we must understand and respect. I am continually flabbergasted by anesthesiologists and nurses who feel obligated to take off the upper part of the patient's nightgown in order to attach the blood pressure cuff and electrocardiograph patches. This is an embarrassing, unnecessary exposure for the female patient. Also, for reasons that are not clear, we often require that patients come to the operating room dressed in only the briefest hospital gown. Children, adolescents, and teenagers should be allowed to wear their underwear or other clothing to the operating room and the clothing should be removed after the induction of anesthesia. It is important to respect modesty and dignity at all ages.

The other concerns of these patients are fear of maiming and fear of death. Regardless of whether or not this is an unrealistic fear, we need to answer their questions appropriately. The last question I ask a child of this age group is "What worries you most?" This gives children an opportunity to verbalize their anxieties. I explain the basic techniques of the control of the anesthetics so they will understand that they will remain anesthetized during the entire operation and not be aware of anything or feel anything until the operation is over. The exception to this is the wake-up technique for scoliosis surgery. The wake-up test is explained to the patient. They are told that they will be asked to move their legs, that they will feel no pain, and that as soon as they move their legs they will be given a medication that will reanesthetize them and that they will stay in the anesthetized state until the end of surgery. For hospitalized patients, the option of patient-controlled analgesia and regional anesthesia is explained. For outpatients the types of analgesia are narcotics and/or regional or local anesthetics. All questions concerning premedication, induction, and postoperative pain relief are directed to the adolescent, who is permitted to make all reasonable decisions.

Fear of Postoperative Pain

One of the major concerns of children of all ages, as well as parents, is postoperative pain relief. For this reason I explain very carefully to both parent and child the options for pain relief. (This is discussed more fully in Chapter 11, Acute Pain Management in Children.) There are a few basics that we need to remember. One is that when regional or local anesthetic techniques are used, when the anesthetic wears off, there may be a painful interlude before other medications become effective. For this reason, for moderately invasive surgery such as hernia repairs or circumcisions, I administer intraoperatively a small dose of morphine (0.05 mg/kg), which will smooth out the offset of the local anesthetic. In addition, particularly in outpatients, the parents are advised to administer an oral analgesic as soon as fluids are tolerated, and before the offset of the local analgesia and the morphine. This usually occurs several hours after the surgery, and there is no rush to administer fluids and/or medications prematurely, which may increase nausea and vomiting in the patient. Another effective analgesic, one that we often forget about, is the use of an ice pack, which can greatly reduce the discomfort of surgical procedures.

The Child at Special Emotional Risk

There are many reasons why a child may be emotionally vulnerable. The child may have had prolonged or repeated hospitalizations, may be mentally retarded, may be a transplant patient (and this part of a transplant family), or may have no parental or family support system. A lengthy hospitalization or frequent repeat hospitalizations can have either a positive or negative effect on a child, depending on the support from the medical staff, the nature of the illness, and the home and parental support. There are times when it becomes impossible for one or both parents to visit the child, because of other children, distance, or finances. Children who have had multiple previous hospital experiences may either have learned to grow with these experiences and understand and trust their caretakers, or for any of a host of reasons, may (appropriately) fear their caretakers. Often a child with a negative history becomes a "silent child." The "silent child" is one with whom communication is almost impossible. Silent children appear to ignore the physician: they watch the television or read a book while the anesthesiologist attempts to discuss the anesthetic with them. Often they know what is coming and they are in the early stages of terror. These are the children who often suffer from nosocomial anxiety and iatrogenic terror. These are the children whose only words are, "No shot, please, no shot." They are difficult to reason with and often are very difficult during induction. In spite of their silence, I continue to explain to them what to expect even though it is a one-way conversation. These are the children who are often quite unapproachable as they arrive in the operating room, so I prepare a "stunning" dose of ketamine (3 mg/kg) to have ready if the child loses control and becomes unmanageable during induction. This will be discussed in detail later.

Patients who represent another special at-risk group are those who have medical conditions that impair communication or that threaten survival. These include retarded children, children with a meningomyelocele (with their many neurosurgical, orthopaedic, and urologic handicaps), and children with organ failure who are in the transplant process. Retarded children are a special problem because of our inability to communicate with them. Children with a meningomyelocele are a challenge because it is difficult to evaluate their mental age. Many of these children are mildly retarded but, because of their repeated and lengthy hospitalizations, have learned the hospital vernacular so well that we may think them more intelligent than they actually are. Commonly on the night before surgery, when preanesthetic rounds are made, they are quite clever and appear to communicate their thoughts and understand the upcoming events. The next morning, however, when the moment of truth arrives, they may be quite fearful and tearful. They really do not want an IV, they do not want a needle, they really do not want anything but to be left alone. Depending on the level and the extent of the meningomyelocele, they may have decreased sensation in their legs. Depending on the age, I usually offer an intravenous or inhalation induction, but if they become very tearful and resistant to either of these, I administer ketamine 3 mg/kg IM in the thigh or calf muscle. Because of the decreased sensitivity of the lower extremity, this represents minimal pain, and if done expeditiously, can be a very humane technique for induction. Because of the location and blood supply, the onset of the ketamine will be delayed, but it will be effective.

Children with severe renal disease have special problems, particularly in adolescence, when they become aware of their sexuality. In addition, they also recognize that survival is in question and that they will need life-long medical care. Unless they have an exceptional result from a transplanted kidney, they will be faced with a lifetime of medical problems. Depending on their age at transplantation, they may also be of short stature.

Parental Involvement in Premedication and Induction

It is difficult if not impossible to discuss premedication without considering the induction of anesthesia. The reason for this is the welcomed movement in pediatric anesthesia to allow and encourage parents to accompany their child to the operating suite and in some hospitals to be present for the induction of anesthesia.[4,5] The parents are the best premedication that any child can have. When parents are allowed to be present for the induction of anesthesia, the vast majority of children need no premedication at all. Many hospitals, however, are still very concerned about turn-around time and there is no question but that getting parents involved with the induction technique can add 3 to 5 minutes.

The types of induction of anesthesia that may be carried out with the parents present vary, depending on the facilities available. In some progressive institutions, arrangements have been made so that the patient or parents may choose from the complete spectrum of induction techniques, including intravenous, intramuscular, rectal, or inhalation inductions. Other institutions with limited facilities may not be able to offer inhalation inductions, but usually the other techniques are possible. Still other institutions, for reasons known only to themselves, do not allow the parents to be present for anything but a tearful and unpleasant separation from their child either in the patient's ward or at the door of the operating room suite. This often resembles an amputation rather than a separation. In the future, the operating suites for both ambulatory and inpatient care should be designed to enable the parents to be present for any of the various types of inductions. In older institutions, facilities should be rearranged so that a small area is available with appropriate oxygen, suction, and monitoring equipment in order that intramuscular, intravenous, or rectal induction can be accomplished with the parents present.

Pediatric anesthesia today is quite similar to obstetric anesthesia of approximately 15 years ago, when the practice was begun of allowing the father or other family member to be present not only during labor but also during birth in the delivery room. There was a great outcry at that time about the medical and legal implications. I can remember some of my colleagues saying, ''If any father comes in the delivery room it will be over my dead body.'' Today, it is more or less expected that the father, or some friend, will be present for the delivery. In some institutions, this person is allowed to be present not only for a routine, uncomplicated delivery but also for a cesarean section, if the choice of anesthetic is regional. I am not suggesting that parents should be allowed to be present for surgery on their child, but I do think that both the parent and the child benefit when the parent is allowed to be present for the induction. It will take time for anesthesiologists to become comfortable with this, but it occurred relatively rapidly in obstetric anesthesia and there is no reason to think that it cannot occur with the same rapidity in pediatric anesthesia. This is not to say that every anesthesiologist should allow the parents to be present for induction in all circumstances; it is an issue of judgment. But we do need to consider what is best for the family and child and start training anesthesiologists that way.

The age groups that benefit most from the parents' presence are the groups from 6 to 8 months to adolescence. The infant up to 6 to 8 months can easily be separated from parents without any degree of unhappiness for the infant and can be induced gently. Likewise, the adolescent or older child with whom one can communicate can be induced with either an intravenous or an inhalation induction with a minimum of unhappiness. Retarded children and retarded adolescents have a special need to have their parents present during the induction of anesthesia. If the parents are not allowed to be present, however, most anesthesiologists believe that there is a place for premedication for children of these ages. Midazolam 0.5 to 0.75 mg/kg PO has become very popular for this purpose. The object of premedication is sedation, and preferably to have the child asleep on arrival in the operating room or shortly thereafter. If parents are not allowed to be present for the induction, they should at least be allowed to stay with their child until it is time for the child to go into the operating room. This greatly modifies the anxiety of both the child and the parent and will allow a greater time for the premedication to become effective and a shorter time for the child to be unhappy.

PREMEDICATION

Sedatives

A peaceful separation of the parent and child is the definition of successful premedication. Unfortunately, at the present time, there is no sedative drug that is successful in 100 percent of children. Most studies of sedatives show a success rate of somewhere between 60 and 70 percent. With higher doses of drugs the percentage certainly increases, but then so do the complications of sedation. Unfortunately, there appears to be a small but significant group of children who are not able to be sedated with the usual doses of drugs. Often these are also the children who need to have an MRI or CT scan, and their pediatricians ask us about types of sedation and other considerations with the intent of avoiding general anesthesia. These children often must make several trips to the MRI or

CT department, where sedation has proven to be inadequate. There are the small number of children who it would appear are impossible to adequately sedate for these procedures and for whom nothing short of general anesthesia is going to be successful. Therefore, this small but significant group of children needs to be identified before they are given enormous doses of sedative drugs in order to accomplish a procedure with "sedation." What is really needed is for an anesthesiologist to take over the management of the child and do what is appropriate; usually this means general anesthesia.

In addition to the selection of the drugs, there are two important factors to be considered when sedatives are given: the route of administration and the timing of administration.

Route of Administration

The route of administration is certainly of more than passing interest to the child. The one thing that children and some adults fear most about the hospital experience is getting a "shot." As a matter of fact, some children become so upset by injections that they lose all trust in their caretakers. Often the desired effect of sedation is completely lost because of the iatrogenic terror that is induced by the injection of a sedative. Fortunately, all sedative drugs can be given orally or rectally (Table 2-1).[6–10]

It is somewhat of a paradox that many times the anesthesiologist recognizes the terror of the needle and orders an oral sedative for an infant or child, and then the surgeon gives intramuscular antibiotics or the pediatrician gives intramuscular steroids or anticonvulsants. The result is that our careful attempts to minimize the trauma to the child are blocked by well-meaning, but not-so-well informed, colleagues. It is very important that we communicate with all of the caretakers of children the need to avoid intramuscular injections before surgery. The patient can use small sips of water to take antibiotics, steroids, or anticon-

Table 2-1. Oral and Rectal Sedatives

Oral premedication
    Outpatient
    Meperidine 1.5 mg/kg
    Valium 0.2 mg/kg
    Atropine 0.02 mg/kg
    Inpatient
    Meperidine 3.0 mg/kg
    Pentobarb 4 mg/kg
    Atropine 0.02 mg/kg

For inpatient or outpatient
    Midazolam 0.5–0.75 mg/kg

Rectal premedication
    Midazolam 0.3 mg/kg

vulsants. In the case of prophylactic antibiotics for children with a history of rheumatic fever or a congenital heart defect, some pediatricians and surgeons have offered the argument that they need a blood level of the antibiotic before surgery. There are no data to support this argument. We can place an IV immediately following the induction of anesthesia, give the antibiotic, and immediately establish the desired blood level. If the physician desires, an oral antibiotic can be given preoperatively. This technique has been used in our institution (Children's Medical Center of the University of Virginia) for the last 10 years and there have been no documented problems.

There has been considerable interest in what have been called the "alternate routes" for the administration of several of the sedative drugs.[11-17] These methods include nasal instillation or sniffing and the oral route in the form of a fentanyl lollipop.[14] These methods have provoked considerable controversy among parents, clinicians, and consumer advocacy groups. On the positive side is the ease of administration. On the negative side is the incidence of nausea and vomiting with the fentanyl lollipop and the potential airway difficulties with nasal sufentanil. The main emotional issue on the negative side is the association of the sniffing of midazolam or narcotics with the sniffing of cocaine. The concern is that the child will more easily mentally bridge the gap between the medical use of drugs and their recreational use. The same is true for fentanyl lollipops: a recreational activity (i.e., enjoying a sucker) is mixed with a highly addicting narcotic (i.e., fentanyl) and used for sedation. For the child who requires sedation, the classic concept of swallowing a drug or taking it in an intramuscular or rectal form is not so easily confused with the concept of recreational drug use. The final chapter has yet to be written on this issue but it is hoped that the guidelines will originate from a medical base, with the needs of parents and children as the primary concern, rather than from a political base, where the motivational factors may be someone's "cause" for political advancement.

Timing of Sedation

Another point to consider is the length of time required for a drug to become effective, which in turn determines how far in advance of surgery the medication must be given. Most oral medications, such as diazepam, demerol, chloral hydrate, and pentobarbital, take 1 hour from the time of administration to reach peak effect. Midazolam takes approximately 10 to 15 minutes to become effective, and is considered a rapid-acting sedative. Because midazolam in an oral preparation is not available in the United States as of 1989 the parenteral form must be used and the flavor improved by mixing it with a small amount of apple juice. However, it should be remembered that midazolam does not last as long as the other above-mentioned drugs, which will often last for 2 to 4 hours. Sedation will last for approximately 30 to 45 minutes after reaching the peak effect. It is important to remember that the child should not be disturbed during the 30- to 60-minute time period that it takes for the drugs to become effective. Another point to remember is that in the usual, busy hospital, it will probably take 15 to 20 minutes for the nurses on the ward or in the ambulatory surgery

Table 2-2. Dosage of Anticholinergics (mg/kg)

	IV	IM	PO
Atropine	0.01	0.02	0.02
Glycopyrrolate	0.01	0.01	0.05

department to administer the medication after the anesthesiologist calls for it. Therefore, the anesthesiologist should allow extra time after calling for a medication to be given before sending for the patient.

If adequate time cannot be allowed for a sedative to become effective, the sedative should be omitted. The reason is twofold: It sometimes is difficult to convince a child that taking the medication is in his or her best interest, and the unhappiness and possible struggle over the administration of the medication leaves the child crying and upset. So, the result of poor timing is a child who may not only be not sedated but who also may be very upset at our belated efforts to do so. When sufficient time is allowed for the drug to become effective, the parents can calm the child and the medication will have a chance to be effective.

Anticholinergics

In the past, it was routine to administer an anticholinergic to patients of all ages. A difference of opinion has developed about whether or not this should be a routine order. In the infant up to 6 months of age the use of anticholinergics does seem to be justified. The dosages are listed in Table 2-2.

Anticholinergics are administered for two reasons: to block the vagus nerve and to decrease secretions. Bradycardia may occur owing to hypoxia, use of succinylcholine or volatile anesthetics, and laryngoscopy. In children under the age of 6 months, bradycardia is defined arbitrarily as a heart rate below 100 beats/min (Table 2-3). At first glance this arbitrary rate may appear to be a bit high. Because of the high degree of vagal tone, especially with hypoxia, bradycardia occurs rapidly. If the heart rate drops rapidly from 160 to 130 beats/min and then over the next 30 seconds to 100 beats/min, it is best to take action at that heart rate, since the next decrement may be to a rate of 60 to 80 beats/min.

Table 2-3. Heart Rate at Various Ages (beats/min)[a]

Age	Average	Range
0–24 hours	145	70–200
1–11 months	130	80–180
1–3 years	110	80–130
4–8 years	100	75–115
8–12 years	88	70–110

[a] Composite of several pediatric texts; awake and sleeping.

The trend and the speed of the trend may be more important than the actual rate. If bradycardia develops during or after induction, three major causes must be considered: hypoxia, vagal stimulation, and a concentration of the volatile agent that is too high. The most serious cause is hypoxia. The development of the pulse oximeter has allowed us to differentiate between hypoxia and other potential causes of bradycardia. The cardiac output of an infant is rate limited, and therefore if bradycardia develops (rate of 100 beats/min), ventilation should be ensured with oxygen, atropine 0.02 mg/kg IV or glycopyrrolate 0.01 mg/kg IV given, and the volatile agent turned down (or off), according to the blood pressure. Any time the heart rate or blood pressure drops the IV should be opened fully. This will more rapidly deliver any drugs administered as well as give a fluid bolus.

Sudden Onset of Bradycardia and/or Hypotension

In an infant under 6 months of age, if after the above measures have been taken the blood pressure is below 40 mmHg and the heart rate below 100 beats/min, or if the heart rate suddenly drops down to a range of 60 to 80 beats/min, the sequence presented in Table 2-4 should be followed. If an IV is not in place, the drugs need to be administered through the endotracheal tube or intramuscularly. A larger (double) dose should be given when these routes are used. If the heart rate is 60 to 80 beats/min instituting heart massage until the rate is above 100 beats/min and the blood pressure is at least 40 to 60 mmHg must be considered because at a low heart rate the circulation may be insufficient for the delivery of the administered drugs. The sequence in Table 2-4 is suggested for a sudden decrease in heart rate and/or blood pressure in any age group.

Use of the pulse oximeter and the capnograph has clearly demonstrated that many episodes previously attributed to hypoxia are not due to hypoxia at all. They appear to be due to an arrhythmia that is related to either vagal stimulation or some as-yet unrecognized mechanism. The problem may well be an anaphylactic/anaphylactoid reaction (see Ch. 3). At any rate, immediate therapy needs to be undertaken before the circulation becomes inadequate and hypoxia occurs. One of the reasons that the various pharmacologic agents may not be effective in the face of bradycardia is a low cardiac output that results from bradycardia. If this is suspected to be the case, external massage should be done in order to improve the circulation, from the standpoint of oxygenation as well

Table 2-4. Sequence for Rapid Decrease in Blood Pressure and/or Heart Rate

1. Discontinue anesthetics
2. Ventilate with oxygen
3. Bolus balanced salt solution
4. Epinephrine 5 μg/kg IV
5. Notify surgeon

as delivery of the pharmacologic agents. If in doubt, external cardiac massage should be done. A 1-ml tuberculin- or insulin-type syringe is quite adequate for measuring the small doses of epinephrine that are needed for infants, children, or adults.

Anticholinergics in Older Infants and Children

There are currently two (and perhaps more) opinions concerning the routine administration of anticholinergics, particularly if succinylcholine is to be administered, to patients 6 months to 1 year of age. Succinylcholine may cause a transient bradycardia in a small number of patients. However, the bradycardia is usually short lived and responds to the completion of laryngoscopy and the initiation of ventilation. The presence of hypoxia will certainly magnify the problem. Before the advent of the pulse oximeter, the state of oxygenation was unknown, and it was difficult to differentiate between the presence of hypoxia and the vagal stimulating effects of succinylcholine or of laryngoscopy. Therefore, one opinion was that all patients, regardless of whether or not they will receive succinylcholine, need an anticholinergic to block the vagus, dry secretions, and prevent the occasional case of bradycardia. The upper range of age for this practice has never been established. The other opinion is that because the incidence of bradycardia is low, and is often due to laryngoscopy and therefore lasts only for a brief period (30 to 45 seconds) and responds to the completion of laryngoscopy and the resumption of ventilation, anticholinergics should be administered only if the bradycardia persists longer than 45 to 60 seconds.

With regard to older infants and children, another difficult question to address is whether or not to administer an anticholinergic before a second dose of succinylcholine. If a second dose of succinylcholine is required, chances are good that hypoxia may well be present, and the conservative approach is to oxygenate the patient adequately and give an anticholinergic. I prefer glycopyrrolate to atropine because the tachycardia with glycopyrrolate use is not as great. The aim of giving anticholinergic drugs for blocking the vagus is to prevent bradycardia and maintain a relatively normal heart rate, not to elicit a tachycardia. At times after atropine administration the heart rate in an infant may exceed 180 or 190 beats/min. This tachycardia serves no useful purpose and may result in an increase in blood pressure and an increase in bleeding.

Another indication for anticholinergics is the drying of secretions. Again, there are two schools of thought on their use. The first is that anticholinergics are benign, while secretions may not be, and therefore it is a good idea to administer anticholinergics to all patients. The second opinion is that in children 6 months to 1 year of age the use of anticholinergics should be more selective, depending on the needs of surgery and the condition of the patient. It is my practice to follow this latter approach in the administration of anticholinergics and administer them according to the needs of the patient and the type of surgery.

Specific Indications for Anticholinergics

There are several circumstances in which the administration of anticholinergics may be extremely helpful.

Patients With a Sensitive Airway

Patients with a sensitive airway (e.g., those with allergic rhinitis, asthma, or a respiratory infection) have a tendency to cough and to develop laryngospasm and apnea because of the sensitivity of the airway and the presence of secretions. Administering a drying agent reduces the quantity of secretions but does not increase their viscosity.[18] In addition, the anticholinergics will dilate the large airways and reduce airway resistance (Fig. 2-1).[19] This can be of particular value in patients with bronchial hyperreactivity who are going to have general anesthesia.

Patients With a Difficult Airway

Patients with a difficult airway often seem to have excessive secretions, either because of the nature of the airway or because of the instrumentation that is done during intubation. Regardless, the conservative approach for these patients is to administer an anticholinergic in an attempt to prevent the problem. Once secretions are present, it takes what seems to be an interminable time for even

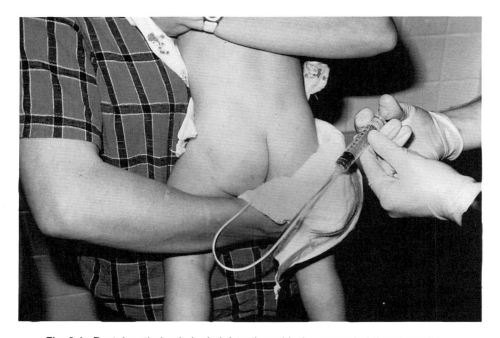

Fig. 2-1. Rectal methohexital administration with the parent holding the child.

high doses of anticholinergics to reduce the secretions. Patients undergoing cleft palate repair appear to have increased secretions, and a drying agent is very useful in this group of patients.

Patients Undergoing Bronchoscopy and Laryngoscopy

Bronchoscopy and laryngoscopy are associated with an increase in the amount of secretions and, in addition, may elicit a vagal reflex, which may cause bradycardia. Therefore, it is quite helpful to administer anticholinergic agents to these patients. It is better to administer the agents either preoperatively or immediately after the IV is started rather than wait for secretions to develop during the procedure and then try to treat them. This latter technique is often met with frustration.

Oral Anticholinergics

Anticholinergics can be given in an oral form, however, there is a decrease in the absorption of these agents in the stomach, so more of the agent must be given. The effective oral dose of atropine is approximately double the parenteral dose. It is effective in 10 to 15 minutes. Only 20 percent of glycopyrrolate is absorbed in the stomach, so the oral dose should be increased by a factor of 5. Compared with atropine, glycopyrrolate has a lesser effect on increasing the heart rate and is the preferred anticholinergic for patients with congenital or acquired heart defects in whom a severe tachycardia would result in a decreased ventricular filling or myocardial perfusion time. Another advantage of glycopyrrolate is that it does not cross the blood-brain barrier because of its quaternary ammonium structure, and hence has no central nervous system (CNS) effects. Scopolamine is an anticholinergic that does cross the blood-brain barrier, and it does have the CNS effects of sedation, amnesia, and sometimes hallucinations, which is why its use is limited. The hallucinations can be treated with physostigmine. The dose of physostigmine is 0.5 mg IV administered slowly over several minutes. Glycopyrrolate is a more effective drying agent than atropine and has a longer duration of action.[19] The injectable form can be mixed in water and taken orally.

Antiemetics

Incidence of Postoperative Nausea and Vomiting

There is a great deal of interest in the problem of postoperative vomiting after any type of surgery, but particularly after strabismus surgery. There is a growing body of literature on the incidence of vomiting and its treatment with various antiemetic drugs.[20-25] The incidence of vomiting without antiemetics ranges from 41 to 85 percent. It is not clear why there should be such an enormous difference in the incidence of postoperative nausea and vomiting but it is probably due to many of the subtle and difficult to recognize differences in clinical practice. Nonetheless, there are multiple studies that report a reduction in the incidence of postoperative vomiting with the use of antiemetics. The most frequently chosen antiemetic is droperidol, and in the case of strabismus surgery a dose of 75 μg/kg is the current recommendation. Even when similar doses of droperidol are administered there are still great differences in the incidence of postoperative vomiting. The incidence in one study was approximately 22 percent including predischarge and postdischarge vomiting.[25] In another study of droperidol using the same dose, the incidence of predischarge vomiting was 36 percent and the incidence of postdischarge vomiting was 32 percent.[23]

It is difficult to compare studies on nausea and vomiting completely because of differences in the time period being studied. Some studies report the occurrence of nausea and vomiting in the recovery room or in the predischarge area and other studies involve data obtained by contacting the parents 24 hours after discharge to see if the child had nausea and vomiting after returning home. Therefore, in comparing studies, it is very important to attempt to determine exactly the time period that is being studied. At times this is difficult to do.

There are many subtle differences in the anesthetic management of patients. It was noted in one of the studies that droperidol caused the children to be more difficult to arouse in the immediate postoperative period, resulting in a delay in being able to give them oral fluids. Another factor that has been suggested to be of importance is the administration of narcotics, which is thought to increase the incidence of postoperative vomiting. There is no consensus about any of these issues because it is so difficult to recognize and control subtle and little-appreciated differences in clinical management when evaluating postoperative nausea and vomiting. It is of interest that in one of the above studies of droperidol 6 of 69 control patients had to be admitted to the hospital because of vomiting. A recent study of the complications following ambulatory surgery reported a 0.9 percent incidence of admissions.[26] Of these patients, approximately one-third were admitted because of protracted nausea and vomiting. It is the requirement of that particular institution that all patients be able to ambulate as well as take oral fluids before discharge. This issue will be discussed later.

In our medical center, in the past 6 years, in over 1,000 cases of strabismus surgery by the same surgeon, no patient has been admitted for vomiting. Some of our children do experience nausea and vomiting in the recovery room and after being discharged. We do not routinely administer any antiemetics such as droperidol either as a premedication or during the intraoperative period. If the child has more than two or three episodes of postoperative vomiting in a 1-hour period, an antiemetic (droperidol 75 μg/kg) is given, but this is unusual. The anesthetic technique we use involves no premedication, either a methohexital (Brevital) or an inhalation induction with the use of succinylcholine modified by a nondepolarizer for intubation, and halothane and nitrous oxide for maintenance of anesthesia. We do not routinely administer an anticholinergic. Our usual plan for postoperative analgesia regardless of the type of surgery is a combination of regional or local anesthesia plus small doses of titrated narcotics. Local anesthetics are of limited usefulness in pain relief for strabismus surgery since their duration of action is relatively short. Strabismus surgery is usually associated with little postoperative pain, although the occasional child will have it. For that reason, narcotics are withheld until the postoperative period, and given as needed. If the surgery is known to be painful, then regardless of whether or not regional anesthesia is used, small doses of narcotics are given intraoperatively for analgesia and sedation in the immediate recovery period. The narcotics used are primarily titrated doses of morphine (0.05 mg/kg) and fentanyl (1 μg/kg). The narcotic doses are repeated until the patient is comfortable. My usual preference is for morphine since most surgery results in pain that is going to last for many hours, and it is well known that morphine lasts longer than fentanyl.

Methods to Reduce Postoperative Nausea and Vomiting

As suggested before there may be subtle, unrecognized differences in anesthesia practice that account for the differences in outcome. One of these subtle differences may be the requirement in some institutions that patients be able to retain oral fluids as well as ambulate before they are discharged from the outpatient facility.[26] Ambulation, particularly when the child has had a narcotic, increases the incidence of vomiting. For that reason, in our practice ambulation is not encouraged or required. Patients are advised that they should remain very quiet for several hours after surgery. In addition, we do not have the requirement that a patient be able to drink and retain fluid before they are discharged from the ambulatory surgery unit. One of the difficulties in treating patients is deciding when they will be able to tolerate oral fluids. Thirst is not an indicator of the ability to tolerate fluids. It has been our impression that the presence of hunger is a good indicator that the patient is able to tolerate oral fluids. For that reason, and because often the child is discharged before oral fluids can be administered, we tell the parents that oral fluids may be administered after the child indicates hunger. It is difficult to determine hunger in children who are under age 3, therefore in this age group we wait at least 2 to 4 hours postoperatively before beginning fluids. Infants under 6 months of age seem to have a lower incidence of nausea and vomiting, therefore in this age group if the child appears to be otherwise awake and healthy and is crying in a manner that is interpreted by either the nurses or the mother to indicate hunger or thirst we then allow them small amounts of sugar water or juice as tolerated.

For older children, the routine after they say they are hungry is to allow small amounts of clear fluids such as apple juice or a soft drink, wait 20 minutes, allow another increment of fluid, and so on. After a period of 1 hour the diet is increased. If the child vomits, the parents are instructed to wait another hour before fluids are administered. Generous quantities of balanced salt solution are administered intravenously during the perioperative period, and therefore we do not worry about dehydration for the first 10 to 12 hours postoperatively. This is why we feel confident in telling the parents not to feed their child until he is hungry, even if it may be the morning after surgery. It should be remembered that ice chips are fluids. If the child's mouth is extremely dry, then we suggest that they allow the child to rinse his mouth. Parents are instructed to call their doctor, an emergency room, or one of our physicians if there is persistent vomiting.

Drugs to Reduce Gastric Volume and Increase Gastric pH

Regurgitation and aspiration is a rare but potentially serious problem.[27] Between 10 and 24 percent of anesthetic deaths in adults are due to aspiration of gastric contents.[28,29] Aspiration continues to be one of the leading causes of death in obstetric patients. For whatever reason, the occurrence and dangers of regurgitation and aspiration are reported to be far less in children.

The critical factors for the development of pulmonary injury in adults are a gastric pH below 2.5 and a volume of gastric fluid greater than 25 ml. In the pediatric patient, the child is considered to be at risk with a similar pH and a gastric volume of 0.4 ml/kg. A combination of these factors is believed to provide a sufficient volume and low-enough gastric fluid pH so that aspiration will result in the development of the pulmonary acid aspiration syndrome. As a practical matter aspiration in children is rare. However, there is a group of patients who would appear to be theoretically at a higher risk for regurgitation and aspiration. These patients include children with a difficult airway, a full stomach, an intestinal obstruction, or a sensitive airway. The mechanism for regurgitation and aspiration in children with a sensitive airway is obstruction secondary to secretions, or in the case of a difficult airway, anatomic obstruction. With the combination of coughing, positive-pressure ventilation (which fills the stomach with gas), and various airway maneuvers, the child is at risk to regurgitate and aspirate. For that reason there has been considerable interest in the administration of either cimetidine alone or cimetidine in combination with metoclopramide.[30,31]

Cimetidine is an H_2-receptor blocker. It has the capacity to increase the gastric pH and reduce the gastric volume. It is absorbed quite adequately from the stomach and achieves peak blood levels in 45 to 60 minutes. It has a long list of potential complications, but they have not been reported with any consistency. Cimetidine is known to reduce the metabolism of other drugs, such as lidocaine, owing to an associated reduction in liver blood flow. The clinical significance of this fact has not yet been fully defined. Cimetidine 7.5 mg/kg PO has been found to be quite effective in reducing the gastric volume and increasing the gastric pH in pediatric patients between the ages of 4 months and 14 years.[30]

Metoclopramide is the other drug that has been recommended as part of the preanesthetic prophylaxis of acid aspiration. Metoclopramide is a dopamine antagonist. Structurally, it is related to procainamide. Its pharmacologic actions are based on three effects: an acceleration of gastric emptying, an increase in the tone in the lower esophageal sphincter, and a depression of the vomiting center in the brain stem. It has no effect on gastric pH. Its major action is to decrease the volume of gastric contents. For this reason it has not been shown to have a high degree of reliability when used alone. A study in adults reported the effects of combining cimetidine and metoclopramide.[31] The most favorable regimen for modifying the risk factors in this study was cimetidine the night before and a combination of cimetidine and metoclopramide the morning before surgery.

In summary, it would appear that the risk of regurgitation and aspiration in the pediatric population is very small, and there appears to be no compelling evidence that would require routine pharmacologic prophylaxis since these drugs also have potential complications and side effects that may be greater than the very low risk of aspiration pneumonia. At the same time it should be recognized that there are certain patients who are at risk (i.e., those having a difficult airway or a full stomach). These patients require the anesthesiologist's extreme attention to detail.

INDUCTION OF ANESTHESIA

The presence or absence of the parents during the induction of anesthesia plays an important part in the choice of induction technique.

Induction With the Parents Present

Benefits of Allowing the Parents to Be Present

One of the major advantages of the parents' presence is that it allows a very close interaction between the anesthesiologist and the family. The anesthesiologist is not a phantom who the parents may never see. The interaction of the anesthesiologist with the family is important for a number of reasons, not the least of which is that it develops lines of communication that minimize misunderstanding and thereby minimize the possibility of medicolegal activity should there be a bad outcome or complication. The parents benefit from the situation because they get to see the loving, tender care that their child receives during the induction of anesthesia. Many parents remember (often negatively) when they had surgery as a child and when there wasn't such a tender and loving induction of anesthesia. The presence of the parents during induction has virtually eliminated the need for sedative premedication. There are still rare circumstances where the parents desire and the child needs some form of sedation, however, the vast majority require and desire nothing.

Most infants under the age of 6 to 8 months are quite content to accompany the anesthesiologist to the operating room with minimal separation problems—the parents may have a problem with separation but the infant usually does not. Children 6 to 8 months to adolescence and those who are retarded and their parents are the group who benefit most from allowing the parents to be present for the induction of anesthesia. Older children and their parents are given the option of having the parent present for induction or of going alone to the operating room. Some of the adolescents enjoy the idea of being able to cope by themselves. The options and techniques of induction are discussed with the parents and with the child.

Parental Involvement and the Induction Area

There are three different scenarios for allowing the parent to participate in the induction of anesthesia with their child. In the first scenario, where separate induction facilities are not available, the parents are allowed to don a sterile gown and mask and accompany their child into the operating room, where the induction is accomplished. In the second scenario an area of the recovery room or the holding area may be used for a limited range of inductions. In this situation, it is usually not possible to have an anesthesia machine in the room so induction is limited to an intravenous, rectal, or intramuscular technique. The rectal technique employs methohexital and the intramuscular technique ketamine; they will be discussed later. When an IV is in place the technique used to accomplish a gentle separation from the parents is that of heavy sedation of the child with thiopental (Pentothal) 2 mg/kg rather than full induction, which usually requires 5 to 7 mg/kg and may result in apnea and the need for airway intervention, and can be quite disturbing to the parents if they are not prepared for it. In addition, it is logistically simpler to use heavy sedation with thiopental and maintain spontaneous ventilation and then transport the child to the operating room. Before thiopental is given, I advise the parents that thiopental can be a very quick-acting agent and that the child might fall asleep or be heavily sedated very rapidly, because I do not want the parents to be shocked or surprised by what is about to occur. Thiopental 2 mg/kg is administered in a rapidly running IV. In the vast majority of children this will induce either heavy sedation or a sleep state. It is important to then rapidly but calmly transport the child into the operating room while the nurse or other assistant guides the parents to the waiting room. It is important to leave the thiopental syringe connected to the IV tubing or immediately available in case additional sedation is needed. On occasion, an inordinate delay in leaving the parents allows the thiopental to redistribute and the child to rouse. Titrating further doses of thiopental 1 to 2 mg/kg will manage the situation until arrival in the operating room, where the induction can be completed with either more thiopental or nitrous oxide and halothane.

Even though these rooms do not have an anesthesia machine, they do need to be equipped with suction, oxygen, and monitors. At our institution a mobile anesthesia cart is in every operating room. The appropriate drugs, endotracheal tubes, largyngoscopes, and other equipment are prepared as for the operation and the cart is taken to the induction area so that this equipment is available should the need arise. After the induction or sedation the cart accompanies the child from the induction area into the operating room.

The third scenario is that of a full-service induction room equipped with an anesthesia machine in which all of the various induction techniques are available. When a full-service induction room is available, the anesthesiologist needs to make a decision about the type of induction and whether or not the child will be intubated for the procedure. There are two possible choices: (1) to sedate or induce anesthesia in the induction room and then move the child to the operating room, where an IV is started and the remainder of the induction and/

or intubation is completed or (2) to complete the induction and intubate in the induction room and then move the patient completely ready for surgery into the operating room. The choice of which method to use depends on two factors: (1) the experience and confidence of the anesthesiologist and (2) the logistics of the operating room and surgeons. Some anesthesiologists feel comfortable taking a child from an induction room to the operating room when he is heavily sedated or has had an inhalation induction. Others need to have an IV in place and the airway controlled with an endotracheal tube. Their major concern is that they will lose control of the patient on the way from the induction room to the operating room or that the patient will pull out the IV, become obstructed, and awaken, and any of a whole host of nightmares ensue. These are all understandable, but are more likely to happen to the inexperienced anesthesiologist. Leaving the thiopental syringe in the IV tubing in the case of a thiopental induction or sedation will allow more thiopental to be administered during transport in the event that this occurs. Also, if an inhalation induction has been done and the patient is transported without an endotracheal tube or gas supply in place, it is important that the nitrous oxide be discontinued for a period of 3 to 4 minutes and 4 to 5 percent halothane administered with mild assisted ventilation so that the child is sufficiently anesthetized but yet breathing spontaneously so that he can maintain his own airway. The transport technique of these patients is quite important and requires three people, two to push the stretcher and one to bring the anesthetic cart with the equipment. In some institutions the stretcher is equipped with oxygen and an anesthesia machine, eliminating many of the concerns in this situation. For those who do not have this available monitoring the patient with a precordial stethoscope as well as a pulse oximeter for the trip from the induction room to the operating room is suggested. It is my preference, in general, to transport the child to the operating room without starting the IV and without intubation and to complete the induction, IV, and intubation in the operating room. This technique of induction speeds up the turn-around time in the room since most surgeons do not begin to scrub and prepare for surgery until they see the patient on the operating table. This they have learned from long experience while waiting for their anesthesia colleagues.

Once the patient arrives in the operating room a management decision needs to be made immediately. If the child is sufficiently sedated from the thiopental or deeply enough anesthetized with halothane to be moved from the stretcher to the operating table, this should be accomplished and the induction completed on the operating table. On the other hand, if the child is beginning to rouse or there is any question about the depth of anesthesia, halothane and nitrous oxide should be administered while the patient is still on the stretcher. Once the airway is controlled the patient is moved to the operating room table. If the patient has an IV in place, an additional dose of thiopental can be given before the patient is moved to the operating table. The advantage to this latter technique is that, if the IV is precarious or the patient should rouse and suddenly pull out the IV, a potentially embarrassing scenario is avoided.

Rectal Induction

If the child has no IV, the induction technique then depends on the age. For the child of 6 to 8 months up to 4 or 5 years, either rectal methohexital or an inhalation technique is used.[32,33] Rectal methohexital is becoming a "consumer" anesthetic. If the child is cooperative or even relatively uncooperative, it can be administered gently and quickly while the child is either held by the parent on the shoulder or placed on the stretcher on the abdomen. After the drug is administered, the child is gently and quickly returned to the arms of the parent. It is important to replace the diaper on the child or to have a special pad available since 10 to 15 percent of children will defecate. It is important to keep the parent appropriately protected. Methohexital comes in 500-mg vials. There is no commercial form of rectal methohexital; so a parenteral form is used. The dose is 30 mg/kg, which will induce 95 percent of children within 5 to 10 minutes. It lasts for 60 to 90 minutes. There is considerable literature at the present time about the appropriate concentration to be used.[34] The answers are not clear, but most clinicians would use either a 5 or 10 percent solution, which would mean that there is either 50 mg/ml or 100 mg/ml. We are currently using a 5 percent solution. The advantage of the 5 percent solution is that less residual drug would be left in the bottle and the higher volume would use more surface area in the rectum for the absorption. An appropriate dose of the drug is drawn up in a 10-ml syringe with a small amount of air to clear the drug from the feeding tube. A No. 8 feeding tube lubricated with surgical lubricant or local anesthetic is then attached to the syringe of medication. The syringe and catheter with the methohexital should be hidden from sight of the child since the child will immediately associate the syringe with pain and begin to react rather negatively. The child is placed on the stretcher or held by the mother, the catheter is inserted 5 to 8 cm, and the drug is injected (Fig. 2-1). The syringe and feeding tube should be removed as a unit. Disconnecting the syringe before removing the catheter may result in an undesired aerosol from the catheter should the child cry. A recent study in one clinic would indicate that it is possible to reduce the 1-hour sleep time of methohexital if the catheter is left in place as the child falls asleep and then the residual methohexital aspirated from the rectum.[35] At the present time this technique is not used in our practice. The rectal methohexital is effective in inducing a hypnotic state in approximately 95 percent of children within 5 to 10 minutes. Waiting longer than 10 minutes has not increased our incidence of success. If the child is not asleep at this point several options exist. If sedated and relatively cooperative the child can be taken into the operating room and an inhalation induction performed. If the equipment is available to do an inhalation induction in the same room then that is accomplished. If the child is completely or moderately uncooperative a "stunning" dose of intramuscular ketamine (3 mg/kg) is administered. Children who have been taking phenobarbital and other medications may have induced their liver microsomal enzyme system for the metabolism of barbiturates, and will require larger doses of methohexital. Therefore, these children are initially given 40 mg/kg. In some of these children this dosage has been successful in inducing hypnosis, while in others the technique is unsuccessful and another induction method is used. Methohexital is a hypnotic and not an anesthetic, therefore, before any painful procedure an analgesic must be given. Usually after a methohexital induction an inhalation anesthetic is continued in a routine fashion. However, if an IV is to be started before the inhalation anesthetic, a small amount of local anesthetic should be introduced before the intravenous cannulae.

There is no question that the rectal administration of any drug is subject to a degree of unpredictability in the amount and speed of absorption.[32] However, in spite of this limitation the use of rectal methohexital has greatly changed induction techniques in children younger than 5 years. Many parents are familiar with the technique and request it for their child. On the other hand, there are parents who would prefer that their child not have a rectal medication. Certainly their wishes are to be respected. But overall, this technique has been very successful in helping to reduce or eliminate the separation trauma in infants and children through age 4 or 5.

Rectal methohexital is effective for about 60 to 90 minutes. For the vast majority of cases, it therefore has little impact on any aspect of the perioperative period. In the event of a rapid turnover, such as the insertion or removal of ear ventilation tubes, methohexital will delay the discharge of the child from either the recovery room or the ambulatory surgery clinic. However, the small increase in time delay is certainly well worth the gentle induction. We need to remember that children and parents are not interested in turnover time, elapsed time, and the like. Parents are much more concerned with the psychological well being of their child. I explain to parents the induction options, including the potentially prolonged recovery time, and I have yet to have a parent choose an induction technique based on turn-around time.

Inhalation Induction

One of the most satisfying aspects of pediatric anesthesia is accomplishing a smooth, gentle inhalation induction in the situation where a child may be not completely cooperative but still reachable. In general, parents can be a great asset with induction. Before we begin, I explain to the parents and child what is going to happen during the inhalation induction process. For the older child the primary discussion is with the child and with the younger child the primary discussion is with the parent. The parents are also forewarned that the child may go through an excitement stage, which may or may not be accompanied by the child's feeling that they are falling. If not forewarned, the excitement period may upset the parents. The child and parents are told that the gases and mask will smell a little funny but that various flavors will be used to disguise the smell. There are various commercial products for this purpose. Several flavors are available and the child is allowed to pick the flavor desired. This allows the child to participate in the process. We encourage either the child or the parent to hold the mask. This increases the cooperation of the child. It is important that the room be quiet and that only the parent and the anesthesiologist communicate with the child. High-flow nitrous oxide in a 70 percent concentration is begun. The mask is held 3 or 4 inches away so the child can see that he is not going to hurt by it. We desensitize the child to the mask upon arrival in the surgical suite by giving him a mask to play with. As the child tolerates the nitrous oxide the mask is brought closer to the face. If the child is cooperative, then we encourage placing the mask on the face. Some anesthesiologists paint a picture of a face on the rebreathing bag and encourage the child to blow up the "balloon." The relatively uncooperative child will not be particularly interested in this game, so attempts to force the mask on the face should not be done. At this point one of two situations will exist: either the child will tolerate the mask being placed on the face or he won't. If the child won't tolerate the mask being placed on the face then the induction is continued with 0.25 percent halothane. If it's a girl, I tell her she will be smelling an odor of fingernail polish and if it's a boy, I tell him the odor is that of airplane glue or exhaust fumes from a rocket. Every anesthesiologist has his or her own pet story or way of distracting the child in order to facilitate the induction.

As the child tolerates this concentration of halothane for 20 to 30 seconds, the concentration is then increased up to 0.5 percent, after another 15 to 30 seconds up to 1 percent, and then stepwise as tolerated up to 4 to 5 percent until the child has been induced. As soon as the child has been induced, as indicated by a loss of lid reflex, I thank the parents for their help and ask the nurse or other health care worker to escort them out of the room and to make sure they are alright. As the parents leave, I turn off the nitrous oxide and continue 4 to 5 percent halothane (dialed concentration in a circle system). After 3 minutes, if the child is ready we proceed to the operating room. One of the main fears during an inhalation induction is the occurrence of laryngospasm, which requires urgent attention. Although this is an extremely rare occurrence, contingency plans must be made. This is a ticklish situation for the anesthesiologist but the parents should be told firmly, "We're having a bit of difficulty and we would like to have you leave now so that we can get the situation under control. Someone will come talk to you as soon as the situation has smoothed out." As this discussion is proceeding I usually administer succinylcholine 4 mg/kg IM, turn off the nitrous oxide, apply monitors, and prepare for intubation after control of the airway.

Application of Monitors

One of the problems in pediatric anesthesiology is deciding when to apply the various monitors (i.e., oximeter, stethoscope, ECG leads, and blood pressure cuff). Monitors can usually be applied to small infants, who don't really care what's happening. However, because of motion the monitors usually are not very useful, but they will be in place when the induction is accomplished. Children 6 to 8 months through age 4 or 5 may or may not accept the application of monitors before the induction. If the child is frightened it is best not to apply any monitors since he has a thin thread of courage and the delay while attaching monitors or the fright of attaching monitors may cause the child to slip from cooperative to uncooperative. Therefore, the timing of monitor placement is a judgment call, depending on the cooperation of the child. If in doubt, it is better not to place the monitor and to wait until after induction rather than lose the cooperation of the borderline-cooperative patient.

Intravenous Induction

There are many clinicians who are extremely skilled in the insertion of a small scalp needle in the hand or foot of an infant or child. They prefer this technique for the induction of anesthesia. In this situation thiopental 4 to 6 mg/kg is given while the parent or assistant holds the child.

Ketamine Induction of Anesthesia

Ketamine is discussed with the parents as one of the induction options, particularly if the child is not cooperative. Although it is preferable to avoid injections, inducing the uncooperative child is the one situation in which a rapid injection is the most humane approach. There are several different scenarios for the use of ketamine. Sometimes parents immediately recognize that their child is not going to cooperate and request from the beginning that their child be given ketamine. At other times the option of ketamine is in their mind but they would prefer that another induction technique such as inhalation or rectal methohexital induction be tried. If the induction technique is successful then the issue of ketamine is moot. However, if the situation is out of control, a different approach is needed. Therefore, during the initial phases of a stormy inhalation induction or failed rectal induction, if the child is totally uncooperative or very unhappy in spite of the parents being there and in spite of all the gentleness and negotiation in attempting to get the child to cooperate, then I remind the parents and child of our options and suggest ketamine. By this time in the induction most parents are ready for a change of technique. The dose of ketamine is 3 mg/kg administered in the deltoid muscle. The drug is administered in the deltoid because it has been shown that a higher blood concentration results from injection into the deltoid as compared with injections into the vastus lateralis or the gluteus. I do not wipe the arm with alcohol since this forewarns the child of imminent pain. In addition, I do not feel that alcohol is necessary. The injection is given rapidly and without aspiration. The thumb is placed on the plunger of the syringe, the syringe is held like a dagger, and the child "stabbed" in the arm (Fig. 2-2). The injection can be given in an instant with a minimum of trauma to the child. A 23-gauge needle combines minimal insertion pain with rapid injection capabilities. A 25-gauge needle requires considerable force on the plunger for injection. The child may pull away during the slower injection phase, dislodging the needle and potentially causing mayhem. Anesthesia is induced with ketamine within 2 to 3 minutes. The parents should be warned about the far-away stare and the open eyes. The 3-mg/kg dose has been successful in 100 percent of the patients in our clinic. The use of 5 to 10 mg/kg of ketamine for induction can cause quite a long and unpredictable recovery, which often proves unsatisfactory. In addition, the 5- to 10-mg/kg dose of ketamine may cause postoperative hallucinations and dreams, which occurs much less frequently

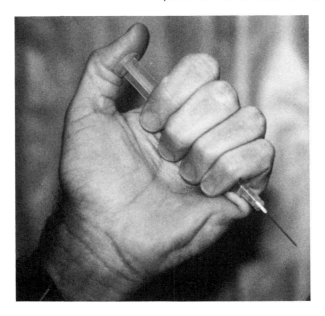

Fig. 2-2. Injection technique for ketamine.

with the smaller doses.[36] After the ketamine induction an IV can be started, usually without the need for local anesthesia. If ketamine is to be continued as the anesthetic, this can be accomplished with small (0.5 mg/kg) titrated intravenous doses. Respiratory depression may occur with a large (2 mg/kg) intravenous dose.[37]

Induction Without the Parents Present

In many hospitals parents are not allowed to be present for the induction of anesthesia. Two different separation points are used. In some hospitals the child is separated from the parents on the ward, at the outpatient clinic, or at the entrance to the operating suite. The child is then often left for what may be agonizing periods of time with or without a caretaker until the operating room is ready. This separation technique resembles an amputation rather than a pleasant separation. In other hospitals the parents are allowed to wait with the child in a holding area until the operating room is ready. This system eliminates the long, lonely wait but does not prevent the inevitable, often painful, separation that young children and parents may experience. It is because of the problems of separation and the lonely waiting period that most people choose to premedicate children when the parents are not allowed to be present for induction. The goal of the premedication is to make the child more cooperative and less fearful and, it is hoped, even sleep. The question of which induction technique to use depends primarily on the age of the child and the degree of cooperation. If the child has an IV in place then certainly there is no question that an intravenous induction is easiest for all concerned. Also because some anesthesiologists are very skilled in the technique of inserting a small scalp vein, anesthesia may be induced in that fashion.

The Uncooperative Child

If the child is unhappy and crying a decision needs to be made about the most humane way to induce anesthesia. If the child is crying but not fighting or out of control either an inhalation induction or the administration of rectal methohexital can be accomplished easily and gently with a minimum of upset to the child. However, if the child is quite upset and uncooperative, the most humane induction technique is the "stunning" dose of ketamine. Unfortunately, there are those who would proceed with a "gorilla" induction, but in my opinion this has no place in pediatric anesthesia. In the "gorilla" induction three or four people physically restrain the child flat on his back on the operating table while the anesthesiologist forces a mask tightly over his face and administers a high dose of halothane to "get it over with quickly" as they say to the child, "Everything is going to be o.k." There is no question in my mind that this is not pleasant for the child or the anesthesiologist—or the gorillas.

The "Steal" Induction

The inhalation induction for the child 6 months to 6 years may present a special problem because the child often does not understand the benefit of surgery but may only remember other unpleasant medical experiences. These are the patients who one hopes are asleep from sedation so that a "steal" induction can be accomplished. In this situation, the child should not be woken to be played with or to have monitors applied. The operating room should be kept quiet. A high flow of 70 percent nitrous oxide is begun and gently blown over the child's face while the child is still asleep in the crib or on the stretcher. Care must be taken not to touch the face at this point since the stimulation will arouse the child. After 1 to 2 minutes then 0.25 percent halothane is introduced and every 30 seconds the concentration is increased by 0.5 percent as tolerated. If the child coughs or breathholds, the concentration of halothane should be turned back one notch for a short period of time until the condition stabilizes and then advanced up to 3 to 5 percent. The side of the face or an eyelash is then touched gently with a finger. If this is tolerated the mask can then be gently applied. At times, the child may rouse from the premedication early in the induction phase. Gentle restraint and reassurance will often win the day. If the child is in ASA category II anesthesia, the stage of altered consciousness and amnesia, then he may need more forceful restraint, which, fortunately, he won't remember. Sometimes, unfortunately, the child will still be in category I and will become extremely uncooperative, struggling and screaming. If this occurs, the option at this point is a "stunning" dose of ketamine. In addition, there are those who would use a gorilla induction.

The Cooperative Child

If the child is not asleep from the premedication then a soft conversation is started as the child is taken from the parents or the bed. A gentle voice and gentle handling are very important. The anesthesiologist may carry the smaller child into the operating room for an inhalation induction. One of the things that these small children do not like is to be forced to lie down. Therefore, I usually hold the child sitting in my lap or sitting on the operating room table. If the child elects to lie down then I let them. On arrival in the operating room it is important to immediately begin the inhalation induction as described above without applying any monitors. Monitors are applied by the circulating nurse as tolerated while the child is being induced. Any inordinate delay in getting the induction started in order to attach the monitors may result in the child losing that thin thread of courage that had enabled him to cooperate in an otherwise frightening experience. Older children are not as frightened and even enjoy being connected to the monitors and seeing the display. The anesthesia equipment should always be checked before the child is brought into the room so that this step does not have to be repeated. The anesthesiologist can monitor the child visually at the beginning of the induction (i.e., watch for movement, talking, breathing pattern, etc). Usually the child will allow a precordial stethoscope to be applied, but if they don't I delay that also. The second monitor to be applied is the pulse oximeter, which can usually be placed early in the induction because it is a painless monitor that requires no pushing or squeezing. As the induction continues, the monitors can be applied in a gentle manner without arousing the child.

Special Circumstances

Some conditions or situations do not fit the usual mold or criteria for the induction technique or the parental participation that has just been described. There are at least four special circumstances, including the anesthesiologist with inadequate training or a different attitude, children in ASA categories III and IV, children with a difficult airway, and children needing emergency surgery.

Training and Attitude of the Anesthesiologist

Some anesthesiologists have minimal or no training in inductions of children with parents present. Others may be afraid of change or, for whatever reason, are unable to change. Therefore, the policy of allowing parents to be present for the induction of anesthesia should never be forced on any anesthesiologist who feels uncomfortable with that situation. Alternatively, the technique of allowing parents to be present for induction is certainly a technique that can be learned, used, and enjoyed by the majority of anesthesiologists.[4,5]

Patients in ASA Categories III and IV

Many anesthesiologists feel comfortable inducing anesthesia with the patient in ASA category I or II while the parents are present but may not feel comfortable doing so with the patient in ASA category III or IV. The paradox is that the ASA category III and IV patients are often those who need, and greatly benefit from, the parents' presence. These include children with leukemia, heart disease, and the like, who unquestionably would benefit from a smooth induction. There is also no question that the induction is more difficult. If an anesthesiologist is willing to allow parents to be present for the induction of children, they should start with patients in ASA category I and II; then, as they develop experience and feel comfortable with the situation, they should consider doing selected ASA category III and IV patients. One example of such a patient is the child with acute upper airway disease who is in respiratory distress. The diagnostic possibilities include acute epiglottitis, croup, or the presence of a foreign body. At times, attempting to separate the parent from the child before proceeding into the operating room may cause a worsening of the child's condition. This happens because the crying and struggling that occur as the parents leave may interfere with the patient's already compromised ventilation. The anesthesiologist then is in a quandary. If he or she feels comfortable with the parents' presence, it may actually be safer for the child to have the parents present for the induction of anesthesia. In the situation of acute upper airway obstruction, the induction is done in the operating room with full equipment and assistance standing by. In this case, the parents wear gowns or operating room attire before entering the operating room. As soon as the early stages of induction are over, the parents are escorted out. In addition, the parents are told that if any difficulty should arise, they must leave when requested. This arrangement with the parents needs to be documented in the chart.

The Patient With a Difficult Airway

Patients with a known or suspected difficult airway are an enormous challenge to the anesthesiologist. These children may be relaxed and cooperative or they may be upset and uncooperative. In general, these children are not sedated for fear that sedation may cause a magnification of the airway problem, which may become manifest on the way to the operating room or in the holding area. Whether or not the anesthesiologist feels comfortable with the presence of the parents is a personal matter. The parents' presence may help to bring about a smooth induction. Separation may cause a relatively stormy induction, resulting in crying and development of airway secretions, which may complicate further the problems of the difficult airway. For a young child, a rectal methohexital induction can be used and the child then placed prone or on his side. Children with a difficult airway may benefit by being premedicated with a drying agent. The choice of induction technique and location depends on the judgment of the anesthesiologist. This is determined by training, experience, and expertise.

Children Needing Emergency Surgery

In general, the child who presents for emergency surgery is assumed to have a full stomach. Often the parents are not allowed to be present for induction. One exception to be considered is the child with a potential open-eye injury. Another is the child with increased intracranial pressure. Patients who have a potential open-eye injury or increased intracranial pressure are at special risk for anything that will cause struggling or crying, because this can cause either a loss of vitreous or a further increase in intracranial pressure. For that reason, these patients need to be treated in a different manner. Unless there is an overwhelming medical reason, any type of invasive laboratory study (e.g., hematocrit or electrolytes) should be avoided. Also, unless medically indicated, this would include the starting of an IV. The details of the induction of the child with a potential open-eye injury will be discussed later in this chapter.

Induction Techniques

The Child With a Full Stomach

The child with a full stomach presents an enormous challenge for the anesthesiologist. First, the anesthesiologist must consider the potential of aspiration in the full stomach. Then, of course, there are innumerable complicating conditions, such as a full stomach with an open-eye injury or a full stomach and increased intracranial pressure. (The child with a full stomach and suspected increased intracranial pressure will be discussed in Chapter 12, Pediatric Neuroanesthesia.) The possibilities seem to be limitless. The various factors that need to be considered in all patients with a full stomach include the position of the child, the induction technique, the intubation technique, and the awakening technique. Most clinicians intubate patients in the supine position while cricoid pressure is applied, the reason being that the head position of the patient should be the one that is most comfortable for the anesthesiologist and the most appropriate for accomplishing a successful laryngoscopy and intubation. Trying new and different techniques in a patient with a full stomach may create more problems than using the familiar techniques with cricoid pressure.

Awake Intubation in Infants

The question of awake intubation and a full stomach is one that elicits a great spectrum of opinions. There are those who think that all infants up to age 3 months should have an awake intubation for surgery, full stomach or not. This is an area that has undergone some rethinking because of several factors, one of which is the concern that in premature infants, the blood vessels of the brain are immature and fragile, and it is thought by some that an awake intubation runs the risk of increasing the pressure in these vessels and rupture leading to intraventricular hemorrhage. Therefore, the opinion of many at the present time is that, except in the moribund infant or the infant with an intestinal obstruction who is actively vomiting, the induction of anesthesia should be accomplished with an intravenous rapid-sequence technique or else begun with an inhalation technique and continued with either administration of intramuscular succinylcholine and intubation or placement of an IV and a modified rapid-sequence technique.

Cricoid Pressure and Ventilation

The subject of cricoid pressure and ventilation always stirs a degree of controversy. There are those who think that ventilation is contraindicated after paralysis and cricoid pressure in a rapid sequence intubation. However, it is my opinion that ventilation after cricoid pressure and paralysis is useful to ensure complete oxygenation, especially if repeat laryngoscopies are required. The need for ventilation should be guided by the oximeter. I often will use the technique of cricoid pressure and ventilation after paralysis in routine cases in order to teach the nurses, residents, and other personnel proper technique so that they are prepared for the true rapid-sequence situation.

Induction in the Patient With a Full Stomach

If the infant has an IV in place, then a rapid-sequence induction can be accomplished. Table 2-5 lists the steps to accomplish a rapid-sequence induction in an infant up to 1 year of age. Preoxygenation is accomplished by blowing a high flow of oxygen from a distance of several inches toward the infant's face. Attempts to place a mask over the face may result in a struggling, fighting infant and completely nullify any benefit of the oxygen.

For children age 1 and older, the sequence is only slightly different (Table 2-6). Atropine or glycopyrrolate is not needed routinely, although for individual cases it may be. Curare 0.05 mg/kg is administered to prevent fasciculation from the succinylcholine. The decision whether or not to use thiopental or ketamine for induction depends on the condition of the patient. If there is a question of the blood volume or if the infant or child is believed to be quite debilitated, ketamine 1 to 2 mg/kg would be the induction agent of choice.

If the infant or child does not have an IV, then rectal methohexital 30 mg/kg can be given with the child on his side or abdomen. An IV is then started using a small amount of local anesthetic. The usual sequence is followed but the thiopental dose is reduced according to the patient's response to the preoxygenation: if no response, then 2 mg/kg; if movement, then 4 mg/kg. Another variation is to give ketamine 3 mg/kg IM, leave the child on his side, start an

Table 2-5. Rapid-Sequence Induction for Infants Up to 1 Year of Age With an IV and Without Increased Intracranial Pressure or an Open-Eye Injury

1. Preoxygenate for 1–2 minutes; apply monitors
2. Atropine 0.01 mg/kg or glycopyrrolate 0.01 mg/kg IV
3. Pentothal 4 mg/kg of ketamine 1 mg/kg
4. Cricoid pressure as soon as tolerated
5. Succinylcholine 2 mg/kg IV
6. Intubation
7. Verify position of tube
8. Release of cricoid pressure
9. Begin maintenance anesthesia

Table 2-6. Rapid-Sequence Induction for Infants and Children Over 1 Year of Age With an IV and Without Increased Intracranial Pressure or an Open-Eye Injury

1. Preoxygenate for 1–2 minutes; apply monitors
2. Curare 0.05 mg/kg
3. Thiopental 4–6 mg/kg or ketamine 1 mg/kg
4. Cricoid pressure as soon as tolerated
5. Succinylcholine 2 mg/kg IV
6. Intubation
7. Verify position of tube
8. Release of cricoid pressure
9. Begin maintenance anesthesia

IV, and then proceed with the above intubation technique. The need for additional thiopental will depend on the patient's response to the mask. There are methods for induction and intubation that do not require the presence of an IV. One technique is to administer succinylcholine 4 mg/kg IM after the induction with either rectal methohexital or ketamine as the child is being oxygenated. As soon as tolerated cricoid pressure is applied and then the rest of the sequence is followed.

Induction in the Patient With a Potential Open-Eye Injury

The field of anesthesiology is similar in many ways to a battlefield in which innumerable land mines have been planted in unknown locations awaiting the unwary. The child with a potential open-eye injury represents one of the more controversial and widely discussed topics in pediatric anesthesia.[38–41] Because of the diversity of opinion it is very difficult to be adamant about a singular technique for the induction of anesthesia and intubation of the patient. One of the major problems in children with a potential open-eye injury or increased intracranial pressure is that any degree of struggling or crying will increase intraocular pressure or intracranial pressure. For that reason, care of these patients should begin before they come to the operating room. Unless the child has some severe systemic illness there is no reason why he should be subjected to any type of painful procedure such as starting an IV or draining blood. These procedures will only upset the child and make him cry, and potentially might cause more harm and defeat the benefits of a smooth induction.

The patient with a potential open-eye injury presents two challenges: first, to perform a smooth induction in a child with a full stomach in order to prevent the aspiration of gastric contents, and second, if the globe is open, to preserve the eye. The parents need to be informed about the potential dangers in a gentle way so that they understand the problems that may face the child and anesthesiologist. This is a situation in which the parents should be allowed to be present in order to assist in preventing a stormy induction.

There are several options for the anesthesiologist. In children aged 1 to 5, rectal methohexital will usually result in a very smooth induction. After the

Table 2-7. Rapid-Sequence Induction for Open-Eye Surgery (or Increased Intracranial Pressure)

1. Induction of choice; start IV. Thiopental as needed
2. Lidocaine 1.5 mg/kg IV
3. Atracurium 0.8 mg/kg or curare 0.05 mg/kg followed by succinylcholine 2 mg/kg
4. Cricoid pressure as soon as tolerated
5. Intubation
6. Verify position of tube
7. Release of cricoid pressure
8. Begin maintenance anesthesia

child is asleep, he is gently laid on a stretcher either on the side or abdomen so that if he regurgitates he won't aspirate. The child is then taken to the operating room, where an IV is started with local anesthesia and a modified rapid-sequence induction is performed. As part of the induction, thiopental 2 to 3 mg/kg and lidocaine 1.5 mg/kg are administered before the muscle relaxant. The object of lidocaine administration is to deepen anesthesia and suppress the cough reflex. If the child is cooperative an inhalation induction is performed and an IV is started and the rapid sequence followed. Another option is to use EMLA cream on the skin 1 hour before the surgery, which will allow an IV to be started without pain. The induction is then performed using thiopental 4 to 6 mg/kg along with lidocaine 1.5 mg/kg, followed by the rest of the rapid sequence. Table 2-7 summarizes the options.

The second major concern after that of regurgitation and aspiration is increased intraocular pressure. There are two potential causes for increased intraocular pressure during intubation, succinylcholine use and laryngoscopy. Succinylcholine is thought to increase intraocular pressure by causing a sustained contraction of the extraocular muscles that lasts from 3 to 5 minutes and is apparently not related to the duration of the neuromuscular block. For that reason, it has been suggested that a nondepolarizing muscle relaxant be given before succinylcholine in order to modify this effect. The literature is replete with studies on the effects on intraocular pressure of the various combinations of nondepolarizing relaxants and succinylcholine. The results of these studies are at variance with each other, some reporting no increase while others report small increases. Consequently, some anesthesiologists prefer to use a nondepolarizing muscle relaxant technique without succinylcholine and thereby avoid the issue. There are equally compelling arguments for either technique, with large series reporting no apparent difference in outcome, although it must be understood that determining outcome in this situation is almost impossible. The advantage of succinylcholine use is a more rapid control of the airway; its disadvantage is the small increase in intraocular pressure that many ophthalmologists do not feel is significant.

The advantage of the nondepolarizing muscle relaxant is that the muscle relaxant itself does not cause an increase in intraocular pressure. There are some dangers and pitfalls that need to be avoided. Laryngoscopy before the muscle relaxant is effective may result in coughing and increased intraocular pressure, therefore it would be useful to monitor the neuromuscular transmission with a nerve stimulator to determine when intubating conditions are appropriate. Also, the stimulation of laryngoscopy can increase intraocular pressure in the lightly anesthetized patient. For that reason, it has been suggested that lidocaine 1.5 mg/kg be combined with whatever muscle relaxant is chosen in addition to the dose of thiopental. There are several potential disadvantages to the use of non-depolarizing muscle relaxants. One of the concerns is that there may be a relatively long time between the administration of the drug and when the conditions are appropriate for intubation. This time interval is important because it is in this period that the airway may be relatively unprotected and aspiration may occur. One of the other concerns with using a nondepolarizing muscle relaxant is that if the patient has a difficult airway, be it recognized or unrecognized, there may be a long period of muscle paralysis and difficulty in maintaining the airway. The use of a medium-acting muscle relaxant such as atracurium or vecuronium has decreased this time period somewhat from that of the previously used pancuronium. There is a new nondepolarizing muscle relaxant, mivacurium, which undergoes hydrolysis by plasma cholinesterase. The advantages of this muscle relaxant are that it has a shorter duration of action and there are no clinically or statistically significant changes in heart rate or blood pressure following its administration. Goudsouzian et al., in a recent study of the neuromuscular and cardiovascular effects of mivacurium in children, reported that there was a 95 percent recovery of the depression of the twitch response in approximately 10 minutes, compared to 23 minutes with vecuronium and 28 minutes with atracurium.[42-44] However, this drug is not as rapid acting as succinylcholine.

Timing of Extubation in the Patient With a Full Stomach

Three things need to be considered in extubating a child with a full stomach: emptying the stomach, awake extubation, and position. Emptying the stomach does not guarantee that the stomach will be empty but it does reduce the quantity of material. When to extubate a child with a full stomach is one of the few issues that anesthesiologists agree on. The answer is when the child is able to protect the airway. This occurs when the child is awake. By awake we usually mean the child is able to reach up and pull out the endotracheal tube, open the eyes, and have purposeful movements; these signs signify the return of the protective airway reflexes. There are times when the child reacts on the airway after the anesthetic is discontinued and before the anesthesiologist thinks that he is awake enough to manage the airway. There are two options. One is to give a small dose of succinylcholine and continue to ventilate the child until more of the anesthetic is removed and the child has recovered more of the airway reflexes. The other technique that has been found quite useful is to administer lidocaine 1.5 mg/kg IV. This will decrease the reactivity of the child to the endotracheal tube and allow protective reflexes to be recovered. At times, even then the child is not awake enough to be extubated, in which case the dose of lidocaine can be repeated. No more than 3 mg/kg of lidocaine should be administered over a 5-minute period, and no more than 6 mg/kg over a 1-hour period. The dose of lidocaine administered to infants under 6 months of age should be reduced to 1 mg/kg because of the limited cardiac reserve and no more than 2 mg/kg over a 5-minute period. These doses are arbitrary but reflect a concern for the decreased cardiac reserve of the young infant.

The position of the child can be quite important in facilitating the removal of secretions and gastric contents should the patient regurgitate or vomit. The child should be placed in the lateral or prone position and then extubated. When possible, these children should be extubated in the operating room. However, at times it is difficult to estimate exactly when the surgery will terminate, therefore the child may not be ready for extubation nor may it be anticipated that the child will be ready within a short period of time. In this situation, the child should be transported to the recovery room and the same type of extubation sequence followed there.

REFERENCES

1. Hopkins CS, Buckley CJ, Bush GH: Pain-free injection in infants. Use of a lignocaine-prilocaine cream to prevent pain at intravenous injection. Anaesthesia 43:198, 1988
2. Steward DJ: Psychological preparation and premedication. In Gregory GA (ed): Pediatric Anesthesia. Vol. 1. Churchill Livingstone, New York, 1989
3. Korsch BM: The child and the operating room. Anesthesiology 43:251, 1975
4. Hanallah RS, Rosales JK: Experience with parents' presence during anesthesia induction in children. Can Anaesth Soc J 30:287, 1983
5. Hanallah RS, Abramowitz MD, Tae HO, Ruttimann UE: Residents' attitudes toward parents' presence during anesthesia induction in children: Does experience make a difference? Anesthesiology 60:598, 1984
6. Brzustowicz RM, Nelson DA, Betts EK, et al: Efficacy of oral premedication for pediatric outpatient surgery. Anesthesiology 60:475, 1984
7. Mattila MAK, Ruoppi MK, Ahlstrom-Bengs E, et al: Diazepam in rectal solution as premedication in children, with special reference to serum concentrations. Br J Anaesth 53:1269, 1981
8. Van der Walt JH, Nicholls B, Bentley M, Tomkins DP: Oral premedication in children. Anaesth Intensive Care 15:151, 1987
9. Saint-Maurice C, Meistelman C, Rey E, et al: The pharmacokinetics of rectal midazolam for premedication in children. Anesthesiology 65:536, 1987
10. Raybould D, Bradshow EG: Premedication for day case surgery. Anaesthesia 42:591, 1987
11. Stanley TH: New routes of administration and new delivery systems of anesthetics. Anesthesiology 68:665, 1988
12. Henderson JM, Brodsky DA, Fisher DM, et al: Pre-induction of anesthesia in pediatric patients with nasally administered sufentanil. Anesthesiology 68:671, 1988
13. Aldrete JA, Roman-de Jesus JC, Russell LJ, D'Cruz O: Intranasal ketamine as induction adjunct in children: Preliminary report. Anesthesiology 67:A514, 1987
14. Feld LH, Champeau MW, van Steenis CA, Scott JC: Preanesthetic medication in children: A comparison of oral transmucosal fentanyl citrate versus placebo. Anesthesiology 71:374, 1989

15. Wilton NCT, Leigh J, Rosen DR, Pandit UA: Preanesthetic sedation of preschool children using intranasal midazolam. Anesthesiology 69:972, 1988

16. Nelson PS, Streisand JB, Mulder S, et al: A comparison of oral transmucosal fentanyl citrate and an oral solution of meperidine, diazepam and atropine for premedication in children. Anesthesiology 70:616, 1989

17. Leiman BC, Walford A, Rawal N, et al: The effects of oral transmucosal fentanyl citrate premedication on gastric volume and acidity in children. Anesthesiology 67:A489, 1987

18. Keal EE: Physiological and pharmacological control of airways secretions. p. 357. In Brain JD, Proctor DF, Reid LM (eds): Respiratory Defense Mechanisms. Part 1. Marcel Dekker, New York, 1977

19. Gal TJ, Suratt PM: Atropine and glycopyrrolate effects on lung mechanics in normal man. Anesth Analg 60:85, 1981

20. Hardy JF, Charest J, Girouard G, Lepage Y: Nausea and vomiting after strabismus surgery in preschool children. Can Anaesth Soc J 33:57, 1986

21. Abramowitz MD, Oh TH, Epstein BS: The antiemetic effect of droperidol following strabismus surgery in children. Anesthesiology 59:579, 1983

22. Lerman J, Eustis S, Smith DR: Effect of droperidol pretreatment on postanesthetic vomiting in children undergoing strabismus surgery. Anesthesiology 65:322, 1986

23. Nicolson SC, Kaya KM, Betts EK: The effect of preoperative oral droperidol on the incidence of postoperative emesis after paediatric strabismus surgery. Can J Anaesth 35:364, 1988

24. Rowley MP, Brown TCK: Postoperative vomiting in children. Anaesth Intensive Care 10:309, 1982

25. Christensen S, Farrow-Gillespie A, Lerman J: Incidence of emesis and postanesthetic recovery after strabismus surgery in children: A comparison of droperidol and lidocaine. Anesthesiology 70:251, 1989

26. Patel RI, Hannallah RS: Anesthetic complications following pediatric ambulatory surgery: A 3 year study. Anesthesiology 69:1009, 1988

27. Hardy J-F: Large volume gastroesophageal reflux: A rationale for risk reduction in the perioperative period. Can J Anaesth 35:162, 1988

28. Edwards G, Morton HJV, Pask EA, et al: Deaths associated with anesthesia. A report of 1000 cases. Anaesthesia 11:194, 1956

29. Dinnick OP: Deaths associated with anaesthesia. Observations on 600 cases. Anaesthesia 11:194, 1964

30. Goudsouzian N, Cote CJ, Liu LMP, et al: The dose-response effects of oral cimetidine on gastric pH and volume in children. Anesthesiology 55:533, 1981

31. Manchikanti L, Marrero TC, Roush JR: Preanesthetic cimetidine and metoclopramide for acid aspiration prophylaxis in elective surgery. Anesthesiology 61:48, 1984

32. Liu LMP, Gaudreault P, Friedman PA, et al: Methohexital plasma concentrations in children following rectal administration. Anesthesiology 62:567, 1985

33. DeBoer AG, Leede LGJ, Breimer DD: Drug absorption by sublingual and rectal routes. Br J Anesth 56:69, 1984

34. Forbes RB, Vandewalker GE: Two percent rectal methohexital for induction of anesthesia in children. Anesthesiology 65:A420, 1986

35. Kestin IG, McIlvaine WB, Lockhart CH, et al: Rectal methohexital for induction of anesthesia in children with and without rectal aspiration after sleep: A pharmacokinetic and pharmacodynamic study. Anesth Analg 67:1102, 1988

36. Sussman DR: A comparative evaluation of ketamine anesthesia in children and adults. Anesthesiology 40:459, 1974

37. Hamza J, Ecoffey C, Gross JB: Ventilatory response to CO_2 following intravenous ketamine in children. Anesthesiology 70:422, 1989

38. Libonati MM, Leahy JJ, Ellison N: The use of succinylcholine in open eye surgery. Anesthesiology 62:637, 1985

39. Bourke DL: Open eye injuries. Anesthesiology 63:727, 1985

40. Rich AL, Witherspoon CD, Morris RE, et al: Letter to editor, re: Use of nondepolarizing anesthetic agents in penetrating ocular injuries. Anesthesiology 65:108, 1986

41. Weiner MJ, Olk RJ, Meyer EF: Letter to editor, re: Anesthesia for open eye surgery. Anesthesiology 65:109, 1986

42. Goudsouzian NG, Alifimoff JK, Eberty L, et al: Neuromuscular and cardiovascular effects of mivacurium in children. Anesthesiology 70:237, 1989

43. Meistelman C, Loose JP, Saint-Maurice C, et al: Clinical pharmacology of vecuronium in children. Br J Anaesth 58:996, 1986

44. Goudsouzian NG, Liu LMP, Cote CJ, et al: Safety and efficacy of atracurium in adolescents and children anesthetized with halothane. Anesthesiology 59:459, 1983

3

CLINICAL PHARMACOLOGY OF INHALATIONAL ANESTHETICS, MUSCLE RELAXANTS, VASOACTIVE AGENTS, AND NARCOTICS, AND TECHNIQUES OF GENERAL ANESTHESIA

Frederic A. Berry

Inhalational anesthetics remain the most popular anesthetic agents for the induction and/or maintenance of anesthesia. This chapter presents a brief overview of the inhalational anesthetics along with the differences within the various anesthetic delivery systems. It includes short discussions of the use of muscle relaxants, vasoactive agents, and narcotics, and concludes with a discussion of techniques of general anesthesia.

INHALATIONAL ANESTHETICS
Nitrous Oxide

Nitrous oxide is a weak inhalational agent. In normal healthy patients, nitrous oxide by itself cannot predictably produce surgical anesthesia since it requires a minimum alveolar anesthetic concentration (MAC) of 105 percent. Its safety is related to its lack of potency, and for this reason other drugs need to be added to achieve the anesthetized state. Nitrous oxide is frequently used in pediatric anesthesia (1) as an induction agent, (2) to reduce the MAC of volatile anesthetics, and (3) in "balanced" anesthesia.

Nitrous oxide is an insoluble anesthetic agent and will rapidly equilibrate in the brain. At the end of 5 minutes the end-tidal concentration of nitrous oxide will be approximately 90 percent of that inspired. This also has clinical significance at the end of anesthesia since the nitrous oxide will off-load rapidly. The rapid clearing of nitrous oxide at the end of surgery is what is responsible for a condition referred to as *diffusion hypoxia*. The rapid efflux of nitrous oxide from the lungs will dilute the inspired oxygen concentration. If the inspired gas is room air, the concentration of inspired oxygen may be reduced significantly, resulting in diffusion hypoxia. For this reason, increased concentrations of inspired oxygen should be given at the end of surgery for several minutes.

Nitrous oxide undergoes very little, if any, biotransformation. It is rapidly eliminated through the respiratory system and the expired gas, with a very small amount being excreted through the skin. Nitrous oxide may be contraindicated if there are large gas pockets within the body. These gas pockets will expand with the addition and equilibration of nitrous oxide. The blood gas partition coefficient for nitrous oxide is 34 times that for nitrogen. Therefore, the nitrous oxide will rapidly equilibrate in any pocket of trapped gas and will cause an expansion of the gas-containing compartment. Nitrous oxide will increase the size of the gas pocket in direct proportion to its concentration, so that 50 percent nitrous oxide will double the gas compartment. Situations in which this may occur include pneumothorax, pneumoencephalography, trapped gas within obstructed loops of bowel or the middle ear.

Of all of the anesthetics that we use today, nitrous oxide probably has the least effect on the circulatory system. Hickey et al. studied the hemodynamic responses of 50 percent nitrous oxide in infants and found a statistically significant depression of systemic hemodynamics, although these changes were believed to be clinically insignificant except perhaps in severely compromised infants.[1] The changes in pulmonary hemodynamics were minimal.

Nitrous Oxide as an Induction Agent and to Reduce the MAC of Volatile Anesthetics

Nitrous oxide is frequently used as the initial anesthetic in inhalational inductions in which a volatile agent is also to be added. In this technique, high-flow (6 to 10 L/min) nitrous oxide in a concentration of 70 percent is used to begin the induction of anesthesia. Nitrous oxide is almost odorless except for a slightly sweet smell. When rubber delivery hoses are used, they often have more odor than the nitrous oxide. Various scents have been used on anesthetic masks to camouflage the odor of the anesthetics. After the child has tolerated the nitrous oxide for a minute or so the volatile agent is added slowly in 0.25 to 0.5 percent concentrations. When the child has tolerated the concentration of the volatile agent for 15 to 20 seconds the concentration is increased by another 0.5 percent. At times the child may breathhold or cough, in which case the concentration should be held constant or reduced temporarily until the reaction to the volatile agent ceases. Then the concentration of the volatile agent can be increased again until induction is accomplished.

Nitrous oxide is used to reduce the MAC of the various volatile agents. In this situation, nitrous oxide is used in a 50 to 70 percent concentration. Since the

MAC for nitrous oxide is 105 percent, whatever concentration of nitrous oxide that is being used will reduce the MAC of the volatile agent by approximately the same percentage. As an example, nitrous oxide in a 50 percent concentration will reduce the MAC of the volatile anesthetic by 50 percent.

Nitrous Oxide in Balanced Anesthesia

Balanced anesthesia refers to a combination of nitrous oxide, narcotics, hypnotics, muscle relaxants, and, recently, regional techniques. When nitrous oxide is used in the balanced technique usually the induction of anesthesia is accomplished with the intravenous administration of a barbiturate, muscle relaxation is accomplished with muscle relaxants, narcotics are given for additional analgesia, and nitrous oxide is administered in a concentration of approximately 70 percent. The advantage of this technique is that the patient recovers very rapidly from the anesthetic as the muscle relaxants are reversed and the nitrous oxide discontinued. The disadvantages of the balanced technique are the limited inspired oxygen potential and that the level of anesthesia achieved is just below the "awareness" level, where slight breaches in technique may allow "awareness" to surface. Also, the light level of anesthesia usually results in an elevated blood pressure, which in some circumstances may be a disadvantage because of increased bleeding and the potential need for blood transfusions. Spinal fusion for scoliosis is discussed later in this chapter as one application of the balanced technique.

Balanced Anesthesia and the Stress Response

Light levels of anesthesia are associated with the *stress response,* which results in the release of antidiuretic hormone. In the postoperative period, if hypotonic intravenous fluids are administered, the increased levels of antidiuretic hormone will cause an increased reabsorption of free water through the distal tubule and collecting duct, resulting in a dilutional hyponatremia.[2] The fluid of choice in the perioperative period is balanced salt solution, which will minimize this problem.

Volatile Inhalational Anesthetics

The volatile inhalational anesthetics are the most frequently used primary anesthetic agents in pediatric anesthesia. The three volatile agents in current use are halothane, enflurane, and isoflurane. Halothane is by far the most popular of the three because of its low cost, ease of administration, and familiarity. The other two have both practical and theoretical advantages, but until their price decreases, they will not replace halothane. A new anesthetic, I-653, is about to appear on the market. I-653 is quite comparable to isoflurane in its cardiovascular effects.[3] It has a very low solubility in blood, extremely low toxicity, little or no metabolism, and because of its low solubility, results in a rapid awakening. At least in experimental animals, isoflurane and I-653 are similar with respect to incidence of epinephrine-induced dysrhythmias and increases in blood pres-

Table 3-1. Metabolism of Inhalational Anesthetics

Anesthetic	Absorbed Anesthetic Recovered as Metabolites (%)
Nitrous oxide	0.004
Isoflurane	0.17
Enflurane	2.4
Halothane	20.0

sure and heart rate.[4] Sevoflurane is another new volatile anesthetic agent that is currently undergoing clinical trials and that has many of the same characteristics. With all the good news, there must be bad news, and the bad news is its price. With cost containment and the enormous negative balance of payments, it is highly unlikely that I-653 or sevoflurane at least in the near future will find much of a market.

Metabolism of Volatile Anesthetics

One theoretical advantage of isoflurane and enflurane is the low degree of metabolism that these drugs undergo compared with halothane (Table 3-1). As a practical matter, this is not very important in short surgeries but may be for long surgeries or those performed on the obese patient.

Induction of Anesthesia Using Volatile Agents

Another theoretical advantage of isoflurane is that is it more insoluble than halothane (blood gas partition coefficient 1.4 vs. 2.3), which means that the alveolar concentration will rise more rapidly toward the inspired concentration and hence the patient should be induced more rapidly and should awaken more rapidly. This theoretical advantage for induction has never been realized in practice since isoflurane is more pungent than halothane, and the pungency provokes coughing and breathholding, which prolongs induction and causes episodes of desaturation.[5] The use of nitrous oxide will reduce the pungency. Still, halothane for the great majority of pediatric patients remains the gentlest of the volatile agents. Fisher et al. compared halothane, enflurane, and isoflurane in outpatient anesthesia.[6] The children in the study were not sedated, and all three agents were administered with nitrous oxide. The results of the study demonstrated that halothane has the fastest induction time with the lowest incidence of excitement. Isoflurane has the highest incidence of coughing and laryngospasm on induction, and the highest incidence of coughing on emergence and in the recovery room. The conclusion of the study is that in a busy outpatient practice, its rapid and smooth induction makes halothane the agent of choice. There is a growing trend toward using halothane for the induction of anesthesia and then switching to isoflurane for the maintenance period for long surgeries or for those performed on the obese patient. The greater solubility of halothane compared to isoflurane in these cases will result in a longer off-loading time of halothane compared to isoflurane. The other disadvantage of halothane is that since it undergoes a higher degree of biotransformation, there is the potential for a relatively prolonged excretion of its metabolic products.

Further Comparisons of Inhalational Agents

The next part of this chapter compares the effects of the inhalational agents on the circulation, respiration, and muscle relaxation. The effects on intracranial pressure are covered in Chapter 12, Pediatric Neuroanesthesia. The majority of the reported studies were done on healthy, unsedated adult volunteers in the absence of disease, drugs, and surgical stimulation. This fact needs to be kept in mind when transferring the data to the patient who has a concurrent disease and is receiving various medications.

Effects of Inhalational Agents on the Circulatory System

The effects of inhalational agents are discussed with special emphasis on cardiac output, blood pressure, and peripheral vascular resistance. What the anesthesiologist really would like to know is what is happening to myocardial performance (i.e., cardiac output). Cardiac output can be measured clinically but, in general, it requires invasive techniques. Echocardiography, a noninvasive technique, has been used to assess ventricular function in children during both isoflurane and halothane anesthesia. Although it is primarily a research tool, there has been progress toward the clinical application of intraoperative echocardiographic measurements of cardiac performance.

Cardiac Output

In adult volunteers there is a dose-dependent reduction in cardiac output with enflurane and halothane (Fig. 3-1). The values for the anesthetic agents are given in end-tidal MAC levels. Isoflurane at 1 to 2 MAC does not cause

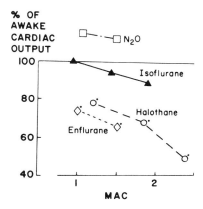

Fig. 3-1. Neither isoflurane nor nitrous oxide depressed the cardiac output below its awake levels in volunteers. In contrast, both halothane and enflurane decreased the output significantly (asterisks), and did so to a greater extent at deeper levels of anesthesia. (From Eger,[65] with permission.)

a reduction in cardiac output. In healthy adult patients and older children nitrous oxide is associated with an increase in cardiac output, which is thought to be due to a weak sympathomimetic effect of this drug. The studies on infants (7 to 15 months) demonstrated that the cardiovascular effects of adding nitrous oxide to isoflurane and halothane were similar to equianesthetic concentrations of isoflurane and halothane in oxygen (1.5 MAC).[7] The reason for this difference is thought to be the normal sympathetic response in adults and older children. It has been shown that the infant has an immature sympathetic nervous system and that this is reflected by the lack of blood pressure response.

The decrease in cardiac output demonstrated with halothane and enflurane closely parallels the changes in blood pressure. Barash et al. studied ventricular function in children during halothane anesthesia and reported a dose-dependent depression of ventricular function.[8] The changes found in their study were believed to be both rate dependent and due to myocardial depression. Figure 3-2 shows these effects. The values of halothane in the figure are inspired, not end-tidal, concentrations of halothane. The administration of atropine 0.2 mg caused a rapid increase in all the rate- dependent variables, resulting in an increase in

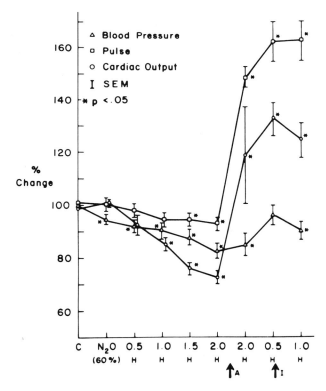

Fig. 3-2. Changes in blood pressure (triangle), pulse rate (square), and cardiac output (circle) with increasing concentrations of halothane. A, atropine; I, intubation. (From Barash et al.,[8] with permission.)

cardiac output. However, the other indices of myocardial performance, such as the ejection fraction and the left ventricular end-diastolic volume, still showed depression. Studies in children 2 to 7 years old using echocardiographic assessment of ventricular function during isoflurane and halothane anesthesia suggest that there is little if any reduction in ventricular function at 1.3 MAC (end-tidal concentrations) of isoflurane, whereas there is significant depression of ventricular function at 1.3 MAC (end-tidal concentrations) of halothane.[9] There was little change in heart rate but there was a progressively significant fall in mean blood pressure with both agents.

Echocardiographic studies demonstrate that there is a difference between the cardiac output effects of isoflurane and halothane in infants and small children (up to 32 months).[10] Both isoflurane and halothane will decrease cardiac output, stroke volume, and ejection fraction. When both groups were given a 15 ml/kg fluid bolus of lactated Ringer's solution the halothane group had a further reduction in ejection fraction and stroke volume, although they increased in the isoflurane group, suggesting a greater cardiovascular reserve with isoflurane in infants and children.

Arterial Blood Pressure

The inhalational agents cause a dose-related decrease in arterial blood pressure. The effects of nitrous oxide, halothane, enflurane, and isoflurane on blood pressure are depicted in Figure 3-3.

Peripheral Vascular Resistance

The inhalational anesthetics have different effects on systemic vascular resistance. Halothane has little effect, whereas isoflurane and, to a lesser extent, enflurane produce a dose-dependent reduction in calculated systemic vascular

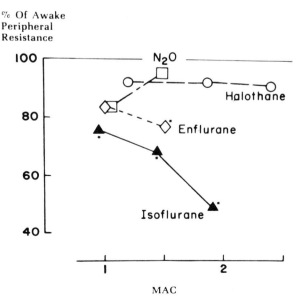

Fig. 3-3. Isoflurane, halothane, and enflurane, but not nitrous oxide, decrease the arterial blood pressure from its preanesthetic value in a dose-related fashion (asterisks indicate a significant change). (From Eger,[65] with permission.)

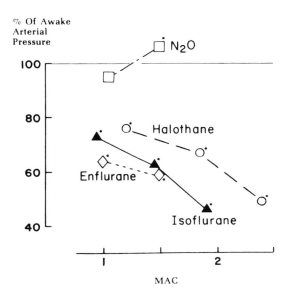

Fig. 3-4. Isoflurane and, to a lesser extent, enflurane cause peripheral vasodilation, while halothane and nitrous oxide do not (asterisks indicate significant changes from awake values). (From Eger,[65] with permission.)

resistance (Fig. 3-4). There is a common clinical misconception that halothane reduces peripheral resistance because of the cutaneous vasodilatation that occurs.

Baroreceptors

There is a dose-dependent depression of baroreceptors with the volatile inhalational anesthetics. This has been demonstrated with halothane in the preterm infant by Gregory.[11] In studies of both adult dogs and humans, isoflurane preserves the baroreflex better than either halothane or enflurane.[12] However, as reported by LeDez and Lerman in preterm infants and by Murat et al. in neonates, there is significant depression of the baroreflex control of heart rate at 1 MAC isoflurane.[13,14] Murat et al. have demonstrated a marked depression of the baroreceptor reflex control of heart rate by fentanyl in newborn infants.[15] This has significant clinical application. One of the compensatory responses of the infant for hypotension is activation of the baroresponse, which increases the heart rate. Therefore, the clinical significance of this finding is that changes in blood volume (i.e. hypovolemia) will not be signalled by an increase in heart rate nor will the neonate be able to compensate for the hypovolemia by increasing the heart rate in an attempt to maintain adequate cardiac output during hypovolemia.

Effects of Inhalational Agents on Ventilation and Muscle Relaxation

The volatile anesthetic agents have a dose-dependent effect on ventilation. The respiratory pattern changes to a regular rhythm, the rate increases, and the tidal volume decreases in the anesthetized state. Exhalation becomes an active process that results in an increase in abdominal muscle tone during exhalation. This is the reason that when ventilation is controlled and the $PaCO_2$ is below the apneic threshold the abdominal muscles are more relaxed. This will reduce or in some cases eliminate the need for muscle relaxants. The effects of anesthetics on the CO_2 response curve are well known, as there is a dose-dependent depression. There is a greater effect of anesthetics on the hypoxic ventilatory drive than on the response to hypercarbia. Knill and Clement examined the effects of subanesthetic doses of halothane (0.15 to 0.30 percent inspired) on the peripheral chemoreflex pathway in adults and found a profound depression of the peripheral chemoreflex pathway via the depression of the carotid bodies.[16] The subjects of the study were somewhat drowsy, but they were coherent and had full recall of the experiment. One of the actions of the peripheral chemoreflex pathway is to protect the body from hypoxia. When the carotid bodies are stimulated by hypoxia, a cascade of protective physiologic defenses are activated. These defenses, an increase in minute ventilation, hypertension, and a favorable redistribution of cardiac output are the result of tachypnea. In the unanesthetized state, there is also central nervous system arousal. The clinical implications are clear—not only for small infants but for all patients. This is why most anesthesiologists intubate almost all young infants and leave them intubated until they have recovered their protective airway reflexes. The drowsy postoperative patient may have sufficient residual anesthesia to depress the peripheral chemoreflex pathway, which may cause hypoventilation owing to their hypoxic and depressed respiratory protective reflexes. The period of recovery in the postanesthesia room as the child eliminates the anesthetic from the system is critical. The pulse oximeter may be of value in monitoring the child who is still unconscious or semiconscious from anesthesia.

The Anesthetic Requirements of Infants

The initial studies of Gregory et al., Nicodemus et al., and Cameron et al. demonstrating age-dependent MACs have been supplemented in the premature infant and neonate by Lerman et al.[17-20] These studies demonstrated that the 1- to 6-month-old infant has the highest anesthetic requirement. Table 3-2 is a

Table 3-2. 1 MAC Requirement[a]

	Isoflurane	Halothane
Preterm		
32 weeks[b]	1.28	0.55
32–37[b]	1.41	
Full-term, 0–1 month old	1.6	0.87
Full-term, 1–6 months old	1.87	1.2
Full-term, 6–12 months old	1.8	
Full-term, 1–5 years old	1.6	1.0
Young adults	1.28	0.87

[a] End-tidal concentrations.
[b] Gestational age.

composite of the various studies of anesthetic requirement. All of the MAC determinations of isoflurane and halothane are end-tidal determinations.

Three possible reasons are postulated for the low MAC in the neonate: (1) elevated progesterone levels, (2) immature central nervous system, and (3) a combination of high circulating β-endorphins and an immature central nervous system.[21-23] MAC in the term-pregnant patient is reduced approximately 30 percent, and this is thought to be related to the circulating levels of progesterone. The progesterone from the mother passes into the fetus, and levels are measurable for the first 10 days of neonatal life. The immature central nervous system of the neonate is responsible for his lower appreciation of pain or, conversely, his high threshold to elicit the pain response. In addition, it has been shown that neonates have higher circulating levels of β-endorphins than do adults. Normally the β-endorphins do not cross the blood-brain barrier and, therefore, have little effect on the central nervous system. However, it has been postulated that in neonates the immature central nervous system and immature blood-brain barrier might allow passage of the β-endorphins, which therefore results in a lower MAC.[23]

Drug Interactions With Volatile Anesthetics

Dosage Requirements for Nondepolarizing Muscle Relaxants Used With Volatile Anesthetics

There is a dose-dependent reduction in the dose of nondepolarizing muscle relaxant needed when volatile anesthetic agents are being used (Fig. 3-5). The dose of nondepolarizing muscle relaxant should be titrated with a nerve stimulator. This not only results in a more satisfactory dose response of muscle relaxant during the surgical procedure but also assists with determining the adequacy of the reversal of muscle relaxants at the conclusion of surgery.

Volatile Anesthetics, Epinephrine Solutions, and Dysrhythmias

Johnston et al. reported on the comparative interaction of epinephrine with enflurane, isoflurane, and halothane.[24] Their patients were all adults in ASA category I or II, and ventilation was controlled to maintain a $PaCO_2$ between 30 and 40 mmHg. One group of the halothane patients received epinephrine 1:200,000 in a 0.5 percent lidocaine solution. The patients were anesthetized with the various volatile agents and the anesthetic concentrations were adjusted to 1.25 MAC. The 50 percent effective dose (ED_{50}) of epinephrine was determined. The ED_{50} was defined as the appearance of three premature ventricular contractions (PCVs) at any time during or immediately following epinephrine injection. The results of that study are indicated in Figure 3-6. The ED_{50} for epinephrine and halothane in adults is 2.1 μg/kg, while the ED_{50} for halothane, lidocaine, and epinephrine is 3.7 μg/kg. The ED_{50} for enflurane and isoflurane

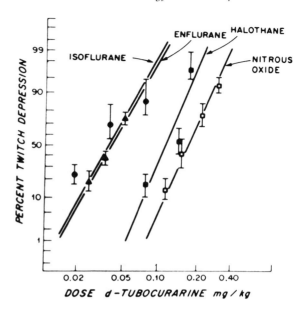

Fig. 3-5. Anesthesia was produced in normocapnic patients with a balanced technique or with 1.25 MAC enflurane, halothane, or isoflurane. Halothane potentiated the effect of d-tubocurarine more than did the balanced technique with nitrous oxide. Isoflurane and enflurane, in turn, produced a greater potentiation (by a factor of 2 or 3) than did halothane. (From Ali and Savarese,[66] with permission.)

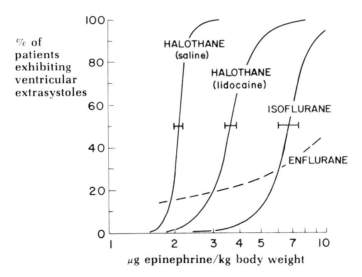

Fig. 3-6. Patients were given 1.25 MAC enflurane, halothane, or isoflurane in oxygen. For halothane, the ED_{50} was 2.1 µg/kg when the medium for epinephrine injection was saline, and 3.7 µg/kg when the medium was 0.5 percent lidocaine. For isoflurane, the ED_{50} was 6.7 µg/kg (epinephrine in saline). The curve for enflurane is flatter than that for halothane or isoflurane: a few patients given enflurane developed extrasystoles at relatively low doses of epinephrine. (From Eger,[65] with permission.)

is considerably higher. Sevoflurane and I-653 have been found to have similar properties to isoflurane with respect to epinephrine-induced dysrhythmias.[4]

There is a major difference between the interaction of epinephrine and halothane in children compared to adults. The report by Ueda et al. in spontaneously breathing children concluded that a mean dose of epinephrine of 7.8 µg/kg given together with lidocaine could be used safely.[25] In the study of Karl et al., doses of epinephrine up to 15 µg/kg were used in normocarbic and hypocarbic pediatric patients who did not have congenital heart disease without any increase in dysrhythmias.[26] Some of the patients in their series had lidocaine administered with the epinephrine while other did not. The reasons for this difference between adults and children are not clear. It is believed by most investigators that the addition of lidocaine to the epinephrine solution increases the margin of safety since the lidocaine will treat the ventricular dysrhythmias caused by the interaction. As a practical matter, it would appear that the dosage recommendation for children receiving halothane should be 10 to 15 µg/kg of epinephrine and that if dysrhythmias develop they should be treated with intravenous lidocaine 1.5 mg/kg. The use of the pulse oximeter has aided greatly in ruling in or out the presence of hypoxia and its role in the causation of dysrhythmias. At this point, it would seem appropriate to discuss in a brief manner the occurrence of dysrhythmias during anesthesia and some of the considerations that go into their diagnosis and management.

Dysrhythmias During Anesthesia

Dysrhythmias are frequent in usual anesthetic practice. The occasional PVC is not a problem. Bigeminy and multifocal PVCs are relatively frequent dysrhythmias that are seen during induction and at the beginning of surgery, and usually are due to light anesthesia. The use of pulse oximetry and end-tidal CO_2 monitors can rule in or out and assist in correcting the more bothersome causes of dysrhythmias, which are hypoxia and/or hypercarbia ($PaCO_2 > 60$ mmHg). If the cause of the dysrhythmia is light anesthesia, then it usually can be corrected by increasing the ventilation and halothane concentration. If this is unsuccessful within a few minutes, then lidocaine 1.5 mg/kg should be administered to deepen anesthesia and decrease myocardial irritability. If halothane is the anesthetic, there may be interaction between the halothane and the elevated catecholamines. Therefore, switching agents to isoflurane or enflurane will terminate the dysrhythmia if this is the etiology.

Mitral Valve Prolapse Dysrhythmias

Mitral valve prolapse has been reported as a cause of intraoperative dysrhythmias in children. Mitral valve prolapse is being recognized more frequently and at an earlier age. The major pathophysiologic changes are structural alterations in the mitral valve leaflet secondary to myxomatous degeneration and abnormal cardiovascular regulatory mechanisms secondary to sympathetic nervous system imbalance. The result is a cardiovascular system that is sensitive to adrenergic stimulation and volume depletion. A longer discussion of mitral valve prolapse is found in Chapter 16, Miscellaneous Potholes. The anesthetic management should include:

1. Careful psychological preparation of the patient and family
2. Sedative premedication
3. Omitting drugs, such as anticholinergics, that cause tachycardia
4. Maintaining an adequate circulating blood volume to decrease the chance of prolapse
5. Titrating intravenous doses of propranolol for control if ventricular ectopia occurs, and if ectopia persists, switching to agents other than halothane (i.e., isoflurane or enflurane)
6. Administering intravenous antibiotics for endocarditis prophylaxis

Complications With Volatile Inhalational Anesthetic Use

Complications with use of volatile inhalational anesthetics include hepatitis and renal failure secondary to inorganic fluoride. Malignant hyperthermia also can be triggered by volatile agents. This will be discussed in Chapter 15.

Hepatitis

The patient who develops jaundice in the postoperative period presents an enormous quandary for the anesthesiologist.[27,28] Although there may be many causes of postoperative jaundice the one that the anesthesiologist is most concerned about is hepatotoxicity caused by a volatile anesthetic. There is good evidence to suggest that halothane hepatitis is a multifactorial disease. In clinical practice one might see two different entities. The one form presents shortly after anesthesia, and is a mild form of toxicity. This form has been well studied in animals through various manipulations of drugs, hypoxia, and other factors. The other form is a fulminant type of toxicity; it usually has a delayed onset of several days to a week and is often lethal. Current thinking strongly suggests that the latter form of hepatotoxicity has an immunologic basis. Approximately 20 percent of halothane undergoes biotransformation during anesthesia. During biotransformation some of the halothane is oxidatively metabolized to a trifluoroacetyl halide moiety. This compound is able to acetylate endogenous liver protein, resulting in a hapten that is immunogenic. Antibodies are then produced against this hapten resulting in a immune response. Recent excitement has developed because patients with halothane hepatitis have been shown to produce an antibody that reacts with trifluoroacetylate albumen. Christ et al., in a series of animal experiments, have demonstrated a hypersensitivity basis for the hepatitis of the volatile anesthetics.[29] They were able to demonstrate enflurane hepatitis and the apparent cross-sensitization between halothane and enflurane, which involves the development of covalently bound liver microsomal adducts. The frequency of the development of hepatotoxicity depends on the degree of metabolism. The metabolism of halothane (20 percent) is much greater than that of enflurane (2.5 percent), which is also much greater than the metabolism of isoflurane (0.17 percent). There have been varying case reports of the development of what would appear to be enflurane or isoflurane hepatitis, although the occurrence is much less frequent than with halothane.[30]

Hoft et al. reported the development of halothane hepatitis in three pairs of closely related women.[31] A genetic predisposition to developing halothane hepatitis is poorly expressed in children, which may be one reason why children have such a low incidence of halothane hepatitis compared to adults. The incidence in adults ranges from 1 in 10,000 to 1 in 35,000, whereas in the study by Wark the incidence in children was 1 in 82,000 patients.[32]

Clinical Considerations in Halothane Hepatitis

There are certain patients who have a greater predisposition to develop halothane hepatitis. These include patients who have undergone repeated anesthetics, obese patients, and female patients. These factors are not thought to be a major problem in children. A high percentage of adult patients who have developed fatal or severe halothane hepatitis have a history of the previous halothane anesthetic resulting in a mild degree of hepatitis characterized by pyrexia and/or malaise. Whitburn has found the same history in children.[33] Therefore, it would appear that a careful history and attention to previous records would help to further reduce the extremely low incidence of halothane hepatitis. One of the difficulties in using a history of temperature alone to signify hepatitis is that approximately 20 to 25 percent of patients will have a postoperative fever of varying duration regardless of anesthetic technique. Therefore, it is important when establishing the occurrence of "hepatitis" following anesthesia that documentation be based upon alterations in hepatic enzymes as well as by pyrexia. If there is any questionable history after a halothane anesthetic then alternative techniques should be used.

Renal Toxicity

Inorganic fluoride in high serum concentrations (50 μM) has been associated with renal damage. The most infamous example of this is seen in methoxyflurane use. The only currently used volatile anesthetic that produces potentially significant concentrations of inorganic fluoride is enflurane. However, as a practical matter the inorganic fluoride levels with enflurane do not usually achieve the levels that are associated with renal damage. Obese patients will achieve a higher level of inorganic fluoride after enflurane use than nonobese patients, as shown by Strube et al.[34] This is thought to be secondary to their large amount of fat tissue, which traps more of the anesthetic and allows for more metabolism of the enflurane. It would appear to have no clinical consequences, however. Hinkle recently reported the inorganic fluoride levels after enflurane use in a group of children aged 1 to 9 years and found that, compared to adults, the inorganic fluoride level peaked earlier (1 hour vs. 4 hours) and the serum levels were lower (10.5 μM vs. 17 μM).[35]

MUSCLE RELAXANTS

The anesthesiologist has a pharmacy full of muscle relaxants to choose from. The choice of muscle relaxant is often based on which muscle relaxant was popular during the anesthesiologist's training period. However, the choice should be made according to the speed of onset, the length of action desired, the cardiovascular and other systemic effects, and the cost.

Succinylcholine

In the past several years succinylcholine has been the subject of much controversy and misunderstanding. One case report suggests that succinylcholine should be reevaluated for elective pediatric anesthesia.[36] This last statement can certainly reasonably be made about every drug that we use in anesthesia, and succinylcholine is no exception. Each drug has advantages and disadvantages. It is my opinion that the advantages and disadvantages of succinylcholine (Table 3-3) are such that it is my most frequent choice for routine intubation. However, there are patients in whom the drug should not be used; these patients as well as the alternatives to succinylcholine will be addressed in this chapter.

Pharmacology

Succinylcholine is a depolarizing muscle relaxant that is composed of two acetylcholine molecules linked through an acetate methyl group. Succinylcholine imitates the role of acetylcholine in stimulating nicotinic and muscarinic receptors. It is this stimulation that produces the desirable and some of the undesirable actions of succinylcholine. Nicotinic receptors are found in the neuromuscular junction, where the action of succinylcholine produces a profound short-lived depolarizing block. Stimulation of muscarinic receptors in the sinus node by succinylcholine may occasionally cause slowing of the heart rate. Stimulation of the autonomic ganglia, a more frequent side effect, results in an acceleration of the heart rate. If pretreated with anticholinergics the patient may exhibit neither of these effects. Before the advent of the pulse oximeter it was difficult at times to separate the bradycardia of succinylcholine from the bradycardia of hypoxia or the bradycardia caused by laryngoscopy and intubation. The development of the pulse oximeter has done two things: (1) allowed mon-

Table 3.3. Advantages and Disadvantages of Succinylcholine

Advantages	Disadvantages
Speed of onset	Myalgias
Profound relaxation	Potassium flux
Short duration of action	Burns, trauma, etc.
Intramuscular administration	Muscular dystrophy
Cost	Prolonged block (phase II)
	Excessive doses
	Atypical cholinesterase
	Malignant hyperthermia

itoring of the patient's oxygenation and (2) as a result of this, improved oxygenation at the time of laryngoscopy and intubation, which has reduced the incidence of bradycardia. Although now it is difficult to differentiate the bradycardia of succinylcholine from that of laryngoscopy, if the bradycardia resolves immediately after the endotracheal tube is inserted, the laryngoscope removed, and the first few breaths of oxygen taken, this suggests that the bradycardia was due to the activation of the vagal reflex by the instrumentation. The bradycardia of succinylcholine rarely requires treatment.

Advantages of Succinylcholine

When given intravenously succinylcholine causes a rapid onset of profound relaxation within 30 to 60 seconds.[37] Because of this rapid, prolonged relaxation, succinylcholine is generally acknowledged as providing the best conditions for intubation in the shortest time of any of the muscle relaxants. In addition, because of its rapid metabolism by cholinesterase, succinylcholine has a short duration of action. For these reasons succinylcholine is an excellent muscle relaxant for routine intubation. In addition, it is an excellent choice for very short (i.e., up to 5 minutes) laryngoscopies and bronchoscopies. Another advantage of succinylcholine is that it is the only muscle relaxant that is currently administered intramuscularly. In addition, succinylcholine is inexpensive. In the past cost was rarely considered important, but it will be quite important in the future.

Succinylcholine and Open-Eye Injuries

Succinylcholine use in the patient with an open-eye injury is controversial. A discussion of its use in these patients is presented in Chapter 2.

Intramuscular Succinylcholine

One of the unique features of succinylcholine is that it can be used intramuscularly. Intramuscular succinylcholine is used in two situations: (1) for rapid airway control after an inhalation induction and (2) for the establishment of an airway after laryngospasm. Some clinicians hesitate to attempt to intubate a child without vascular access. However, vascular access may be difficult in small infants and children. There are skilled practitioners who are able to obtain vascular access while the anesthesiologist maintains the airway, however, this situation does not always exist, and often the anesthesiologist is the most skilled. Therefore, when a difficult vascular access is anticipated, shortly after the induction of anesthesia with halothane-nitrous oxide, succinylcholine 4 to 5 mg/kg should be administered in the deltoid muscle and the nitrous oxide discontinued.[38] The deltoid muscle is used because it allows a more rapid uptake of drug than either the thigh or the buttock. It takes approximately 2 to 3 minutes for intramuscular succinylcholine to produce relaxation, and the relaxation will last from 15 to 25 minutes. The airway is then established and the patient placed on a ventilator. Then the anesthesiologist can seek vascular access while the surgeon is prepping. The advantage of this technique is that it allows control of the airway during often-prolonged attempts at vascular access. Hannallah et al. report very little cardiovascular effect with intramuscular succinylcholine.[39]

Succinylcholine and Laryngospasm

Perhaps the most important use for intramuscular succinylcholine is in the child who is undergoing an episode of laryngospasm during an inhalation induction, with airway obstruction, hypoventilation, and desaturation. Laryngospasm is accompanied by apnea, so the problem may rapidly become a vicious cycle of apnea and obstruction, leading to a complete inability to ventilate the patient. I have a very low threshold for administering succinylcholine to patients who are experiencing varying degrees of laryngospasm. At times it is difficult to differentiate between upper airway obstruction and laryngospasm. Therefore, if the diagnosis is uncertain, the use of an oral airway and/or positive pressure and other airway maneuvers are certainly indicated in order to unobstruct the airway. Some clinicians believe that positive pressure can "break" laryngospasm. However, in the case of laryngospasm, it is my experience that excessive positive pressure (greater than 10 to 15 cmH$_2$0) will only make the laryngospasm worse. Laryngospasm will break because of pharmacologic intervention or because of hypoxia. It is better to have a very low threshold to administer intramuscular succinylcholine and establish an airway while the child is still oxygenated in the early stages of laryngospasm than to persist in the use of the previously described maneuvers (positive pressure, etc.) Often the result is a child with complete obstruction and progressive desaturation, which is accompanied by the alarming tones of the oximeter. Administration of succinylcholine 1 mg/kg IV or lidocaine 1.5 mg/kg IV is the first step in the early development of laryngospasm, but if there is no intravenous access the only alternative route is the intramuscular use of succinylcholine. Another risk of laryngospasm in the obstructed patient with hypoxia is the development of postobstructive pulmonary edema (see Chapter 13).

Succinylcholine and the Difficult Airway

Another advantage of succinylcholine is that if the patient has an unexpected difficult airway and intubation is impossible after administration of succinylcholine, because of its rapid metabolism the duration of muscle relaxation will be short. Within 3 to 5 minutes the effects of succinylcholine will be gone and the patient will recover muscle and airway reflexes.[37] If a longer-acting muscle relaxant were used in this situation, the period of difficult airway management (and terror) would be much longer.

Disadvantages of Succinylcholine

Succinylcholine and Myalgias

Patients who have undergone general anesthesia often have muscle pain. Myalgias, particularly in the ambulatory patient, may be debilitating. Therefore, it would seem appropriate to minimize this muscle pain. It should be recognized, however, that patients who have undergone general anesthesia and surgery will often have muscle pain even if they have not received succinylcholine. It has been shown that the muscle fasciculations thought to be associated with the myalgias can be minimized and in some cases eliminated with the use of a nondepolarizing muscle relaxant such as curare. Curare 0.05 mg/kg should be administered approximately 3 minutes before the succinylcholine for maximum effectiveness. This will not only reduce the muscle pain, but will also greatly reduce the incidence of myoglobinemia and myoglobinuria that have been reported in children. There is also a documented decrease in the increase in serum creatinine phosphokinase associated with the administration of succinylcholine.[40] For a long time it was thought that children do not fasciculate, hence there would be no reason to be concerned about myalgias in this age group. However, in my clinical experience I have seen several children between the ages of 2 and 4 years who complained after operation of muscle pain. The pretreatment with a nondepolarizing muscle relaxant should begin in patients at the age of ambulation.

Succinylcholine and Potassium Flux

Some of the clinical problems with succinylcholine were not immediately recognized after its approval for clinical use. These problems include hyperkalemia in burn and trauma patients and those with Duchenne muscular dystrophy, among others. The major issue of potassium flux is that when there has been neuromuscular disease or other trauma that results in tissue destruction and denervation, there is an increase in the number of acetylcholine receptors. Succinylcholine activates more acetylcholine receptors, resulting in an increase in the release of potassium (potassium flux) and hence varying degrees of hyperkalemia. Mild hyperkalemia may only be associated with electrocardiographic (ECG) changes and perhaps with minor cardiac dysrhythmias; unfortunately, at times the hyperkalemia may result in cardiac arrest and death. In patients with a severe injury such as a burn, or crush injury, succinylcholine can be administered the first 24 to 48 hours after injury and before the receptors increase. However, after that, nondepolarizing muscle relaxants should be used. There are no studies documenting when there may be a clinically significant increase in the acetylcholine receptors nor are there any studies to document how long they remain.

Succinylcholine and Duchenne Muscular Dystrophy

There has been an enormous amount of confusion about the association of muscular dystrophy and malignant hyperthermia. There are multiple case reports that indicate an association between the two, but in many of these case reports neither the diagnosis nor the association has been established by techniques for making the diagnosis of malignant hyperthermia that are acceptable today.[41] In one case report the diagnosis was made by the calcium uptake test.[42] The major reason to avoid succinylcholine in patients with muscular dystrophy is because of the problem of potassium flux, not because of malignant hyperthermia. Also, halothane should be used with caution in patients with muscular dystrophy because these children may well have cardiac involvement.

Succinylcholine and Prolonged Blockade

At times succinylcholine is followed by prolonged neuromuscular blockade. The most frequent causes of a prolonged blockade are excessive doses of succinylcholine or an atypical cholinesterase level. Succinylcholine is metabolized by plasma pseudocholinesterase. Approximately 1 in 3,000 patients will have an atypical cholinesterase and will remain paralyzed for 2 to 3 hours following the normal doses of succinylcholine. Therefore, it is useful to use a nerve stimulator if there is any question about whether or not the succinylcholine block has terminated. My usual practice is to use a succinylcholine-facilitated intubation, and if further muscle relaxation is needed to use a nerve stimulator to titrate incremental doses of a nondepolarizing muscle relaxant.

Succinylcholine and Masseter Muscle Tone

If in the 1960s and 1970s anesthesiologists were asked to choose the most feared clinical problem it would have been malignant hyperthermia. There was no known treatment for the disease and the mortality rate approached 50 to 60 percent. For a long time it was a mystery disease because of its infrequent occurrence, the lack of a specific diagnostic test, a lack of understanding of the metabolic derangements and their treatment, and the fact that malignant hyperthermia did not occur with every exposure to the anesthetics. It was natural then for clinicians to look for associations of clinical signs with the various anesthetic agents that would allow for the early suspicion of malignant hyperthermia, the discontinuation of surgery, and, one would hope, the successful aborting of an episode of malignant hyperthermia. One of the earliest articles by Donlan et al. reported on a series of three patients in whom it was believed there was a high degree of suspicion of malignant hyperthermia.[43] These patients had received succinylcholine and developed masseter spasm. Review of this original paper with our current knowledge would suggest that two of the three patients did not have malignant hyperthermia. One was suspected of having malignant hyperthermia because of a positive calcium uptake test. Many other papers appeared in the literature concerning the association of masseter spasm and malignant hyperthermia susceptibility, and objective criteria were sought to determine what this relationship was. Schwartz et al. and Carroll et al. reported a very high incidence of an increase in tone in the masseter muscle, which they called *masseter spasm* (1 to 2.3 percent of all children receiving a combination of succinylcholine and halothane), and were concerned that this might herald the early onset of malignant hyperthermia.[44,45] In the series by Schwartz et al. all 12 patients who underwent the calcium uptake test were found to be positive. The calcium uptake test that they used has proved not to be reliable in making the diagnosis of malignant hyperthermia. At any rate, none of the patients in either series developed malignant hyperthermia. Rosenberg and Fletcher tested a large group of patients who had masseter spasm following administration of succinylcholine.[46] He performed a muscle biopsy and caffeine and halothane contracture testing and found that 50 percent of these patients had a positive biopsy. These patients were called *malignant hyperthermia susceptible*. Therefore, with these two pieces of information (that 50 percent of patients with masseter spasm will have a positive muscle biopsy and that up to 2.3 percent of children who are exposed to halothane and succinylcholine will develop masseter spasm) the next logical step was to conclude that succinylcholine must be a bad drug. The numbers, however, have not borne this suspicion out.

There are two possible solutions to the question of what masseter spasm really is and possibly what it means: (1) the response of the muscle to succinylcholine and (2) the dosage of succinylcholine. One of the pharmacologic observations that has not been appreciated is that after the intravenous administration of succinylcholine there is an increase of 6 to 25 percent in baseline muscle tone before the profound relaxation.[47] This increase in baseline muscle tone, in my opinion, is the source of much of the confusion in trying to sort out the issue of masseter spasm (or masseter muscle rigidity, trismus, jaw stiffness, or whatever the clinical enigma is called). Van der Speck et al. suggested that increases of masseter muscle tone and malignant hyperthermia were not the same thing and that we needed to reevaluate what the increase in masseter muscle tone really means.[48,49] The problem is that determining the tone of the masseter muscle is a subjective exercise. There are no objective criteria that we use clinically to evaluate or document masseter muscle tone.[50] What is masseter muscle spasm to one observer may not be to another. Van der Speck has suggested, furthermore, that perhaps there is a tonic response of the masseter muscle similar to that of ocular muscle. Gronert has suggested that we need to reevaluate the problem of masseter spasm, or what he refers to as *trismus*.[51] He feels that in the face of trismus the anesthetic can continue without triggering agents and the patient evaluated for malignant hyperthermia. If the studies indicate the hypermetabolic state of malignant hyperthermia, then anesthetics are discontinued and dantrolene is administered. The development of an increase in muscle tone or cardiac dysrhythmias that are not easily controllable with lidocaine suggest that the patient is undergoing a hypermetabolic episode (i.e., malignant hyperthermia) and that the anesthetic needs to be abandoned and treatment for malignant hyperthermia begun.

One of the pressing clinical issues facing the anesthesiologist, then, is what to do if the patient apparently develops trismus after the administration of succinylcholine. Rosenberg believes that if a patient develops trismus following succinylcholine, regardless of the findings (or lack of findings) the anesthetic needs to be immediately stopped and the patient treated with dantrolene for malignant hyperthermia, and that at a later date a muscle biopsy needs to be done for malignant hyperthermia.[52] I disagree with the recommendations of Rosenberg and agree with Gronert that we need to have a more objective evaluation of trismus and the clinical condition of the patient. If there is any question about an increase in masseter muscle tone then an end-tidal CO_2 monitor should be used and the patient carefully followed. Trigger agents should be discontinued and other anesthetic agents used. If the procedure is short (i.e., under 15 minutes) then it can usually be completed without any consequence. However, if cardiac dysrhythmias occur or if there is a general increase in muscle tone then the surgery should be immediately stopped and the patient evaluated for malignant hyperthermia with blood gases and plans made to treat with dantrolene. The 1- to 1.6-mg/kg dose may well result occasionally in incomplete relaxation of the masseter muscle.

The other possibility for confusing the status of the masseter muscle tone is the dosage of succinylcholine that was used in these studies. Meakin et al., who determined the dose-response curves for succinylcholine in neonates, infants, and children,[47] confirmed that infants are more resistant to the neuromuscular blocking effects of succinylcholine than older children, and that the older children are more resistant to the neuromuscular blocking effects of succinylcholine than adults. Therefore, it was their recommendation that a larger dose of succinylcholine be used for neonates, infants, and children, and that an intubating dose of 3 mg/kg be used for neonates and infants, and a 2-mg/kg dose be used for children. When one reads the earlier studies on the association of masseter spasm and succinylcholine the doses of succinylcholine are in the range of 1 to 1.6 mg/kg, which is below the recommended dose of Meakin et al. This insufficient dose may well explain the relatively high incidence of increase in masseter muscle tone.

Nondepolarizing Muscle Relaxants

The anesthesiologist of today has a whole array of nondepolarizing muscle relaxants to choose from. Table 3-4 gives their duration of action and cardiovascular effects. There has been an ongoing search for a nondepolarizing muscle relaxant that would mimic succinylcholine's short onset and rapid offset but none of its disadvantages. Mivacurium is undergoing clinical trials: Goudsouzian et al. have reported a 95 percent twitch depression in 90 seconds and a 95 percent recovery of the depression of twitch response in approximately 10 minutes, with

Table 3-4. Cardiovascular Effects and Length of Action of Muscle Relaxants

Drug	Autonomic Ganglia	Cardiac Muscarinic Receptors	Histamine Release	Blood Pressure Effect
Succinylcholine[a]	Stimulates	Stimulates	None	0
Atracurium[b]	No effect	No effect	Slight	↓
Vecuronium[b]	No effect	No effect	None	0
d-Tubocurarine[c]	Blocks	No effect	Moderate	↓ ↓
Metocurine[c]	Blocks weakly	No effect	Slight	0
Pancuronium[c]	No effect	Blocks weakly	None	↑ ↑

[a] Short-acting.
[b] Intermediate-acting.
[c] Long-acting.

no cardiovascular side effects.[53] This may be the drug of choice in the future for its short duration of relaxation and as an alternative to succinylcholine.

There is little difference between the medium-acting muscle relaxants, atracurium and vecuronium, except for cost, which is subject to change, and their metabolism by the infant, which is not. Atracurium is the medium-acting muscle relaxant of choice in the infant under 1 year of age because of the infant's ability to metabolize it. Vecuronium in this age group is considered a longer-acting muscle relaxant because of the infant's inability to metabolize it.

Atracurium has certain advantages over vecuronium when used for intubation. Vecuronium has no cardiovascular effects, so if intubation is done with light levels of anesthesia the child may have a hypertensive response to the procedure. On the other hand, atracurium is associated with histamine release and may cause a reduction in blood pressure, which will help to counter or neutralize the hypertensive effects of laryngoscopy and intubation.

NARCOTICS

Narcotics are major perioperative drugs for most infants and children. They have been particularly useful as an adjunct in managing the critically ill neonate and infant.[54,55] A problem has surfaced with the use of high-dose fentanyl (25 to 50 μg/kg) in the neonate.[56,57] The problem is that of extremely low clearance of the fentanyl, which results in the need for ventilatory support for up to 40 hours after operation in infants who had no respiratory impairment secondary to either the surgery or disease. A recent study by Gauntlett et al. investigated the pharmacokinetics of fentanyl in neonatal humans and lambs.[57] At least two factors affect the clearance of fentanyl during the neonatal period. These are postnatal age and the type of surgery. The type of surgery may well affect intraabdominal pressure, which may reduce liver blood flow. The liver is the primary organ of metabolism of fentanyl. Either the immaturity of the neonatal liver or alterations in liver blood flow could be the causative factor for this decreased metabolism. Therefore, in neonates, it would be appear that a combination of volatile agent, regional anesthesia, and small dose of narcotic (i.e., under 3 μg/kg) would reduce the need for postoperative ventilation that may be required with high-dose narcotics. On the other hand, if the infant will require postoperative ventilation for other reasons, then the dose of narcotic is no longer a major concern.

ANAPHYLACTIC/ANAPHYLACTOID REACTION TO ANESTHETIC AGENTS

An *anaphylactic* reaction is a life-threatening allergic reaction initiated by an antigen that binds to IgE antibodies. This type of reaction requires prior exposure to the antigen. An *anaphylactoid* reaction is clinically indistinguishable from an anaphylactic reaction. The difference is the inability to prove an antibody involvement in an anaphylactoid reaction. The diagnosis of IgE-mediated reaction is by skin testing with antigens and by radioallergosorbent testing (RAST). Since they are clinically indistinguishable and are treated the same, they will be discussed as one clinical entity.

The pathophysiology is degranulation of mast cells and basophils, which releases histamine and the chemotactic factors of an anaphylactic/anaphylactoid reaction. This leads to the release of further chemical mediators that adversely affect the circulatory, respiratory, and cutaneous systems. The affected circulatory system is characterized by vasodilatation and increased capillary permeability; the respiratory system by bronchospasm and upper airway edema; and the cutaneous system by flushing and urticaria. The onset of symptoms may be immediate or delayed up to 20 minutes. These reactions have been reported with many of the anesthetic agents as well as the surgical equipment that we use, therefore this complication needs to be in the differential diagnosis of sudden hypotension and bradycardia.[58]

There is a misconception that an anaphylactoid reaction is always accompanied by the triad of findings that includes cutaneous manifestations, pulse and blood pressure changes, and bronchospasm. However, it should be remembered that severe cardiovascular changes can occur with no cutaneous or respiratory tract findings (Table 3-5). Initially it may be difficult to make a diagnosis of an anaphylactic/anaphylactoid reaction because the only system that may be involved is the cardiovascular system. This is why patients who develop a sudden bradycardia and severe hypotension should be treated with epinephrine 5 μg/kg IV as the initial treatment. Depending on the response of the patient, the doses may or may not need to be repeated. It is advisable to avoid the administration of calcium and β-blockers since these drugs will continue the degranulation. A full-blown reaction may need to be treated for a prolonged period of time (i.e., 2 to 6 hours or longer) and require very large doses of intravenous epinephrine. In these situations, consideration should be given to starting an epinephrine drip. Intravenous steroids and diphenhydramine may be useful as secondary therapy in these reactions, but the first-line drug is epinephrine. The other immediate therapeutic measures would be to give a large fluid bolus of balanced salt solution and continue its administration until the circulation has stabilized as well as to increase the inspired concentration of oxygen.

There has been a great increase in the reporting of severe intraoperative an-

Table 3-5. Signs of Anaphylactic/
Anaphylactoid Reaction
(% of Patients Involved)

Tachycardia	94
Circulatory collapse	92
Widespread flush, edema	79
Bronchospasm	39
Cardiac arrest	14
Bradycardia	6
Dysahythmias	4

aphylaxis owing to latex.[59,60] Latex is the natural form of rubber that contains a protein capable of producing an anaphylactic reaction. The largest number of cases so far reported have been children who have undergone multiple procedures. It is much more frequent in children with a meningomyelocele who not only have undergone multiple surgical procedures, but who also have had bladder catheterizations with latex catheters. Patients at increased risk are those who have had mucous membrane and/or peritoneal surgery during which the surgeon wore latex gloves. These reactions may be very difficult to identify if there is not a high index of suspicion. They may occur any time during the surgical procedure and have no apparent relationship to any drug or any other manipulation that has been performed. Some present primarily with cardiovascular signs and symptoms, others with respiratory or cutaneous reactions.

Incidence of Anaphylactic/Anaphylactoid Reactions

The drugs most frequently involved in an allergic problem during anesthesia are antibiotics. This is followed by protein, fentanyl, thiopental (Pentothal), and the muscle relaxants. The incidence of allergic reactions has never been completely documented in the United States, but in Australia and Great Britain the incidence is somewhere between 1 in 5,000 and 1 in 10,000. Compared to the incidence of malignant hyperthermia, which is 1 in 15,000 in children and 1 in 50,000 in adults, these severe allergic reactions are much more frequent. This fact needs to be kept in mind both when considering the causes of hypotension and bradycardia as well as when balancing the risk:benefit ratio of succinylcholine. The mortality and morbidity from these severe allergic reactions is considerable. The reported mortality rate in the British series is 4.3 percent, and there is a 5.6 percent rate of irreversible brain damage. The problem with treating these allergic reactions is that they are difficult to recognize and require intervention with what may at times be large doses of epinephrine as well as fluids and an increase in oxygen concentration.

TECHNIQUES OF ANESTHESIA
Stress Response and MAC

The basis for administering anesthesia to a child should be the clinical status of the child and the MAC required to provide anesthesia. If a patient is moribund, hypotensive, and in extremis, certainly resuscitation is in order and the use of anesthetic agents is minimal. As the patient responds to resuscitation anesthetic agents are titrated according to the condition of the patient. This should be the general philosophy for all patients regardless of age.

Once it is recognized that an infant or child needs anesthesia the main questions at that point are what type of anesthetic to administer and how much will it take to induce the "anesthetized state." There has been a recent development of interest in the "stress response." It has been suggested that patients who have a blunted "stress response" have a better outcome.[61-63] The complete nature of the "stress response" has not been fully characterized but in general it refers to the humoral response of the body to the stress of anesthesia and surgery, and is identified by increases in plasma epinephrine, norepinephrine, glucagon, aldosterone, corticosterone, antidiuretic hormone, and β-endorphins. The pathophysiologic results of perturbations in the stress hormones are alterations in energy stores and redistribution of blood flow from unessential organs to the heart, brain, and lungs, which can alter the demands of the circulatory system as well as alter the liberation and metabolism of the free radicals. There are volumes of studies of outcome data for patients undergoing various types of surgical procedures that compare anesthetic techniques to reduce the stress hormones by the use of narcotics and other drugs versus standard anesthetic techniques in which the primary anesthetic is inhalational. Perhaps in the future we will know how to immediately measure stress hormones so that we can alter our anesthetic technique to maintain whatever the perceived ideal level of stress response would be. Therefore, the previous classic triad of general anesthesia, which was thought to consist of hypnosis or loss of consciousness, analgesia, and muscle relaxation, may now include another factor of equal importance, the control of the stress response.

Where does that leave the anesthesiologist today? The only option available to the anesthesiologist today is to know the various MACs at different age levels and the anesthetic techniques that will accomplish what we consider to be the anesthetized state as reflected in the MACs. MAC is usually defined as the minimal alveolar concentration at which 50 percent of the patients move (or don't move) in response to a surgical incision. Varying concentrations and combinations of inhalational agents and narcotics have been used to achieve this level. The inhalational anesthetics are capable of achieving the MAC of anesthesia by themselves, although it requires 105 percent nitrous oxide to arrive at the MAC. Narcotics can significantly reduce the MAC for inhalational agents, but with the exception of sufentanil, they do not appear to be able to provide a 1 MAC anesthesia as we define the term. Narcotics are thought to have a ceiling effect regardless of the dose of the narcotic. One of the problems with determining the MAC of narcotics is that at the higher dosage levels, the patient either can't maintain spontaneous ventilation or has a "wooden" chest, which interferes with determining MAC. It is paradoxical that while the stress response may be completely blunted by narcotics the patient may still have awareness. The concept of "MAC awareness" may become much more important as we arrive at a definition of the ideal anesthetic state.

Blood Pressure Control and Anesthesia

Once the anesthesiologist has determined the amount of anesthetic agent that is required to provide at least a 1 MAC anesthesia, attention can be turned to other clinical considerations. One of these is blood pressure control. There is general agreement that the usual patient ought to remain either normotensive or in an induced state of hypotension. For non- blood-losing operations iso- or normotension is certainly a reasonable goal. However, with increasing degrees of blood loss, there are increasing advantages to establishing a state of induced hypotension. The advantages of reducing blood pressure and thereby reducing blood loss are (1) a reduction in the need for transfusions and (2) a reduction in bleeding in the surgical field, which increases the speed and/or quality of the surgery. The past 5 years have been marked by an increasing awareness of the problems associated with blood transfusions (e.g., AIDS) as well as the subsequent development of anesthetic and surgical techniques to minimize blood loss, recycle blood, and thereby minimize the risk of transfusions. In this light the manipulation of blood pressure by using various anesthetic agents is certainly a desirable goal. If there is to be minimal or no blood loss, any of the agents can be used as long as the patient doesn't move and is unaware. However, if blood loss and transfusions are a concern, anesthetic techniques to reduce blood pressure and blood loss must be used. The inhalational agents, muscle relaxants, narcotics, and various ancillary drugs can be used to reduce blood pressure. Table 3-4 lists the hemodynamic effects of the nondepolarizing agents. These pharmacologic factors should be considered when managing the blood pressure.

Hypotensive Anesthesia

The "wake-up" test is one application of hypotensive anesthesia. The wake-up test is performed following the surgical manipulation of the spinal cord during correction of scoliosis. The concern is that the correction in the curvature of the spinal column will impinge upon the circulation of the spinal cord, resulting in a deficit. The object is to be able to rapidly wake up the patient at the appropriate time and have the child follow the simple command of moving the legs. Balanced anesthesia is the preferred technique. Balanced anesthesia in this situation consists of a thiopental 5 to 7 mg/kg induction, nitrous oxide in a concentration of 60 to 70 percent, and morphine 0.2 to 0.3 mg/kg IV or fentanyl 5 to 10 μg/kg IV. The choice of muscle relaxants is quite important. Pancuronium is a mild vagolytic drug known to cause varying degrees of stimulation of the adrenergic nervous system, leading to an increase in heart rate and blood pressure. For this reason, it is a poor choice as a muscle relaxant when hypotensive anesthesia is desired. The muscle relaxants of choice are curare, atracurium, or vecuronium depending on the length of the surgery. Curare and, to a lesser extent, atracurium will produce a dose-related release of histamine. Histamine is a vasodilator and will reduce the blood pressure for several minutes. There is minimal histamine release in children under 2 to 3 years of age. In older children, dividing the curare dose into several increments will modulate the histamine release and the hypotension. Hydralazine in 0.1-mg/kg increments or sodium nitroprusside 2 to 3 μg/kg/min will augment the hypotension. Hydralazine is given incrementally every 10 minutes until the desired blood pressure is achieved. Sometimes the baroresponse to the hypotension may result in a reactive tachycardia, which will increase the blood pressure. In this event, a β-blocker such as propranolol can be titrated in doses of 0.01 mg/kg in order to control the heart rate. Another very useful agent is labetalol, which is both an α- and a β-blocker. The usual desired mean blood pressure is in the range of 45 to 60 mmHg. When a volatile agent is used for hypotension 1 to 2 MAC are used with the varying adjuncts to arrive at the desired levels of blood pressure.

In summary, the pharmacologic approach to hypotensive anesthesia is usually a two-phase process. The initial phase is the administration of the hypotensive agent (i.e., sodium nitroprusside or hydralazine) and so on. The body often attempts to overcome the hypotensive state by a series of compensatory steps such as the activation of the renin-angiotensin-aldosterone response or the baroreceptor response, which results in tachycardia and an increase in arterial blood pressure. Phase two is the administration of pharmacologic agents to block these compensatory mechanisms. A knowledge of the compensatory responses greatly enhances the ability of the anesthesiologist to manipulate the pharmacologic agents appropriately in order to create the desired control of the blood pressure.

Blood Volume and Anesthesia

The previous sections describe anesthetic techniques for use when the patient's blood volume and circulation are normal. At times, however, either the patient will be hypovolemic or his exact volume status will not be known. In those situations, the anesthetic agents are chosen according to the ability to support the blood pressure and the blood volume. Patients who are moribund and/or in shock require resuscitation with minimal if any anesthetic agent. As they respond, a small dose of ketamine or narcotic can be administered, and then the other anesthetic agents added according to the response. Pancuronium would be the muscle relaxant of choice in the hypovolemic patient since it is both vagolytic and sympathomimetic. It has been a very useful muscle relaxant in the initial management of the trauma patient or the patient with a reduced blood volume. However, because of its hypertensive cardiovascular effects, it is certainly not a good agent to use in patients who are normotensive and normovolemic. Ketamine is a very useful anesthetic agent for patients with a marginal circulation because of its ability to produce the anesthetized state as well as its activity as a weak vasopressor.

In summary, the anesthesiologist needs to have a game plan when considering the goals for the anesthetic management of the patient. Blood pressure control is certainly one of the major goals. All anesthetic agents and adjuncts can be thought of in light of their ability to alter blood pressure.

Extubation and Postoperative Ventilation

Another major consideration when administering anesthesia to a child is postoperative ventilation. For purposes of this discussion children can be divided into two basic groups: (1) those in whom extubation is anticipated at the end of or shortly after the end of surgery and (2) those in whom a period of postoperative ventilation is anticipated. If extubation is anticipated at the end of surgery or shortly thereafter in the recovery room, the anesthetic agents need to be tailored to that end. On the other hand, if the patient is going to undergo a period of ventilation of several hours or days, the choice of anesthetic agents, including muscle relaxants, narcotics, and other drugs, is not as important.

Extubation at the End of Surgery

If extubation is anticipated at the end of surgery or shortly thereafter, the anesthetic agents need to be titrated accordingly. It is my opinion that children under the age of 1 year and most older children should be extubated while in the awake or relatively awake stage, recognizing that the definition of "awake" is arbitrary. The basis of the concept is that an awake infant has protective reflexes and can maintain the airway. However, in this age group it is difficult to determine exactly how awake they are. In the older child, the awake state is much easier to determine. Often the child will respond to the command to open the eyes or will make a purposeful movement to remove the endotracheal tube. The infant is more difficult to judge. The criteria that I use are whether the child (1) opens the eyes, (2) makes a purposeful movement for the endotracheal tube, and (3) have protective airway reflexes. At times the small infant will not open the eyes; therefore, if the infant is crying, I judge him to be in the awake state even if the eyes are closed, since crying is a purposeful activity. Planning for an extubation at the end of surgery begins an hour or so before the end of surgery, depending on the length of the operation. If the operation is short and nondepolarizing muscle relaxants are used, atricurium is the relaxant of choice. On the other hand, if the case has been going on for an hour or so and a longer-acting nondepolarizing agent such as curare has been used, for the last 30 to 40 minutes of the anticipated surgery a switch to atracurium with the dosage titrated by a nerve stimulator will greatly assist in making the reversal of the muscle relaxant considerably easier. The inhalational agents are slowly decreased over the last 10 to 20 minutes. Suctioning of the airway is done early (i.e., before turning back any anesthetic, etc.) so that manipulation of the airway is avoided at the end of surgery. Also, the bovie pad is not placed on the back of the child, since at the termination of surgery the circulating nurse may well jackknife the child on the neck to remove the pad, thereby stimulating the airway. I use nitrous oxide in a concentration of 70 percent at the end of surgery to allow the reduction of the inhalational agent. The muscle relaxants are reversed in the last 5 or so minutes of surgery according to the nerve stimulator. I prefer edrophonium 1 mg/kg for the reversal of muscle relaxants, since it will have a peak effect in 2 minutes, whereas neostigmine (0.6 mg/kg) will require 8 to 10 minutes to achieve 90 percent reversal (Fig. 3-7).[64] When the surgeon informs me that he is approximately 1 to 2 minutes from the termination of surgery, I turn off all anesthetic agents and use high-flow oxygen to purge the circuit and provide a high F_IO_2 for the infant. Also, 30 to 45 minutes before the end of surgery, I administer a small dose of narcotic such as morphine 0.05 μg/kg to smooth out the termination of surgery and to provide analgesia for the infant. Even if a regional technique was used, a small dose of morphine will smooth this period out. Usually, however, I do not administer morphine to infants who are in the neonatal period. If the infant opens the eyes and reaches

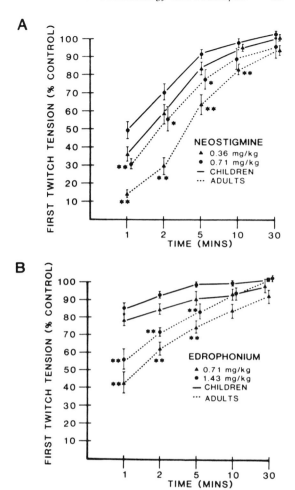

Fig. 3-7. Recovery of first-twitch tension as a percentage of control in pediatric patients (pooled data) compared with adults after neostigmine **(A)** and edrophonium **(B)**. Significant differences between adults and pediatric subjects are seen after the same dose of antagonist: $*P < 0.05$. $**P < 0.01$. (From Meakin et al.,[64] with permission.)

for the endotracheal tube, extubation is performed in the operating room. At times, it is difficult to tell when the child is ready for extubation. Therefore, for this group of infants, the volatile anesthetic agents are decreased rapidly toward the end of surgery. Small doses of narcotics such as morphine 0.05 mg/kg are added as the volatile agent is reduced or discontinued. A nerve stimulator is used to determine the reversal of the muscle relaxant at the end of surgery.

Timing of Extubation

There are times when all of the anesthetic agents have been discontinued and the muscle relaxants have been reversed, and yet the protective reflexes are not judged to be sufficiently recovered for the child to have complete airway control. However, if extubated while coughing and breathholding the child may go rapidly into laryngospasm. One technique to smooth over this situation is to use intravenous lidocaine, which will deepen the anesthesia and allow the patient to return to spontaneous ventilation, and thereby allow removal of the inhalational anesthetic agent. These are difficult judgments to make. It should be remembered that coughing and apnea with an endotracheal tube in are laryngospasm and apnea with an endotracheal tube out; apnea is part of the reflex of laryngospasm. These episodes can truly test the mettle and patience of the anesthesiologist. It is my opinion that if in doubt the endotracheal tube should remain in and lidocaine administered intravenously. It is even better to administer the lidocaine in the last several minutes of the case if the possibility of extubation is in question. The dose of lidocaine in the infant under 6 months of age is 1 mg/kg. In the older infant and child the dose is 1.5 mg/kg. The dose of lidocaine can be repeated once in 5 minutes for a total dose of 2 to 3 mg/kg in 5 minutes. At times, the anesthesiologist may become impatient and wish to extubate the patient in the operating room. When there is any question about whether or not to extubate it is has been my approach to leave the patient intubated, transport him to the recovery room with an oxygen supply, and then perform the extubation in an unhurried fashion in the recovery room. Anesthesiologists feel a little inept if they have to remain in an operating room with an intubated patient with everybody standing around shifting quietly and sometimes complaining not so quietly about the anesthetic technique.

Laryngospasm

If the child goes into laryngospasm either in the operating room or in the recovery room certain steps need to be immediately taken. These include having available intravenous succinylcholine or intramuscular succinylcholine, airway equipment, and a bag and mask for positive-pressure ventilation. The era of the pulse oximeter has certainly assisted greatly in the management of these patients. As soon as the oxygen saturation drops below 90, if the patient is still in complete laryngospasm and apneic, I administer succinylcholine 1 mg/kg IV because I know that within 30 to 60 seconds the oxygen level will continue to drop and the pulse rate will begin to drop along with the blood pressure. If no IV is present, intramuscular succinylcholine 4 mg/kg is given. It is important not to wait until there is a drop in the pulse rate or blood pressure because uptake of the succinylcholine will be reduced and the onset of paralysis delayed. If the pulse rate has dropped below 80 to 90 beats/min in an infant or below 60 beats/min in a child, then external cardiac massage should be considered until there is a recovery of ventilation and circulation. I always leave ECG patches on an infant regardless of the level of consciousness until the infant is in the recovery room. The reason for doing this is that one never knows when some disaster will occur. The presence of the ECG patches allows an immediate attachment of the ECG. The precordial stethoscope should be used for the transportation of any child to the recovery room. It will provide information not only while in transit but in the recovery room as the monitors are being attached and the child assessed.

Postoperative Ventilation

When postoperative ventilation is anticipated or desired it is usually because the surgical procedure is extensive or because of the underlining condition of the patient. Most of these patients will be taken to an intensive care unit, which in most hospitals requires somewhat of a steeplechase run. For that reason, the patient should be kept anesthetized and paralyzed for the trip to the intensive care unit. There is nothing more frightening than having a child extubate himself in an elevator. At any rate, any transport from the operating room to a far-away unit of the hospital should include equipment for monitoring and establishment of an airway. Sufficient assistance should accompany the patient to ensure adequate support should disaster strike en route.

ANESTHESIA GAS DELIVERY SYSTEMS

Anesthesia gas delivery systems can be classified primarily as (1) nonrebreathing systems or (2) rebreathing systems. Both have advantages and disadvantages. The nonrebreathing systems are reputed to be simple and have a low resistance, which allows the infant to breathe spontaneously. The types of nonrebreathing systems include the Jackson Reese modification of the Ayers T-piece and the Bain circuit. They require a fresh gas flow of approximately 100 to 150 ml/kg/min. The disadvantages of the nonrebreathing system are that the high fresh gas flow becomes very expensive when isoflurane is used. In addition, temperature control is more difficult because of the high flows and humidification is cumbersome to add to the circuit. There is the concern of pollution of the operating room. As a result, the simple nonrebreathing circuit has become complicated by the addition of humidifiers, scavenging systems, and other systems.

In my opinion, the rebreathing anesthetic delivery systems have more advantages than disadvantages. The usual anesthesia machine and circuit can be modified for pediatric use by the addition of infant breathing tubes and a 0.5-ml or 1-L bag. This allows a very rapid changeover from an adult to a pediatric system. The advantages of using a standard anesthesia machine are that it is very easy to set up, the FIO_2 is monitored, the airway pressures are monitored, a ventilator is available, the gases are scavenged, and a humidifier is easily added to the circuit. There have been no studies to indicate that there is any greater problem in letting an infant breathe spontaneously with a semiclosed system as opposed to a nonrebreathing system. It is evident that the choice of anesthesia apparatus is related more to personal preference than science. Now that end-tidal gas sampling is becoming generally available the enormous potential savings by using a low-flow semiclosed system might encourage an increase in its use. This is particularly true when an agent such as isoflurane is used.

Another extremely important concept when comparing nonrebreathing and rebreathing circuits is to understand exactly what concentrations of anesthetics are found in the various parts of the circuit and being delivered to the patient. The three concentrations that are of importance to the anesthesiologist are the dialed concentration, the inspired concentration, and the end-tidal concentration. In a nonrebreathing system the dialed concentration is essentially the same as the inspired concentration. Therefore, any change in the dialed concentration results in an immediate change in the inspired concentration. In a circle system, the relationships between dialed concentration and the inspired concentration are quite different. The inspired concentration is the result of a mixture of the dialed concentration in the fresh gas flow and the end-tidal concentration of the expired gases in the rebreathing circuit of the circle. The differences between the dialed concentration and the inspired concentration are due to several factors: (1) the ratio of fresh gas flow to minute ventilation, (2) the length of time that the anesthetic has been administered, (3) the 5- to 7-L dead space within the anesthesia circuit. At the beginning of the induction phase of anesthesia, the dead space and rapid uptake can be modulated by increasing the fresh gas flow. The differences between dialed and inspired concentrations are much greater during the first 15 to 20 minutes of induction. After the first 30 minutes, as tissue uptake begins to equilibrate, the end-tidal concentrations increase significantly, and the differences become smaller. In a circle system in a case lasting 1 to 2 hours there is usually a 10 to 20 percent difference between the dialed concentration and the inspired concentration, and between the inspired concentration and the end-tidal concentration.

The use of end-tidal gas sampling has also brought into question what gas concentrations should be recorded on the anesthesia record. It is evident that from an anesthetic standpoint the most important is the end-tidal concentration, because this is the anesthetic concentration that is anesthetizing the patient. The dialed concentration is relatively unimportant when the end-tidal concentration is known. For instance, during the initial induction phase often a dialed concentration of 4 to 5 percent halothane is used but the inspired and end-tidal concentrations are much lower. In cases of bronchoscopy and laryngoscopy, where there is air entrainment and dilution of the anesthetic gases, the anesthetic management may require a dialed concentration of 3 to 4 percent halothane for long periods of time. However, an end-tidal measurement would indicate a much lower concentration of anesthesia in the patient. The use of end-tidal gas sampling has also brought about a new understanding of the uptake and distribution of anesthetics. It is important when reading studies of the inhalational agents to understand the type of anesthetic system that was being used during the administration of the anesthetic agent and exactly where the reported anesthetic concentrations were measured. These differences need to be kept in mind when evaluating anesthetic agents and adopting them into practice. The issue of the dialed concentration of anesthetic has come up in legal cases with the purposeful confusion by the plaintiff's expert as to the concentration of anesthetic within the child.

REFERENCES

1. Hickey PR, Hansen DD, Stafford M, et al: Pulmonary and systemic hemodynamic effects of nitrous oxide in infants with normal and elevated pulmonary vascular resistance. Anesthesiology 65:374, 1986

2. Burrows FA, Shutack JG, Crone RK: Inappropriate secretion of antidiuretic hormone in a postsurgical pediatric population. Crit Care Med 11:527, 1983
3. Weiskopf RB, Holmes MA, Eger EI II, et al: Cardiovascular effects of I-653, in swine. Anesthesiology 69:303, 1988
4. Weiskopf RB, Eger EI II, Holmes MA, et al: Epinephrine-induced premature ventricular contractions and changes in arterial blood pressure and heart rate during I-653, isoflurane, and halothane anesthesia in swine. Anesthesiology 70:293, 1989
5. Phillips AJ, Brimacombe JR, Simpson DL: Anaesthetic induction with isoflurane or halothane: Oxygen saturation during induction with isoflurane or halothane in unpremedicated children. Anaesthesia 43:927, 1988
6. Fisher DM, Robinson S, Brett CM, et al: Comparison of enflurane, halothane, and isoflurane for diagnostic and therapeutic procedures in children with malignancies. Anesthesiology 63:647, 1985
7. Murray D, Forbes R, Murphy K, Mahoney L: Nitrous oxide: Cardiovascular effects in infants and small children during halothane and isoflurane anesthesia. Anesth Analg 67:1059, 1988
8. Barash PG, Glanz S, Katz JD, et al: Ventricular function in children during halothane anesthesia: An echocardiographic evaluation. Anesthesiology 49:79, 1978
9. Wolf WJ, Neal MB, Peterson MD: The hemodynamic and cardiovascular effects of isoflurane and halothane anesthesia in children. Anesthesiology 64:328, 1986
10. Murray D, Vandewalker G, Matherne P, Mahoney LT: Pulsed doppler and two-dimensional echocardiography: Comparison of halothane and isoflurane on cardiac function in infants and small children. Anesthesiology 67:211, 1987
11. Gregory GA: The baroresponses of preterm infants during halothane anaesthesia. Can Anaesth Soc J 29:105, 1982
12. Kotrly KJ, Ebert TJ, Vucins E, et al: Baroreceptor reflex control of heart rate during isoflurane anesthesia in humans. Anesthesiology 60:173, 1984
13. LeDez KM, Lerman J: The minimum alveolar concentration (MAC) of isoflurane in preterm neonates. Anesthesiology 67:301, 1987
14. Murat I, Lapeyre G, Saint-Maurice C: Isoflurane attenuates baroreflex control of heart rate in human neonates. Anesthesiology 70:395, 1989
15. Murat I, Levron JC, Berg A, Saint-Maurice C: Effects of fentanyl on baroreceptor reflex control of heart rate in newborn infants. Anesthesiology 68:717, 1988
16. Knill RL, Clement JL: Site of selective action of halothane on the peripheral chemoreflex pathway in humans. Anesthesiology 61:121, 1984
17. Gregory GA, Eger EI II, Munson ES: The relationship between age and halothane requirements in man. Anesthesiology 30:488, 1969
18. Nicodemus HF, Nassiri-Rahimi C, Bachman L, Smith TC: Median effective doses (ED$_{50}$) of halothane in adults and children. Anesthesiology 31:344, 1969
19. Cameron CB, Robinson S, Gregory GA: The minimum alveolar concentration of isoflurane in children. Anesth Analg 63:418, 1984
20. Lerman J, Robinson S, Willis MM, Gregory GA: Anesthetic requirements for halothane in young children 0–1 months and 1–6 months of age. Anesthesiology 59:421, 1983
21. Palahnuik RJ, Schnider SM, Eger EI II: Pregnancy decreases the requirement for inhaled anesthetic agents. Anesthesiology 41:82, 1974
22. Molliver ME, Kostovic I, Vanderloos H: The development of synapses in cerebral cortex of the human fetus. Brain Res 50:403, 1973
23. Moss IR, Conner H, Yee WFH, et al: Human β-endorphin-like immunoreactivity in the perinatal/neonatal period. J Pediatr 101:443, 1982

24. Johnston RR, Eger EI II, Wilson C: A comparative interaction of epinephrine with enflurane, isoflurane, and halothane in man. Anesth Analg 55:709, 1976

25. Ueda W, Hirakawa M, Mae O: Appraisal of epinephrine administration to patients under halothane anesthesia for closure of cleft palate. Anesthesiology 58:574, 1983

26. Karl HW, Swedlow MD, Lee KW, Downes JJ: Epinephrine-halothane interactions in children. Anesthesiology 58:142, 1983

27. Brown BR, Gandolfi AJ: Adverse effects of volatile anaesthetics. Br J Anaesth 59:14, 1987

28. Cousins MJ, Gourlay GK, Knights KM, et al: A randomized prospective controlled study of the metabolism and hepatotoxicity of halothane in humans. Anesth Analg 66:299, 1987

29. Christ DD, Kenna JG, Kammerer W, et al: Enflurane metabolism produces covalently bound liver adducts recognized by antibodies from patients with halothane hepatitis. Anesthesiology 69:833, 1988

30. Eger EI II, Smucker EA, Ferrell LD, et al: Is enflurane hepatotoxic? Anesth Analg 65:21, 1986

31. Hoft RH, Bunker JP, Goodman HI, Gregory PB: Halothane hepatitis in three pairs of closely related women. N Engl J Med 304:1023, 1980

32. Wark HJ: Postoperative jaundice in children. The influence of halothane. Anaesthesia 38:237, 1983

33. Whitburn RH, Sumner E: Halothane hepatitis in an 11-month-old child. Anaesthesia 41:611, 1986

34. Strube PJ, Hulands GH, Halsey MJ: Serum fluoride levels in morbidly obese patients: Enflurane compared with isoflurane anaesthesia. Anaesthesia 42:685, 1987

35. Hinkle AJ: Serum inorganic fluoride levels after enflurane in children. Anesth Analg 68:396, 1989

36. Delphin E, Jackson D, Rothstein P: Use of succinylcholine during elective pediatric anesthesia should be reevaluated. Anesth Analg 66:1190, 1987

37. Foldes FF, McNall PG, Borrego-Hinojosa JM: Succinylcholine: A new approach to muscular relaxation in anesthesiology. N Engl J Med 247:596, 1952

38. Liu LMP, DeCook TH, Goudsouzian NG, et al: Dose response to intramuscular succinylcholine in children. Anesthesiology 55:599, 1981

39. Hannallah RS, Oh TH, McGill WA, Epstein BS: Changes in heart rate and rhythm after intramuscular succinylcholine with or without atropine in anesthetized children. Anesth Analg 65:1329, 1986

40. Cozanitis DA, Erkola O, Klemola UM, Makela V: Precurarisation in infants and children less than three years of age. Can J Anaesth 34:17, 1987

41. Wilhoit RD, Brown RE, Bauman LA: Possible malignant hyperthermia in a 7-week-old infant. Anesth Analg 68:688, 1989

42. Kelfer HM, Singer WD, Reynolds RN: Malignant hyperthermia in a child with Duchenne muscular dystrophy. Pediatrics 71:118, 1983

43. Donlon JV, Newfield P, Sreter F, Ryan JF: Implications of masseter spasm after succinylcholine. Anesthesiology 49:298, 1978

44. Schwartz L, Rockoff MA, Koka BV: Masseter spasm with anesthesia: Incidence and implications. Anesthesiology 61:772, 1984

45. Carroll JB: Increased incidence of masseter spasm in children with strabismus anesthetized with halothane and succinylcholine. Anesthesiology 67:559, 1987

46. Rosenberg H, Fletcher JE: Masseter muscle rigidity and malignant hyperthermia susceptibility. Anesth Analg 65:161, 1986

47. Meakin G, McKiernan EP, Morris P, Baker RD: Dose-response curves for suxamethonium in neonates, infants and children. Br J Anaesth 62:655, 1989

48. Van Der Spek AFL, Fang WB, Ashton-Miller JA, et al: The effects of succinylcholine on mouth opening. Anesthesiology 67:459, 1987
49. Van Der Spek AFL, Fang WB, Ashton-Miller JA, et al: Increased masticatory muscle stiffness during limb muscle flaccidity associated with succinylcholine administration. Anesthesiology 69:11, 1988
50. Berry FA, Lynch CL: Letter to the editor: Succinylcholine and trismus. Anesthesiology 70:161, 1989
51. Gronert GA: Management of patients in whom trismus occurs following succinylcholine (letter). Anesthesiology 68:653, 1988
52. Rosenberg H: Lecture: Malignant Hyperthermia (#266). 40th Annual Refresher Course Lectures and Clinical Update Program, 1989. Presented at the Annual Meeting of the American Society of Anesthesiologists, October 14–18, New Orleans, 1989
53. Goudsouzian NG, Alifimoff JK, Eberly C, et al: Neuromuscular and cardiovascular effects of mivacurium in children. Anesthesiology 70:237, 1989
54. Robinson S, Gregory GA: Fentanyl-air-oxygen anesthesia for ligation of patent ductus arteriosus in preterm infants. Anesth Analg 60:331, 1981
55. Hickey PR, Hansen DD: Fentanyl and sufentanil-oxygen-pancuronium anesthesia for cardiac surgery in infants. Anesth Analg 63:117, 1984
56. Koehntop DE, Rodman JH, Brundage DM, et al: Pharmacokinetics of fentanyl in neonates. Anesth Analg 65:227, 1986
57. Gauntlett IS, Fisher DM, Hertzka RE, et al: Pharmacokinetics of fentanyl in neonatal humans and lambs: Effects of age. Anesthesiology 69:683, 1988
58. Levy JH: Allergic reactions during anesthesia. J Clin Anesth 1(1):39, 1988
59. Gerber AC, Jorg W, Zbinden S, et al: Severe intraoperative anaphylaxis to surgical gloves: Latex allergy, an unfamiliar condition. Anesthesiology 71:800, 1989
60. Swartz J, Braude BM, Gilmour RF, et al: Intraoperative anaphylaxis to latex. Canad J Anaesth (In press)
61. Anand KJS, Hickey PR: Randomized trial of high-dose sufentanil anesthesia in neonates undergoing cardiac surgery: Effects on the metabolic stress response. Anesthesiology 67:A502, 1987
62. Anand KJS, Sippell WG, Aynsley-Green A: Randomised trial of fentanyl anesthesia in preterm babies undergoing surgery: Effects on the stress response. Lancet 1:243, 1987
63. Roizen MF: Should we all have a sympathectomy at birth? Or at least preoperative? Anesthesiology 68:482, 1988
64. Meakin G, Sweet PT, Bevan JC, Bevan DR: Neostigmine and edrophonium as antagonists of pancuronium in infants and children. Anesthesiology 59:316, 1983
65. Eger EI II: Isoflurane (Forane): A Compendium and Reference. Anaquest, Madison, WI, 1984
66. Ali HH, Savarese JJ: Monitoring of neuromuscular function. Anesthesiology 45:216, 1976

4

PRACTICAL ASPECTS OF FLUID AND ELECTROLYTE THERAPY

Frederic A. Berry

The topic of practical aspects of fluid and electrolyte therapy for infants and children can certainly evoke more differences of opinion among pediatricians and anesthesiologists than almost any other subject. The reasons for these differences of opinion are multiple. There are many different methods of calculating fluid and electrolyte requirements. Some of the more common ones are based on weight, body surface area, and caloric intake. The number of formulas for fluid therapy based on these systems is limited only by the number of authors writing on the subject. The overzealous clinical application of these formulas by some clinicians frequently results in an extremely rigid system of fluid therapy on the one hand and an intolerance of other clinicians' formulas on the other. Considering the derivations of the various systems for calculating fluid requirements, and recognizing the biologic variations in children, it becomes clear that the various systems and formulas for fluid therapy are guidelines, and that the fine-tuning of a system must be based on the response of the patient to the fluid therapy. This response is reflected in the patient's

1. State of consciousness
2. Blood pressure
3. Urine output
4. Skin turgor
5. Electrolyte values

METHODS FOR CALCULATING THE REQUIREMENTS FOR FLUIDS AND ELECTROLYTES

A quick review of the various methods for calculating fluid therapy will reveal that they are based on assumptions that require the recognition of biologic variability, variability in measurement, and, in the case of body surface area, a

Table 4-1. A Profile of the 12 Patients of DuBois Used for Estimating Surface Area

Age (yrs)	Sex	Description
2	F	Rickets, pectus
12.5	F	Prepubescent, normal development
18	M	Diabetic; tall and emaciated; 11-day alcohol binge with minimal food
21	M	Measurements 3 months after severe typhoid infection
21.5	M	Tall, thin. On weight-reduction diet
22	M	Tall and thin
26	F	Well-proportioned sculpture model
32	M	Legs amputated at age 6. Stroke 6 years after measurements, leaving residual paralysis
36	M	Cretin. Physical development of an 8-year old
43	M	Bilateral leg amputation 5 years previously. Obese
?	F	Short and fat, age not given

relatively nonpediatric approach to patient selection as the basis for the nomogram that was originally used. The original equations of DuBois and DuBois in 1916, which are the basis for the initial nomograms for calculating body surface area in common usage today, were derived from a series of 12 patients.[1] The determination of body surface area is based on a formula incorporating the height and weight of the patient. Of the original series of 12 patients, 10 were adults and 2 were children (Table 4-1). One child was 2 years of age and afflicted with rickets and pectus excavatum. The other child was a normal, 12-year-old prepubertal female. The remaining 10 patients represent something of an anatomic potpourri. They included two double amputees, a cretin, and a malnourished, diabetic alcoholic. DuBois and DuBois recognized the limitation of the sample population and the large potential standard deviation in the use of the formula. The title of one of their classic papers was "A formula to estimate the approximate surface area if height and weight be known." This hardly sounds like a formula to be carried to the second decimal point. Years later, in 1935, Boyd published an analysis of the various publications on surface area measurement and made with several very interesting but somehow forgotten observations.[2] She calculated the standard deviation in the formula of DuBois and DuBois, and found it to be 18.6 percent for infants under 3 kg and 7.5 percent for individuals over 3 kg. In addition, Boyd compared the equation for weight only and surface area, and found that the standard deviation was only 0.7 percent. This hardly justifies the need for a surface area nomogram and the extra calculations that are necessary. A reflection on the patient selection used by DuBois and DuBois and the standard deviation in their formula would suggest that there is leeway in the calculation and application of any formula based on body surface area or weight, and that any degree of rigidity is completely artificial.[3]

It is evident from this introduction that there are inherent inaccuracies with any formula used to calculate fluid requirements. If certain facts are recognized, though, any formula may be used. The first fact to recognize is that there is variability owing both to normal biologic variability in the human and to accuracies in the measurement of weight, height, or whatever one is measuring. The second fact is that many patients come to the operating room with varying degrees of fluid deficit owing to maintenance and replacement deficits, whereas the formulas for calculating fluid requirements are primarily for determining maintenance fluids and not replacement fluids. The deficit may be due to the patient having had a bowel prep, a fever, bleeding, vomiting, trauma, or some other reason.

The third fact to recognize is that the use of a formula to calculate fluid requirements is strictly a guideline, much as the calculation of a dose of thiopental (Pentothal). When administered the dose may be adequate, or for one reason or another may be inadequate, with more drug being required. This is our dose-response system for the administration of drugs. There is always a normal range given for the dose of thiopental, and the same is true with a "dose" of fluids. The main point to remember is that calculation and administration of the "dose" of fluid is the first step, and the second and most important step is the response of the patient to the fluid therapy. The response occurs in terms of vital signs, urine output, and other findings. Fortunately for the patient and the anesthesiologist, 90 percent of our patients do not need a critical determination of their fluid and electrolyte therapy; the compensatory mechanisms of the body are able to maintain a normal fluid and electrolyte content. However, depending on one's practice, 5 to 10 percent of patients (this is obviously an arbitrary number) need an ongoing analysis of fluid administration. The fluid therapy discussed in this chapter is aimed at this group of patients. The balance of patients can survive with any system, and will therefore be appropriately managed with this system of fluid therapy as well.

DEVELOPMENT OF THE RENAL SYSTEM

The renal system undergoes a very interesting embryologic development.[4] There are three overlapping renal systems: the pronephros, the mesonephros, and the metanephros. The metanephros is the permanent kidney; it begins to develop in the fifth fetal week after the regression of the previous renal systems. By the 34th week of life (2.0 kg) the process of differentiation of the renal tissue is complete. Each kidney produces approximately one million nephrons. After the 34th week all increases in renal size result from the continued enlargement and growth of the nephrons rather than from the formation of new nephrons. The basic renal system in its simplest concept consists of an interface between the vascular system and a selective excretory organ. The interface between these two systems allows a continuous selective processing of blood through filtration, excretion, and reabsorption in order to conserve essential material and as a conduit to discharge the waste materials. Therefore, the basic renal unit consists of three parts: a vascular system to supply blood flow, a conservation and excretory system for processing the blood, and a collecting system for collecting and discharging the urine.

The newborn kidney has similarities to the newborn lung. It has a high vascular resistance, which results in a low blood flow. This low blood flow leads to a low glomerular filtration rate (GFR). This low GFR results in limited renal function in the first 24 hours of life. However, shortly after birth, as systemic pressure increases and renal vascular resistance decreases, there is improvement in renal blood flow and GFR; and by 4 to 5 days there is marked improvement in the ability of the neonatal kidney to conserve fluid as well as excrete an overload. By 1 month of age the full-term infant's kidney will be approximately 70 percent mature. The premature nursery graduate who has bronchopulmonary dysplasia and is receiving furosemide (Lasix) may represent a special problem for the anesthesiologist. First of all, the urine output and specific gravity are not as useful in evaluating the fluid status of the child because they are altered by furosemide. Second, because of the tendency for these infants with residual lung disease to develop interstitial pulmonary edema, very conservative fluid administration is required. Third, furosemide should be continued in the perioperative period in these patients.

FLUID REQUIREMENTS
Maintenance Fluids

Maintenance fluids (which are hypotonic fluids) are required for five basic reasons:

1. Thermoregulation; evaporation from the skin is an essential part of thermoregulation
2. Excretion of solids (waste products via the kidney)
3. Water loss in the stool
4. Water loss from the respiratory tract
5. Growth

It is hoped that the intraoperative period is short enough that this last factor can be ignored! The maintenance fluid requirement will vary depending on the caloric requirements and metabolic rate of the infant or child. In infants up to 1 year of age, the requirement is 6 ml/kg/hr; 1 to 5 years, 4 ml/kg/hr; 6 years to puberty, 1 to 2 ml/kg/hr. For purposes of calculation, an average amount of maintenance fluids is usually used in the perioperative period. The electrolyte requirement for sodium is 2 to 3 mEq/kg/day, and for potassium 1 to 2 mEq/kg/day. Usually potassium is omitted in the perioperative period. The combination of maintenance fluid and electrolyte requirement gives a hypotonic electrolyte solution, the usual fluid being one-quarter to one-third strength saline.

Replacement Fluids

Replacement fluids can be thought of as those fluids required primarily to replace extracellular fluid deficits. Extracellular fluids consist of (1) transcellular fluid, which can be thought of as a specialized type of extracellular fluid, the

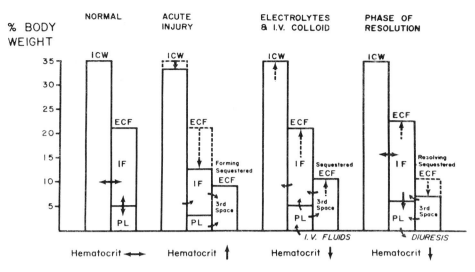

Fig. 4-1. Formation and resolution of third-space fluid. *ICW*, intracellular water; *ECF*, extracellular fluid; *IF*, interstitial fluid; *PL*, plasma. Intracellular water and extracellular fluid are shown in terms of percentages of body weight in the average 70-kg adult male in the first paired columns. With acute injury, operation, infection, or burn, a parasitic third fluid space is formed, the fluid of which is in continuity with the normal extracellular fluid but not available to it. The result, shown in the second figure, is an acute volume depletion of the available interstitial fluid and plasma. Restitution of normal volumes of plasma and interstitial fluid by infusion of electrolyte solutions and colloid is shown in the third figure. The sequestered fluid in the abnormal third fluid space represents additional volume, electrolytes, and body weight. With clearance of the sequestered fluid, shown in process in the fourth figure, the patient receives an autoinfusion of water and extracellular fluid electrolytes, and loses the additional volume through a diuresis of sodium with urine. The arrows show the major direction of flow. (From Randall,[19] with permission.)

best example being that of the gastrointestinal tract; (2) interstitial fluid; and (3) blood. Trauma to the body essentially results in a loss of blood volume and interstitial fluid (Fig. 4-1). The traumatic alteration of the capillary membranes leads to a loss of what is referred to as *third-space fluid*. This fluid is lost from the circulating volume of extracellular fluid, but is still present as far as the patient's weight is concerned. Obstruction of the gastrointestinal tract results in a loss of transcellular fluid. Table 4-2 lists the sodium and potassium contents of the various types of transcellular fluid. The replacement fluid for extracellular fluid is a balanced salt solution (BSS), such as full-strength lactated Ringer's or saline.

In pyloric stenosis, the obstruction results in a loss of pure gastric juice. Other types of intestinal obstruction in which the point of obstruction is below the entrance of the bile duct into the intestine cause a loss of fluid with a sodium content of 120 to 160 mEq/L, a result of the mixture of bile with the other intestinal fluids. There are two steps to be taken in correcting the fluid and electrolyte deficits and continuing losses in pyloric stenosis. The first is to correct the sodium deficit and the second is to replace the gastric fluid that continues

Table 4-2. Electrolyte Concentration of Various Body Fluids

Source	Na (mEq/L)	K (mEq/L)
Saliva	50	2
Gastric	60 ± 30	9.1 ± 4
Bile	145 ± 15	5.1 ± 1.2
Ilium	125 ± 20	5.0 ± 2.1
Diarrhea	60 ± 30	30 ± 15
Cerebrospinal fluid	140 ± 5	4.5 ± 1
Sweat	30 ± 10	

to be lost until the surgical correction. This is very close to the amount of sodium found in BSS and in upper gastrointestinal tract obstruction. It is therefore easier to replace the fluid that is lost with BSS rather than to measure the electrolyte content of the fluid being lost. Diarrhea fluid has a somewhat greater variability in sodium content, depending on the cause of the diarrhea. From a practical viewpoint, this can be replaced with BSS and the extra sodium easily excreted. It must be remembered that there are two steps in calculating the appropriate fluid replacement in gastrointestinal tract obstruction. The first is to calculate the sodium deficit and the second is to provide for the ongoing sodium loss.

Patients with hydrocephalus who have a shunt are occasionally faced with the potential loss of cerebrospinal fluid if the shunt becomes infected and the fluid is drained by externalizing the shunt. The lost fluid contains electrolytes in the same concentrations as in extracellular fluid.

COMPENSATORY MECHANISMS OF THE BODY FOR FLUID AND ELECTROLYTE LOSS

The compensatory mechanisms of the body for fluid and electrolyte loss fall into two basic general categories: (1) definitive compensatory mechanisms and (2) temporary compensatory mechanisms (Table 4-3). The definitive compensatory mechanisms are located within the renal and gastrointestinal systems.

Table 4-3. Compensatory Mechanisms

Definitive compensatory mechanisms
    Renal
    Gastrointestinal
Temporary compensatory mechanisms
    Renal—ADH
    Transcapillary
    Endogenous vasopressors
        Angiotensin II
        Vasopressin (ADH)
        Sympathetic amines

The definitive compensatory mechanisms are those of an increased reabsorption of sodium and water, however, in the surgical patient the main definitive mechanism is through the renal system.

Definitive Compensatory Mechanisms

The body's definitive mechanism for compensating for a loss of sodium and water is the renin-angiotensin-aldosterone system. The sensing device for the activation of this compensatory mechanism is located within the macula densa of the juxtaglomerular apparatus of the kidney (Fig. 4-2). This is the part of the kidney where the distal tubule returns to the glomerulus through the vascular hilum of the glomerulus (i.e., the point where the afferent arteriole enters and the efferent arteriole exits the glomerulus). The mechanism is activated when there is either a low sodium content in the fluid of the distal tubule or a low pressure, or perhaps by some other factor. At any rate, renin is released by the kidney and enters the systemic circulation, where it converts angiotensinogen into angiotensin I. The converting enzyme then transforms angiotensin I into angiotensin II. Angiotensin II has several activities: (1) it is an extremely potent vasopressor; (2) it causes the release of aldosterone from the adrenal cortex; (3) it stimulates the release of vasopressin, or antidiuretic hormone (ADH), from the pituitary; and (4) it causes a compensatory response of increasing fluid absorption within the gastrointestinal system. The most important action at this

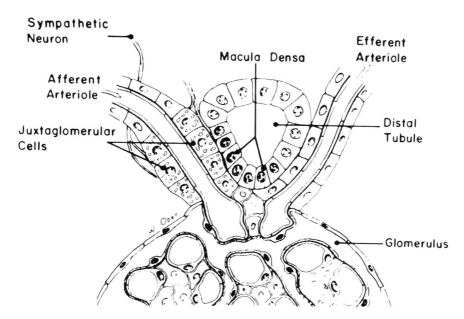

Fig. 4-2. Diagrammatic representation of the renal juxtaglomerular apparatus showing the afferent and efferent arterioles, juxtaglomerular cells, and macula densa. (From Levens et al.,[20] with permission.)

point is that aldosterone, released from the adrenal cortex, enters the systemic circulation, where it has a direct effect on the kidney by stimulating sodium absorption in the distal tubule and collecting duct, with water being reabsorbed with this sodium. This will then isotonically increase the extracellular fluid volume of the body if adequate sodium is administered. As long as the circulating extracellular fluid volume and sodium remains normal, however, the osmoreceptors will be stimulated to maintain the plasma osmolality within the very narrow range of approximately 280 to 290 mOsm/L. The secretion of ADH is thus inhibited, allowing more water to be excreted in the distal tubule and collecting duct, and the urine to become extremely hypotonic. Aldosterone causes essentially all of the available sodium to be reabsorbed. In older infants and children the urine sodium will drop to less than 5 mEq/L. In the neonate the urine sodium may be as high as 20 to 25 mEq/L. The indications of an activation of the renin-angiotensin-aldosterone system is a decrease in urine output as well as urine sodium. The clinical history is useful at this point; in a small infant or child the parents will notice a reduction in the number of times that the diapers become wet and in addition will notice that the urine has become more concentrated.

Temporary Compensatory Mechanisms

At times, the loss of blood or extracellular fluid exceeds the quantity or quality of replacement administered, resulting in a decreased circulating plasma volume. The body's temporary compensatory mechanisms will then be activated to maintain the circulation. Under such conditions the volume receptors take precedence over the osmoreceptors. This is discussed in more detail later in the chapter. If the volume loss threatens to reduce the blood volume from normal, the various endogenous vasopressor substances will be released. These include the sympathetic amines (epinephrine and norepinephrine), vasopressin (ADH), and angiotensin II. Because all clinicians are aware of the actions of epinephrine and norepinephrine, they will not be discussed here. ADH is released when there is a volume challenge. It is released as a definitive compensatory mechanism if there are osmotic alterations in the plasma. In addition, vasopressin, through its vasopressor action, has a very active role in maintaining the blood pressure when there is a volume challenge. Angiotensin II is part of the cascade when the renin-angiotensin-aldosterone system is activated, and is the most potent vasoconstrictor that the body releases.

Transcapillary refill is another temporary compensatory mechanism that the body activates to help maintain a normal circulating plasma volume. Transcapillary refill refers to the translocation of extracellular fluid from the interstitial fluid of the body to the plasma compartment. The interstitial fluid acts as a volume buffer to increase the plasma volume. As seen in Figure 4-3, there is an ongoing exchange and turnover between the plasma volume and the interstitial fluid volume. However, with unreplaced extracellular fluid loss, the fluid movement from the interstitial fluid to the plasma volume is greater than that in reverse, with the result that the reduced plasma volume is augmented. The loss

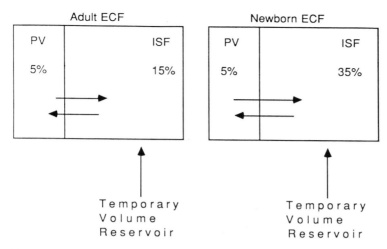

Fig. 4-3. Extracellular fluid volume demonstrating that interstitial fluid (*ISF*) is a temporary volume reservoir for the plasma volume (*PV*).

of interstitial fluid volume causes a reduction in skin turgor. A loss of skin turgor represents a significant loss (more than 5 percent of the body weight) of fluid and electrolytes from the body, which must be replaced with a BSS. This type of fluid replacement requires a bolus of 25 ml/kg of BSS and the reevaluation of volume. There is a limit to the amount of transcapillary refill that can occur. The interstitial fluid volume can constrict by about 20 to 30 percent of its original volume. Further losses of extracellular fluid volume will reduce the circulatory plasma volume, resulting in hypovolemia and hypotension. The early sign of hypovolemia is orthostatic hypotension. If the volume loss continues and the hypovolemia becomes greater, hypotension in the supine position will occur. Supine hypotension represents a blood volume loss of at least 20 to 25 percent of the total blood volume.

APPROPRIATE SECRETION OF ANTIDIURETIC HORMONE AND HYPONATREMIA

Appropriate Secretion of Antidiuretic Hormone

At times there are unrecognized or unappreciated losses of sodium (i.e., through bleeding, third-space losses, vomiting, etc.) combined with the administration of hypotonic fluid (e.g., 0.25 percent saline in 5 percent dextrose). The subtle and sometimes not so subtle loss of sodium exceeds the required sodium replacement. The renin-angiotensin-aldosterone system will have already been activated, resulting in the absorption of all the available sodium. Since the sodium content of the body determines the extracellular fluid volume, this volume loss activates volume conservation. The baroreceptor then takes precedence over the osmoreceptor, and the ADH mechanism is activated. This decreases the permeability of the distal tubule and collecting duct to water, thereby increasing free water reabsorption. This reabsorption will in turn hypotonically re-expand the extracellular fluid volume and hence dilute the plasma sodium. This condition is referred to as a *dilutional hyponatremia* in response to the appropriate secretion of ADH. The degree of hyponatremia is related to the extent of the sodium deficit as well as the volume of hypotonic fluid administered. The early signs of hyponatremia (a serum sodium level of 120 to 125 mEq/L) are mainly lethargy and nausea and vomiting, which further complicate the situation. When the sodium level goes below 120 mEq/L, central nervous system irritability may lead to a decreased level of consciousness, seizures, nausea and vomiting, and the risk of aspiration. This condition is referred to as *acute symptomatic hyponatremia*, and can lead to severe neurologic problems, including death.

Acute Symptomatic Hyponatremia

Acute symptomatic hyponatremia is in general a postoperative problem.[5] However, the reason that it is being discussed at this point in the chapter is because the pathophysiology of the compensatory mechanisms has just been discussed and I feel it would be appropriate to have a full discussion at this juncture.

Acute symptomatic hyponatremia is a medical emergency, resulting in a patient who is at risk for vomiting, aspirating, seizures, and hypoxia. The initial treatment of any seizure is supportive, while the diagnosis is being made. Airway control and oxygenation are needed. Small intravenous doses of diazepam (0.1-mg/kg increments up to 0.3 mg/kg) should be administered to control the seizure if the seizure continues. The patient may require intubation if the seizures continue or if the sedation and postictal state result in the patient's inability to protect their airway. Any patient who has a seizure in the perioperative period should have a serum sodium and glucose determination to evaluate the possibility of hyponatremia and hypoglycemia. The patient who has a seizure in the perioperative period and who has been receiving hypotonic fluids such as 0.25 or 0.5 percent saline should also be treated immediately with sodium bicarbonate as described below. One cannot wait for 30 to 40 minutes while the serum sodium is being determined.

Postoperative hyponatremia is the most frequent postoperative electrolyte disturbance.[6] It usually takes from 3 to 24 hours to develop since it requires the ongoing losses of sodium along with the administration of hypotonic fluid. The pathophysiology of the problem is that as the osmotic pressure of the plasma decreases because of the dilutional hyponatremia an osmotic gradient is developed between the extracellular and intracellular fluid compartments. Mother nature cannot tolerate such a gradient and therefore water passes from the extracellular fluid space into the intracellular fluid space, thereby reducing the intracellular osmotic pressure. The price that is paid for this is an increase in intracranial pressure owing to the swelling of the cell. There is also a disturbance of the cell function owing to the electrolyte disturbances resulting from the dilutional hyponatremia. The treatment of acute symptomatic hyponatremia is to increase the osmotic pressure of the extracellular fluid volume. This is brought about through the administration of a hypertonic solution, which will reverse the osmotic gradient and reduce the intracellular water content. The usually prescribed treatment is 3 percent saline, however, in the vast majority of the hospitals this fluid is kept in the pharmacy, and at best is 30 to 40 minutes from the location at which it is acutely needed. On the other hand, sodium bicarbonate is immediately available in all emergency drug boxes in all locations throughout the hospital. Sodium bicarbonate is a 6 percent solution of sodium. Therefore, the first step in treatment of patients who are suspected of having acute symptomatic hyponatremia is to administer 2 ml/kg of sodium bicarbonate over 1 to 2 minutes. This will increase the serum sodium approximately 6 mEq/L. If symptoms subside and the patient regains consciousness within 15 to 20 minutes then no further bicarbonate is needed. The intravenous fluid administered should immediately be changed to a balanced salt solution. If, however, the patient remains symptomatic and the sodium level remains below 120 mEq/L, then consideration should be given to administering another bolus of sodium bicarbonate.

Chronic Hyponatremia

There is considerable controversy over the treatment of hyponatremia because there has been some confusion in the literature between the treatment of acute symptomatic hyponatremia and the treatment of (relatively) chronic asymptomatic hyponatremia. Chronic hyponatremia is a medical condition in which there is a very slow, but progressive, decrease in the serum sodium value. This may be due to diet, water intoxication, or diuretic use. In these circumstances the slowly developing hyponatremia allows the osmotic pressure gradient to be minimized by readjustment of the osmotic pressure between the extracellular fluid and the intracellular fluid. In acute hyponatremia the ability to adjust the osmotic pressure gradient is overwhelmed by the magnitude of the change. For that reason, acute symptomatic hyponatremia, with its decreased level of consciousness, nausea and vomiting, and seizure activity, requires rapid aggressive therapy to minimize or prevent brain damage. On the other hand, in slowly developing hyponatremia, the period of treatment should also be slowly developing. The rapid correction of chronic asymptomatic hyponatremia is potentially dangerous and may result in a condition known as the *osmotic demyelination syndrome.*[7]

INAPPROPRIATE SECRETION OF ANTIDIURETIC HORMONE

The appropriate secretion of ADH should not be confused with the syndrome of inappropriate secretion of ADH (SIADH). The latter has been reported to be associated with pulmonary disorders such as tuberculosis and pneumonia as well as with other forms of chronic infection, tumors of the lung and duodenum, and central nervous system disorders such as infection, intracranial tumors, and head trauma. As with the appropriate secretion of ADH, SIADH also results in hyponatremia. The differential diagnosis of these two causes of hyponatremia depends on the patient's history and other laboratory findings. With appropriate ADH release, the hyponatremia is associated with marked reduction in the urine sodium concentration. With SIADH, the amount of urine sodium is normal, since there is no alteration in the renal mechanism for regulating sodium balance. The problem in SIADH is that the inappropriate secretion of ADH causes an inappropriate reabsorption of water, leading to a dilutional hyponatremia. The total-body sodium in this situation is within normal limits, whereas in the situation of appropriate ADH release, there is a reduction in total-body sodium. The treatment for the two conditions is obviously quite different. With appropriate ADH release and hyponatremia, the treatment involves giving sodium. With SIADH, the appropriate treatment is to reduce the amount of extracellular water by restricting fluids and/or administering a diuretic such as furosemide or a drug such as demeclocycline.

ASSESSMENT OF FLUID AND ELECTROLYTE STATUS

The preoperative assessment of any patient depends on the history, physical examination, and appropriate laboratory studies. Appropriate laboratory studies cover a broad spectrum; in the healthy patient no laboratory studies are needed, while the severely ill infant or child may require extensive and repeated laboratory studies. The important facts to glean from patient history are the length of time that an infant or child has been NPO and the frequency and concentration of the urine output.

A decrease in urine output and an increase in urine concentration are often the first signs of dehydration. The important, salient features to be obtained from the physical examination are the overall condition of the infant (i.e., its state of alertness, the skin turgor, and status of the eyeballs and fontanelles) and a comparison of its current weight with a previous weight. The laboratory studies of importance include the electrolytes, blood urea nitrogen, and creatinine measurements, the hematocrit, and the specific gravity of the urine. If there is concern about the pulmonary system of the infant or about its acid-base status, an arterial blood gas analysis should be done.

Preoperative Electrolyte Derangements

Hyponatremia is the most frequent serious electrolyte disturbance that occurs in the perioperative surgical patient. The most frequent basis for its occurrence is a loss of body sodium through the several mechanisms that have been described and fluid replacement with a fluid of low sodium content. Asymptomatic hyponatremia secondary to the appropriate secretion of ADH should be treated with administration of a balanced isotonic salt solution.

Calculating Electrolyte Deficits

Two examples of preoperative sodium deficits, and their correction are given below. The first example is an infant who is normovolemic but hyponatremic as a result of an iatrogenic fluid administration. The second is the more familiar situation of a hypovolemic, hyponatremic infant.

In the first case, the 3-month-old, 5-kg infant with pyloric stenosis was admitted for rehydration and surgery. The diagnosis was made in a small community hospital after a 2-day history of projectile vomiting, after which the infant was transferred to a tertiary care hospital for definitive treatment. An IV of 5 percent dextrose in 0.25 percent saline was started. The infant arrived approximately 5 hours later, after having received 250 ml of the solution. The initial sodium level was 125 mEq/L. The infant was well hydrated and had a normal urine output. The electrolyte problem was a sodium deficit.

How does one calculate the sodium deficit in the example given above? The following is a simple method. The sodium space of an infant is the extracellular fluid volume. The extracellular fluid volume of a 3-month-old infant is approximately 30 percent of the body weight (Fig. 4-4). Therefore, this infant had an extracellular fluid space of 1.5 L (0.30 × 5 kg). The average normal sodium value is 140 mEq/L. This infant had a sodium of 125 mEq/L. The deficit is therefore 15 mEq of sodium per liter of extracellular fluid. Since this infant has 1.5 L of extracellular fluid, the sodium deficit is 22 mEq of sodium. Lactated Ringer's solution contains 130 mEq of sodium per liter of fluid, or 13 mEq of sodium per 100 ml of fluid. Therefore, it would take the administration of approximately 200 ml of lactated Ringer's solution to reverse the sodium deficit. This fluid is added to the maintenance fluid requirement of 4 ml/kg/hr (as BSS)

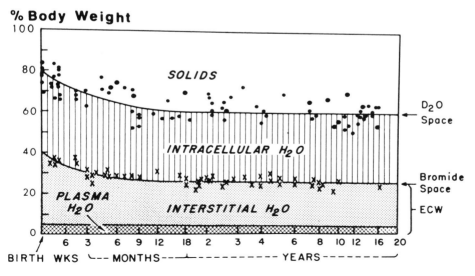

Fig. 4-4. Percent body weight of the various body compartments with age. (Modified from Talbot et al.,[21] with permission.)

to meet the total fluid and electrolyte requirement of this infant (deficit plus maintenance). BSS should be administered at the rate of 125 ml/hr (25 ml/kg/hr) for 2 hours. The electrolyte measurement should be repeated and surgery performed when the serum sodium is 130 mEq/L or over.

The second infant, age 4 months, also had a diagnosis of pyloric stenosis. In this case there was a 4-week history of progressive intermittent vomiting, which was treated by the usual repeated changing of the formula. Over the last week before admission, the infant's vomiting became more protracted and the mother became concerned because the infant was very sleepy and hadn't wet his diaper in 6 hours. The serum sodium was 122 mEq/L. This case involves an infant who has a significant reduction in extracellular fluid volume in addition to a deficit in the sodium content of the extracellular fluid. In this situation, a correction would have to be made for both the extracellular fluid volume and sodium deficit of the extracellular fluid. In this case, the infant was more symptomatic than in the first case, and had a decrease in skin turgor and a decreased level of alertness. The infant had been weighed 4 weeks previously, when the vomiting began, and his weight was 5.5 kg. His current weight is 5 kg, and the deficit in extracellular fluid is therefore approximately 0.5 L. A deficit of 0.5 L of extracellular fluid is equal to 70 mEq of sodium (0.5 L $\times$ 140 mEq/L = 70 mEq). An infant who weighs 5 kg and who has an extracellular fluid deficit of 0.5 L is significantly (10 percent) dehydrated. The total sodium deficit in this situation is calculated by adding the sodium deficit of the extracellular fluid (140 mEq/L $-$ 122 mEq/L = 18 mEq/L deficit) to the volume deficit of the extracellular fluid. The extracellular fluid volume would be 1.7 L $\times$ 18 mEq/L, or approximately 30 mEq of sodium. The total deficit in this situation is approximately 100 mEq of sodium (70 mEq + 30 mEq). This infant should be given a bolus of 25 ml/kg of BSS (5 kg $\times$ 25 ml/kg = 125 ml) over a 20- to 30-minute period, and then 25 ml/kg of BSS (5 kg $\times$ 25 ml/kg = 125 ml) given hourly for the next 2 hours. The electrolyte measurement should then be repeated and the sodium deficit recalculated. At this point the sodium deficit would be approximately 50 percent corrected. In the first situation the infant's volume and sodium deficit would have been corrected after the initial 2 hours of fluid administration, and if the physical examination were normal and the electrolytes returning toward normal (i.e., greater than 130 mEq of sodium per liter), then surgery could be safely performed. However, in the instance of the second, moderately severely dehydrated infant, a sodium deficit would, if the original assumptions were correct, still exist, and it would probably take a total of 6 to 8 hours to return the infant to a more ideal state of fluid and electrolyte balance. The correction of fluid and electrolyte deficits should be accomplished before surgery. The infant should be alert, the skin turgor normal, the fontanelles and eyeballs no longer sunken, the urine output between 1 and 2 ml/kg, the urine specific gravity dropping, and the serum sodium returning toward normal. Anesthesia in infants is difficult enough without complicating the situation with a fluid and electrolyte problem.

The clinical situation of the dehydrated infants just described is at one end of the spectrum of a clinical situation that requires correction before coming to the operating room. At the other end of the spectrum is the infant for elective surgery who is otherwise normal and in whom the only deficit is the result of an NPO period. These patients need no special preoperative fluid therapy. However, children who present with varying degrees of dehydration from being on lengthy NPO regimens should have an IV started intraoperatively even if the case is short. We can minimize some of the problems of the NPO period by being more reasonable about the length of time during which we require infants and children to be NPO.

HOW LONG SHOULD THE NPO PERIOD LAST?

There has been considerable rethinking about the length of the NPO period. This has come about through numerous studies that have demonstrated that our previous prolonged NPO periods were inappropriate. It has recently been shown that administering a clear fluid such as apple juice up to 2.5 hours before surgery as compared with a longer period of being NPO results in the gastric pH remaining essentially the same and the gastric volume decreasing.[8,9]

Infants under 6 months of age, therefore, can continue to have formula or breast milk up until 6 hours before surgery, followed by clear fluid until 3 hours before surgery. Older infants and children are not given milk or food on the day of surgery but can have clear fluids until 3 hours before premedication or until the time at which they arrive in the operating room or induction area for surgery. Hospital-based infants can be awakened in the middle of the night to be given fluids. However, it is unreasonable to expect parents who may be driving long distances to arrive at the ambulatory unit early in the morning to wake their infants up in the middle of the night. The result is that these infants and children often have fairly prolonged periods of being NPO, perhaps as long as 12 to 15 hours, since they've usually been put to bed at 7:00 to 8:00 PM the night before and their surgery may not be until late the next morning or early afternoon. Therefore, in these infants and children, when surgery is scheduled for late in the morning or early afternoon, it is permissible for them to be given clear fluids up until 3 hours before the scheduled surgery. A clear fluid is one that contains no particulate matter. This modification of the guidelines for NPO has resulted in the parents being much happier about not having to battle their small child over the starvation period and a happier child who may have better veins for venipuncture since their fluid status will be normal. The need for this more humane technique to minimize starvation and thirst in the young child was recently brought home when a nurse who was bathing a 3½-year-old child before surgery called the operating room in distress. She was upset because the child drank some of the bath water because he was so thirsty. The bath water contained a soap solution, thus reflecting the degree of desperation that thirsty infants and children are driven to.

INTRAOPERATIVE FLUID THERAPY

There is some question about what type of fluid therapy to give during the surgical period. As noted earlier, the two types of fluids the body requires are maintenance fluids and replacement fluids. Some investigators recommend ad-

Table 4-4. Guidelines for Fluid Administration in Patients Age 3 and Under: BSS

1. First hour: hydrating solution, 25 ml/kg, plus item 3 below
2. All other hours, plus item 3 below
     Maintenance fluid = 4 ml/kg
     Maintenance + trauma = basic hourly fluid
     4 ml/kg + mild trauma, 2 ml/kg = 6 ml/kg/hour
     4 ml/kg + moderate trauma, 4 ml/kg = 8 ml/kg/hour
     4 ml/kg + maximal trauma, 6 ml/kg = 10 ml/kg/hour
3. Blood replacement with blood or 3:1 volume replacement with crystalloid

ministering 0.25 percent saline as a maintenance fluid and BSS as a replacement fluid. It gets rather cumbersome in the operating room to try to administer two different types of fluids at two different rates, and for practical considerations as well as for postoperative reasons I therefore administer BSS as the standard perioperative fluid. The postoperative considerations for fluids are vomiting, unexpected bleeding, and perhaps third spacing of extracellular fluid. It is difficult, if not impossible, to predict which patient will have these varying postoperative problems, but all of these complications require full-strength replacement fluids. If the administration of sodium has been marginal (i.e., 0.25 percent saline) during the surgical period, the patient will have no sodium reserve in the postoperative period in order to cope with these potential postoperative complications. Therefore, it is my opinion that BSS should be used intraoperatively and postoperatively in order to prevent the electrolyte disturbances that may occur. The renal system has an enormous capability to excrete extra sodium and other electrolytes not needed by the body. On the other hand, the kidney cannot create sodium, but can only conserve that which is administered. Tables 4-4 and 4-5 present guidelines for fluid administration during the operative period. The guidelines in Table 4-4 are for infants and children up to age 3, and those in Table 4-5 are for children age 4 and over. The only difference for the two groups is the quantity of hydrating solution used (25 ml/kg vs. 15 ml/kg). If the patient has been receiving intravenous fluid and is adequately hydrated upon arriving in the operating room, no hydrating solution is needed, and the patient's fluid requirements begin at item 2, "All other hours."

The object of giving the hydrating solution is to make up for fluids lost during

Table 4-5. Guidelines for Fluid Administration in Patients Age 4 and Over: BSS

1. First hour: hydrating solution 15 ml/kg, plus item 3 below
2. All other hours, plus item 3 below
     Maintenance fluid = 4 ml/kg
     Maintenance + trauma = basic hourly fluid
     4 ml/kg + mild trauma = 2 ml/kg = 6 ml/kg/hour
     4 ml/kg + moderate trauma, 4 ml/kg = 8 ml/kg/hour
     4 ml/kg + maximal trauma, 6 ml/kg = 10 ml/kg/hour
3. Blood replacement with blood or 3:1 volumen replacement with crystalloid

the NPO period. Rather than expecting the anesthesiologist to calculate the exact deficit for each patient, it is recommended that the volume of hydrating solution for infants 3 years of age and under be 25 ml/kg. In addition, for the first hour, any blood lost must be replaced with either blood or crystalloid in the ratio of 3:1. The child age 4 and over has a lower requirement for maintenance fluids, which is why the amount of hydrating solution given to such patients is smaller (15 ml/kg). If the surgical procedure is rather short (i.e., up to 1 hour), the IV will usually be discontinued within the first several hours after surgery. Therefore, in this situation, it is recommended that fluids be given at the rate of 25 ml/kg/hr for infants and children age 3 and under, and at 15 ml/kg/hr for children 4 years of age and over, for the first 2 to 3 hours after the surgical procedure. This bolus of fluid will replace any deficits that may occur, as well as give the patient a "cushion" during the postoperative period.

Maintenance Fluid During Surgery

Item 2 in Tables 4-4 and 4-5, "All other hours, plus (item) 3," is the blood replacement formula. In order to simplify the maintenance fluid requirement intraoperatively, the same number, 4 ml/kg, has been given for all age groups. Children over age 3 do have a lower maintenance fluid requirement, but using only one figure makes both the memorization of the table and the calculations easier. It should be remembered that these are guidelines. In general, if a surgical procedure is going to last longer than 2 hours and is going to involve significant fluid and blood losses the patient may have a urinary catheter to help to monitor the adequacy of fluid replacement. If the urine output exceeds 1 to 2 ml/kg/hr, the amount of fluid is reduced. If it is less than 1 ml/kg/hr the fluid input is increased.

Replacement Fluid During Surgery

The two major needs for replacement fluids are in (1) blood loss and (2) translocated (third-space) fluid from trauma.

Translocated Fluid

The formula guidelines for translocated fluid call for 2 to 6 ml/kg depending on the severity of trauma. This is an arbitrary figure, but with experience, reasonable estimates of loss can be determined and an appropriate fluid volume administered according to the patient's response. Sometimes more is needed.

Management of Blood Loss

Management of blood loss depends on the condition of the patient and the nature of the surgery.

The Condition of the Patient

If a patient is undergoing volume resuscitation with blood because of a pre-existing condition, any blood lost needs to be replaced with blood until the patient is stable. If an infant is chronically ill and has the anemia of chronic illness, and if the blood loss exceeds 5 percent of the blood volume, transfusion should certainly be seriously considered. The concept of anemia will be discussed below. A helpful guideline in determining the appropriate amount of blood to be administered is the ability to deliver oxygen to the cells. Considerable amounts of blood loss (to be later defined) can be replaced with crystalloid if the patient is able to deliver adequate oxygen to his cells. The delivery of oxygen depends on the cardiovascular system and pulmonary system in addition to the hemoglobin. Patients who have a limited cardiac output and limited ability to saturate their hemoglobin will not tolerate as low a hemoglobin as normal patients. Therefore, patients with these limitations to the delivery or saturation of hemoglobin may require a higher hemoglobin level than that listed in Table 4-6 as acceptable hemoglobin and/or hematocrit. This is seen in infants with cyanotic congenital heart disease who have elevated hematocrits. Sometimes nature overdoes the process and the hemoglobin level is so high that the blood viscosity increases, leading to a reduction in blood flow, sludging, and hypercoaguability. The hemoglobin or hematocrit necessary for optimal tissue blood flow as well as oxygen delivery has not been well defined. However, patients with significant cardiovascular or pulmonary disease would probably benefit from a hemoglobin of at least 10 g/dl (a hematocrit of 30). Patients with normal cardiovascular and respiratory systems can function adequately at a hemoglobin level of 7 or 8 g/dl (a hematocrit of 20 to 25). Clinical judgment must be used when determining the appropriate hemoglobin or hematocrit for the patient in question. Table 4-6 also lists the normal hematocrits for children of various age groups. It should be noted that the newborn infant has an average hematocrit of 54, and that the lowest hematocrit in a full-term infant occurs at the age of approximately 10 to 12 weeks (i.e., a hemoglobin of 10 g/dl and a hematocrit of 30). This results from two factors: a rapid increase in body weight and a lagging ability of the bone marrow to supply adequate red cells. Therefore, at this age, a hematocrit of 30 might not only be acceptable, but might be normal. As the infant grows older the normal values for the hematocrit rise.

Table 4-6. Normal and Acceptable Hematocrits in Pediatric Patients

	Normal Hematocrit		Acceptable Hematocrit
	Mean	Range	
Premature	45	40–50	35–40
Newborn	54	45–65	35–40
3 months	36	30–42	25
1 year	38	34–42	20–25
6 years	38	35–43	20–25

"Normal" vs. "Acceptable" Hematocrit

A "normal" hematocrit would be any hematocrit within the range of 2 SD. An "acceptable" hematocrit is defined either as a hematocrit that is acceptable for the condition of the patient or for the surgical procedure that is to be performed. The hematocrit may or may not be normal according to the guidelines given above for a normal patient, but it may be normal for the condition of the patient (e.g., sickle cell anemia or renal disease). The medical profession is currently trying to define what an acceptable hematocrit is. Table 4-6 gives the results of such an attempt. This is obviously a guideline, and as such is arbitrary. This rearrangement of our priorities and definitions has come about through the fear of AIDS and hepatitis from transfusions. The benefits from reducing the number of transfusions are a reduction in exposure to blood-borne diseases, laboratory errors in cross-matching, and febrile or allergic reactions to blood. At the same time, the risk of a low hematocrit must be appreciated. If the patient has a normal cardiovascular and respiratory system, hematocrits of 20 to 25 are usually tolerated without any particular consequences. As a matter of fact, in chronic renal failure, the acceptable hematocrit might be in the range of 17 to 20. If a 6-month-old infant appears to be otherwise normal but has a hematocrit of 25, this hematocrit may be termed "acceptable," but it is obviously not normal. Therefore, if a patient with a hematocrit of 25 presents for "elective" surgery, two things must be considered: (1) why the patient has a hematocrit of 25 and (2) if the cause of the patient's anemia is known, whether "elective" surgery should be performed. The answer to the second question is a qualified "yes," since it depends on other factors, such as the type of surgery to be done and other potential medical problems of the patient. There are certain surgical procedures, particularly in premature nursery graduates that are considered urgent. These include surgery for the retinopathy of prematurity and surgery for hernia repair. Premature infants have a high incidence of hernias. Hernias that occur in the first year have a higher incidence of incarceration and other potential catastrophes than hernias that appear later in life. This is discussed more fully in Chapter 5, Physiology and Surgery of the Infant. Table 4-7 lists the most frequent causes of anemia. If the cause for the patient's anemia cannot be determined, elective surgery should be postponed until a diagnosis can be made. If the surgery is urgent, it can be accomplished, but there must be an ongoing effort to diagnose the reason for the anemia.

At times, the anemia may require the preoperative administration of blood

Table 4-7. Causes of Anemia

Prematurity
Diet
Underlying medical problems
    Infections
    Malignancies
    Renal disease
    Hemoglobinopathies

in order to permit a safer induction. This is a matter of clinical judgment; there are no magic numbers. In the case of emergency surgery the situation may be so grave that blood administration and the induction of anesthesia must be simultaneous. Patients who are hypovolemic represent a considerable anesthetic risk. The need to press ahead immediately must be balanced with the need for preoperative preparation of the patient.

The Nature of the Surgery

The other determinant of when to replace blood is the nature of the surgery. If the nature of the surgery is such that it may entail major losses of blood that may not be immediately controllable, such as major vascular surgery in any anatomic location, blood should be administered as soon as significant blood loss (5 to 10 percent of blood volume) occurs. If the nature of the surgery is such that bleeding can easily be controlled, such as in operations on extremities or on the gastrointestinal system, blood loss can be allowed to occur, and, within acceptable blood-loss guidelines, can be corrected with crystalloid. The guidelines for acceptable blood loss depend on the age, the starting hematocrit, and the estimated amount of blood loss. The usual amount of allowable blood loss is approximately 25 to 30 percent of the circulating blood volume. The other guideline that has been suggested is a final hematocrit in the range of 20 to 25. This latter guideline may be acceptable for infants age 2 to 3 months and older. A postoperative hematocrit of 30 is suggested for premature infants and infants up to 1 month of age.

Some rather complicated formulas have been used to calculate the acceptable blood loss. These require either an extraordinary memory or a notebook. For clinicians who have neither, the following guidelines are suggested. The allowable blood loss is either a 25 to 30 percent loss of blood volume or until the hematocrit declines to approximately 20 to 25 for infants 2 months and older and to 30 for those under 2 months. The blood volume can be calculated from the body weight. For infants and children, 8 percent of the body weight is the blood volume. Mature males have a blood volume of 7.5 percent of body weight, and mature females, 7 percent of body weight. If the patient is obese, the percentage of blood volume should be reduced by 0.5 percent since fat tissue does not contain as much blood as lean tissue.

As an example, a 1-year-old infant weighing 10 kg will have a blood volume of 8 percent of body weight, or 800 ml. An acceptable reduction of blood volume would be 25 to 30 percent of the blood volume, which is equal to 200 to 240 ml of blood. The clinician needs to estimate or calculate the blood loss as it occurs and replace the blood loss in a 3:1 ratio with a BSS. A 30 percent reduction in hematocrit, if one assumes that the infant's hematocrit is 36, would result in a reduction in the hematocrit of 12, or a final hematocrit of 24. Another example is a 10-kg 1-year-old, who has an iron deficiency anemia, with a hematocrit of 30. Let us assume that this patient has a large hemangioma that has become infected and is beginning to bleed slightly, necessitating surgery on an urgent basis. A 20 to 25 percent reduction in blood volume in this infant would reduce the hematocrit by approximately 6 to 8, and the finishing hematocrit would be 22 to 24. This is an acceptable hematocrit. The allowable blood loss should be discussed with the surgeon preoperatively so that all members of the surgical team can be in agreement about the best way to proceed with replacement and transfusion therapy. In general, when a blood loss of 25 to 30 percent is projected, an arterial line might well be indicated, and serial hematocrits can be determined in order to verify the clinical estimation of the amount of blood loss.

If the anticipated blood loss is greater than 30 percent, it would seem appropriate to allow the patient to hemodilute to a hematocrit in the mid 20s and then to begin to replace blood loss with blood following the hematocrit. In addition, patients with this degree of anticipated blood loss are more easily managed with an arterial line and urinary catheter.

The Place of Glucose in Routine Intravenous Solutions

There has been considerable controversy recently about the administration of glucose in routine intraoperative intravenous solutions.[10] The question that arises is twofold: Is glucose in intravenous solutions necessary or potentially harmful?

Is Glucose Necessary in Intravenous Solutions?

Some investigators believe that glucose is necessary in intravenous solutions to prevent hypoglycemia or that blood glucose determinations need to be obtained if intravenous solutions are given without glucose. This is a matter of opinion that has caused considerable controversy. One of the major difficulties in determining whether or not glucose is required, based on the incidence of hypoglycemia, is that there is a considerable difference of opinion as to exactly what blood level of glucose is defined as hypoglycemia. Based on the various studies in the literature, it is my opinion that hypoglycemia is not a concern in normal children and therefore there is no reason to routinely administer glucose in intravenous fluids. In addition, I do not believe that it is necessary to routinely monitor the blood glucose values in these patients who receive intravenous fluids without glucose. It is becoming the practice of many clinicians to consider glucose a drug and to administer it according to specific indications. Thomas[11] defined hypoglycemia as a blood glucose level below 40 mg/dl, whereas Welborn et al.[12] defined hypoglycemia as a blood glucose level below 50 mg/dl. Unfortunately, the literature is not clear about the definition of hypoglycemia. I consider a blood glucose level below 40 mg/dl in older infants and children as hypoglycemia and a blood glucose level of 30 mg/dl as the lower limit of normal in full-term infants.

There are, however, certain infants and children who may be at risk for developing hypoglycemia. These include infants who have had intrauterine growth retardation, infants of diabetic mothers, diabetics, and infants who have documented hypoglycemia. If there is any question about hypoglycemia, blood glucose levels should then be determined in these patients. In infants and children who have been on hyperalimentation or enhanced glucose regimens, these regimens should be continued while monitoring the blood glucose level during this surgery.

Is Glucose Potentially Harmful in Intravenous Solutions?

There have been a number of studies in experimental animals that have indicated the potential for the augmentation of ischemic brain injury by glucose infusions.[13-16] The concern is that if the central nervous system has recently been exposed to a glucose solution and ischemia occurs, the anaerobic metabolism of the glucose will result in an increase in lactic acid and a decrease in intracellular pH. With reperfusion this combination appears to cause an augmentation of the ischemic central nervous system injury. Without glucose the ischemic injury itself may be only transient and complete recovery is expected. However, the administration of glucose in a number of animal studies resulted in significant clinical impairment of the animal as well as significant histopathologic neurologic deterioration. In some animal studies this has occurred in spite of an insignificant increase in plasma glucose. One study in children has associated high levels of blood glucose during hypothermic circulatory arrest with transient neurologic deficits.[17]

I am familiar with several medicolegal cases in which a child suffered a short ischemic episode, resuscitation appeared to be adequate, and yet the child sustained a severe neurologic injury that was completely unexpected by the surgical team. In all of these cases, a dextrose solution had been administered. Therefore, at the present there is a re-evaluation of the place of routine glucose in intravenous fluids.

In summary, there is no evidence that glucose is required in routine intravenous solutions. Augmentation of ischemic brain injury from glucose would appear to be a greater risk than any of the benefits that have so far been described from its administration in normal patients. We do not routinely administer glucose nor do we routinely check intraoperative blood glucose values.

MONITORING OF THE PATIENT

The basic monitors for all patients are:

1. A precordial stethoscope
2. An electrocardiograph
3. A device for measuring the blood pressure
4. A pulse oximeter
5. Temperature monitoring

Temperature monitoring should be available for all patients, but for very short procedures does not necessarily need to be employed. We do not routinely monitor temperature during computed tomography since the technique of choice, which will be discussed in Chapter 12, is that of rectal methohexital (Brevital) supplemented with various intravenous agents. Intubation is not routinely done and, as a matter of fact, is rarely done. Therefore, the stimulation of either a rectal or an oral temperature probe would interfere with the anesthetic technique.

The need for additional monitors is based on the basic condition of the patient and the surgical procedure being done. Patients having elective surgery in which the blood loss is less than 25 to 30 percent can be monitored with the basic monitors. However, if the patient has a compromised cardiovascular or respiratory system, it might be appropriate to insert a catheter in the bladder to determine the urine output, or an arterial line. At other times, when the patient is essentially sound but having life-threatening surgery, the choice of monitors depends on the degree of difficulty of the surgery, the anticipated problems, the anesthetic techniques, and the need for postoperative monitoring. The selection and use of monitors is certainly a matter of judgment. In surgical procedures in which large losses of blood or major alterations in oxygenation and ventilation are anticipated, or in major surgery where hypotensive anesthesia is desired, the use of a direct arterial line may be of major benefit. The advantages of an arterial line are that it gives an ongoing indication of blood pressure and that it permits sampling for arterial blood gas measurements, hematocrit, electrolytes, and clotting profiles. The guidelines for the administration of fluid and blood must be tempered by the condition of the patient and the patient's response to the surgery and the fluid and blood administration.

Blood Pressure as an Indication of Blood Volume

In infants and young children up to the age of 3 or 4, in whom the sympathetic tone is not fully mature, the blood pressure is a good indication of the blood volume. This statement needs to be qualified, as the blood pressure of an infant and small child will certainly follow the expected pharmacologic responses from the anesthetic agents and be increased or decreased appropriately. However, when the blood pressure has been steady and the anesthetic concentrations unchanged, changes in the blood pressure will reflect changes in blood volume owing to the loss of blood. This indicates a need to increase the blood volume according to the guidelines, as already discussed.

Rapidly Developing Hypotension and/or Bradycardia

One guideline for determining the adequacy of fluid and blood therapy is to follow the patient's vital signs. Blood pressure monitoring is required in all patients regardless of the anticipated fluid and blood needs. If there is hypotension and/or bradycardia of sudden onset, the anesthesiologist must have a checklist of what to do and what the diagnostic possibilities are. The checklist for what to do in hypotension and/or bradycardia of sudden onset is given in Table 4-8. Believe the monitors until you can prove they are inaccurate! There are four major reasons for the sudden development of hypotension and/or bradycardia:

Table 4-8. Steps in Treatment of Hypotension and/or Bradycardia of Suddent Onset

1. Turn off the anesthesia
2. Ventilate with 100% oxygen
3. Bolus fluids and/or blood
4. Epinephrine 5 μg/kg
5. Notify the surgeon

1. Inadequate ventilation resulting in hypoxia
2. Inadequate cardiac output secondary to myocardial depression
3. An inadequate circulating blood volume
4. A vagal reflex

The pulse oximeter has been a boon both for the management of our patients and to determine the etiology of some of their intra- and postoperative problems. In the past, when there was sudden bradycardia and/or hypotension, the primary cause was thought to be hypoxia, which it often was. However, now with an oximeter, we have a monitor that will indicate whether hypoxia is the problem or not. Since the advent of the oximeter and in infants with a normal oxygen saturation, I have seen several instances of bradycardia and hypotension that were not caused by hypoxia but by a vagal reflex. Furthermore, release of traction by the surgeon did not correct the reflex, nor did the administration of an anticholinergic in two of the cases correct the problem. In the past, cases like this would have been attributed to hypoxia and the anesthesiologist charged with negligence.

One of the most important aspects of this checklist is to make sure the patient is ventilated with 100 percent oxygen. This does not mean seeing whether the ventilator is working; it means verifying, with a stethoscope, the movement of oxygen in and out of both of the patient's lungs. A pneumothorax may present as a sudden drop in blood pressure. A disconnect from the ventilator may also cause this development. A precordial or esophageal stethoscope should be present on all patients to monitor ventilation and heart sounds on a continuous basis throughout surgery. Another point to be made when ensuring that the patient is ventilated with 100 percent oxygen is to recheck the flow meters and to be certain that oxygen is being administered. The type of fluid that should be given is BSS. If the blood loss is approaching its acceptable limit, blood should be given in a bolus of 10 ml/kg. If the problem is bradycardia without hypotension, an anticholinergic such as glycopyrrolate or atropine should be administered in a dose of 0.02 mg/kg. If the bradycardia or hypotension does not immediately (within 60 seconds) respond to the glycopyrrolate or atropine, epinephrine should be administered in a dose of 5 μg/kg. If bradycardia is accompanied by hypotension, then epinephrine in a dose of 5 μg/kg should be administered immediately. The definition of bradycardia requiring epinephrine for children under 1 year is a heart rate under 100 beats/min with a blood pressure under 50 mmHg. For the older child, relatively lower pulse rates and the same type of blood pressure are an indication to administer the epinephrine. If the response to this is not rapid, it should be repeated. Anaphylaxis may present as hypotension and bradycardia without any cutaneous or respiratory involvement. Epinephrine is the treatment of choice. If the patient has been receiving blood or there is thought to be some other metabolic derangement resulting in hypocalcemia, the administration of calcium 10 to 20 mg/kg may be beneficial. If the blood pressure does not respond to any of these measures, and if the oxygen saturation is dropping, the ventilation must be rechecked and the position and placement of the endotracheal tube verified in spite of what appear to be normal breath sounds. At times, particularly in small infants, ventilation of the stomach may sound quite similar to ventilation of the lungs. Listening to the stomach as well as the lungs may also provide invaluable information about placement of the endotracheal tube in spite of this problem. If ventilation is in doubt, the patient must be laryngoscoped and the tube placement checked. If the tube placement is in doubt, the patient should be extubated, ventilated with a bag and mask, and reintubated. If the blood pressure continues downward and drops below 50 percent of the control blood pressure, external cardiac massage should be begun. There should be a low threshold for initiating external cardiac massage.

The surgeon should be notified as soon as any unexplained decrease in blood pressure and/or bradycardia occurs. The two reasons for this are that the surgeon may have observed something or done something that the anesthesiologist does not yet known about. There may be a large volume loss within the thoracic or peritoneal cavity, traction of viscera, or distortion of a major blood vessel such as the vena cava. The surgeon deserves to know about the crisis so as to be able to assist in the diagnosis of the problem and the resuscitation of the patient.

Slowly Developing Hypotension

Some of the causes for slowly developing hypotension are:

1. Anesthetic overdose, either relative or absolute
2. Hypercarbia
3. Hypoxia
4. Inadequate fluid volume
5. A low ionized calcium
6. Obstruction of major blood vessels

If there is a gradual downward trend in the blood pressure, the anesthesiologist has time to review the possibilities. The first thing to ensure is that the patient is receiving adequate oxygenation, which has been made rather easy by the pulse oximeter. The second is to make sure that there has not been a drift in the flowmeters, resulting in an actual or relative overdose of anesthetic. The third is to recalculate the blood and fluid loss to determine if a subtle but significant loss has occurred and produced a mild hypovolemic state. If the patient has been receiving a large number of blood transfusions, consideration should be given to the administration of calcium. The initial dose is between 10 and 20 mg/kg. When a slow downward trend occurs in the blood pressure, the surgeon should be notified for the same reasons as when there is sudden hypotension. In any situation in which there are unexpected findings such as hypotension, tachycardia, or bradycardia, monitoring of the patient should be intensified. This might include determining blood gases, hematocrit, and electrolytes.

Elevated Blood Pressure and Pulse Rate

At times, the blood pressure and/or pulse rate slowly or rapidly increases above control levels during surgery. A partial list of the possible reasons for this includes light anesthesia, hypercarbia, hypervolemia, and, rarely, the malignant hyperthermia syndrome, or a pheochromocytoma. A systematic approach is useful to determine both the diagnostic possibilities to be considered and the diagnostic steps to be taken when this happens. The anesthetic system, oxygen delivery, and patient's ventilation are at the top of the list. The use of end-tidal CO_2 and a blood gas analysis may help clarify the problem. The reader is referred to Chapter 15 for a discussion of the malignant hyperthermia syndrome.

Pulmonary Edema

Pulmonary edema is rare but may develop during the course of surgery or appear in the postoperative period. During surgery it should be suspected when there is decreased pulmonary compliance, coarse breath sounds, and pink frothy endotracheal secretions. In the postoperative period pulmonary edema should be suspected in the intubated patient if there is delayed awakening from anesthesia, airway irritability, pink frothy endotracheal secretions, and tachypnea. After extubation, the signs and symptoms that suggest pulmonary edema are delayed awakening, excessive coughing and secretions, dyspnea, tachypnea and retractions. Unexplained oxygen desaturation is suggestive of pulmonary edema during both the operative and postoperative periods. The major causes of pulmonary edema include:

1. Postobstructive pulmonary edema
2. Cardiogenic pulmonary edema secondary to underlying congenital or acquired heart disease
3. Aspiration pulmonary edema
4. Pulmonary edema secondary to volume overload

Refer to Chapter 13 for a discussion of postobstructive pulmonary edema, and to the end of this chapter for a discussion of the treatment of fluid overload.

POSTOPERATIVE FLUIDS
Routine Cases

One of the major controversial areas of fluid and electrolyte management occurs in the postoperative period. If the patient has had a routine anesthetic and is undergoing surgery of short duration, the question is when to discontinue the intravenous fluids and when to start oral fluids. For outpatients the answer may be more difficult; for inpatients the answer is simple: the IV is left in place until it can be determined that the infant or child is able to take oral fluids. The question that has to be answered is, "When is the appropriate time to try oral fluids?" The answer is, when the patient's stomach and gastrointestinal system can absorb the fluids and when there will be a minimal chance that the patient will vomit from the administration of oral fluids. There is no magic formula and no magic time. The guidelines I use to determine readiness for oral fluids for patients who are old enough is the ability to say that they're *hungry*. This may take hours or the rest of the day. When patients are hungry, this generally means that the gastrointestinal system is active and ready to absorb fluids. Thirst is not a sign that the patient is ready to absorb oral fluids. Sometimes the state of thirst is confused with the state of hunger. Most patients who are thirsty naturally request something to help alleviate the dryness and thirst. Well-meaning care-takers often know the patient should not have fluids, but for some reason give them ice chips. Ice chips are fluid. If the patient has been nauseated and vomiting, the ice chips will often prolong the process. If the patient has not yet been nauseated and vomited, the ice chips will often initiate the process. Moreover, as soon as the ice chips melts and the water is swallowed, the patient's mouth is just as dry as before. The best way to treat a dry mouth is to allow the patient to rinse the mouth but not swallow. For ambulatory patients the IV is continued in the immediate postoperative period at a rate of 15 to 25 ml/kg/hr. The same criterion for oral fluid intake is followed (i.e., hunger). If the patient is not hungry before being ready for discharge, then oral fluids are still not attempted. The IV is discontinued and the patient discharged with instructions to start oral fluids slowly only when *hungry*. This may be late at night or the next morning.

When oral fluids are first started they are given in small amounts, such as 1 to 2 ounces. Then 15 to 20 minutes is allowed to elapse in order to see if the fluids remain in situ. If they do, further small increments of fluid are given. If the patient becomes nauseated or the hunger disappears, the fluid should be temporarily discontinued until hunger returns. The type of fluids to be admin-istered are fluids such as soft drinks and apple juice. Water and milk are not good choices at this point. Then alimentation is increased to crackers, soup, and so on, and then on to a regular diet as tolerated.

Restarting Glucose Solutions

In the postoperative period there is little danger of ischemia occurring owing to anesthetic difficulties and if the patient is awake and recovering satisfactorily from anesthesia, glucose can be started as indicated.

Complicated Cases

The more complicated the patient and the problem, the more important the postoperative fluid and electrolyte balance becomes. The one factor that needs to be remembered about surgery is that closure of the abdomen does not mean that there is a cessation of fluid loss into the operative area. Additionally, in major surgery there is bound to be a slow, continuous loss of blood from tissues that have been incised. The amount of blood and fluid loss depends on the extent of the surgery. The postoperative fluid requirements of the patient include maintenance fluids and replacement fluids. Maintenance fluids should be given at a rate of 4 ml/kg/hr, administered as BSS; the replacement fluid needs depend on fluid loss either through bleeding, third spacing, or vomiting. The amount of fluid administered is guided by the patient's urine output, the blood pressure, the presence of orthostatic hypotension, and so forth. The renal system will sensitively reflect, along with the baroreceptors and osmoreceptors, the balance between the blood and fluid that is being lost and that which is being replaced. As long as the fluid and electrolytes being administered equal or exceed those lost, the renal system will be able to cope with the situation and quite easily excrete any overload. On the other hand, if an inadequate sodium concentration is administered in the face of continued sodium losses, the patient's compensatory mechanisms will become activated, resulting in alterations in the serum sodium, and in some cases acute symptomatic hyponatremia. Replacement fluids should be given as long as replacement-type fluids are being lost. Some surgeons and anesthesiologists immediately change all intravenous solutions postoperatively to 0.25 or 0.5 percent normal saline or some other hypotonic and hyponatremic solution, thereby incurring the rare but potentially devastating problem of acute symptomatic hyponatremia.

One of the earliest signs that fluid loss is exceeding fluid replacement is a decrease in urine output. The three basic reasons for this decrease are heart failure, renal failure, and an inadequate replacement fluid volume. If a patient has a normal cardiovascular system and the urine output was normal in the preoperative and intraoperative periods, there is absolutely no reason to believe that there has been a sudden onset of either renal or cardiac failure. In the vast majority of clinical circumstances, the problem is inadequate fluid administration. There are two approaches to solving the problem of a decrease in urine output. The most appropriate is a fluid challenge with BSS, even if there is a concern about renal failure. Any pre-existing renal disease sufficient to result in a postoperative decrease in urine output would certainly have been determined preoperatively. Patients with renal disease need an adequate volume of fluid in order to help clear the solute load, since they lose the ability to concentrate as well as dilute the urine. In the vast majority of cases the reason for a decrease in urine output is a decrease in extracellular fluid, which requires a fluid challenge with BSS. The volume administered should be 15 to 20 ml/kg over a 20-minute period. There are still a few clinicians who think that patients with a decreased urine output need a diuretic. The problem with this approach to a decrease in urine output is that it treats only the symptoms and not the cause. On the other hand, if the patient has been given what appears to be adequate fluids, the urinary catheter has been checked and found functional, then a small dose of diuretic may be indicated.

At times, due to the head-down position, coughing, or something else, the eyelids of the patient may become edematous, and this may confuse the issue of fluid balance. Edema of the eyelids rarely indicates fluid overload; in extreme circumstances it may accompany fluid overload and cardiac failure, but this is the exception rather than the rule.

If the fluid bolus is unsuccessful in increasing the urine output, a more extensive reassessment of the situation is in order. Blood gases, blood chemistries, and the hematocrit should be determined; a chest x-ray should be taken to see if the heart appears normal and whether or not there is early pulmonary edema. An assessment of the cardiovascular status of the patient should be made. A central venous pressure (CVP) line may be helpful in evaluating the capacitance system and right ventricle. If the CVP is below 15 cmH_2O, a repeat fluid bolus of 10 ml/kg can be administered while carefully monitoring the CVP. If the CVP reaches 15 to 18 cmH_2O and there is still no urine output, consideration should be given to the to the insertion of a Swan-Ganz catheter to assure normal filling pressures. At present, this is practiced only in the older child, and very infrequently.

A popular misconception is that postoperative surgical patients should weigh what they weighed preoperatively. I have often been told by surgical and pediatric colleagues that I have overloaded a patient with fluids, based on the fact that the patient had a weight gain. If a patient has had extensive traumatic surgery, and fluid resuscitation is appropriate, they will gain weight. Surgery causes trauma and injury to capillaries, and leads to the third spacing of extracellular fluid, which results in the need to replace the translocated extracellular fluid with BSS and a weight gain. As the injured tissue repairs itself, the integrity of the capillary bed returns and the extra fluid will be diuresed, without colloid or diuretics.

A question that often arises is, "What type of fluids should the patient have in the postoperative period?" The most frequent complication of anesthesia and surgery is vomiting, and when patients vomit, they are effectively losing BSS. It is most difficult to predict which patient will have this complication, and BSS would therefore seem to be the appropriate fluid to administer postoperatively. In addition, if the patient has any degree of tissue trauma or blood loss, the BSS will serve as a replacement fluid for the fluid lost. If hyponatremic and hypotonic fluids are administered, the renal system can maintain a normal fluid and electrolyte balance by excreting the extra free water. For the patient with normal kidneys and mild losses this presents no difficulty. However, for patients who have unexpected losses and protracted nausea and vomiting, the challenge of the situation may exceed the ability of the renal system to compensate for the electrolyte loss, leading to the release of ADH. This state, the appropriate secretion of ADH, which has already been described, produces varying degrees of hyponatremia.

Burrows et al. reported a stress-related release of ADH in a group of patients undergoing corrective posterior spinal fusion surgery for idiopathic scoliosis.[18] All of these patients were awakened intraoperatively to assess whether or not the spinal cord was intact, and for this purpose the patients had a nitrous oxide narcotic anesthetic. This form of surgery produces a high degree of stress that results in the appropriate release of ADH. If hypotonic solutions are administered, the ADH release will encourage the reabsorption of water, resulting in varying degrees of hyponatremia. However, if isotonic solutions are administered, the serum sodium values will remain normal. The patients in their study reflected what might be expected from this physiologic response. Of their 24 patients, 20 received hypotonic intravenous solutions in the immediate postoperative period, and all of them experienced a significant decrease in serum sodium (6.2 ± 2.9 mEq/L).

TECHNIQUES OF FLUID ADMINISTRATION
Administration Sets

The usual packaging of fluid is in 1-L containers, and this is certainly appropriate for the child 10 years of age and older. The macrodrip administration sets (which give 13 drops/ml) are also appropriate, since they allow a more rapid rate of administration. One concern in the fluid therapy of infants and children is the accidental administration of a large bolus (the entire liter) of fluid in a short period. This is a extremely rare occurrence in a busy surgical suite. This fluid dose is easily tolerated by the 10-year-old child, but would be less well tolerated by the smaller child or infant. For this reason, pediatric buretrols of 100 or 150 ml with a microdrip (60 drops/ml) have greatly increased the safety of fluid administration, and their use is encouraged in children under 10 years of age. The administration sets can be filled with the amount of fluid the infant is to receive in 2 to 4 hours. Even if the IV is allowed to run unobserved and all of fluid is administered, it rarely would result in a problem. For small premature infants, the safety of the system can be further increased by the addition of a constant-infusion pump, which allows precise control of the fluid administered. These pumps do have drawbacks, however: they are expensive, take up space, and can malfunction.

Continuous-Flush Systems for Monitors

The other area of fluid administration that presents a potential problem involves the continuous-flush system used in the various cardiovascular monitors, such as the arterial line, central line, and Swan-Ganz catheter. Most continuous-flush systems administer 1 to 3 ml/hr of a heparinized flush solution to prevent clotting of the catheter. All of these devices have a rapid-flush mechanism for clearing the line following blood sampling. The rapid-flush mechanism can deliver a fairly broad range of fluid volumes that are insignificant in a large patient but may be quite significant in a smaller one (i.e., a 3-kg infant). The answer to this problem is to use a constant-infusion pump rather than the continuous-flush device to maintain patency of the catheter.

TREATMENT OF FLUID OVERLOAD

From time to time, either relative or actual fluid overload may occur. When the anesthesiologist is faced with the situation of a patient whose blood pressure is low and getting lower, the assumption must be that the vascular volume is inadequate and that volume resuscitation is required. This is particularly true when the surgical procedure involves large amounts of fluid and blood loss. Therefore, the anesthesiologist gives large volumes of fluid in order to ensure that the patient's vascular volume has been adequately replaced. On occasion, this may result in either a relative or an actual fluid overload of the patient. At times the patient may have underlying cardiac disease, yet it is hard to differentiate between the problems of a pump and the problems of an adequate preload. If the patient has cardiac disease, it might be helpful to consult the pediatrician or cardiologist, particularly if it occurs in the postoperative period. It may be appropriate to consider the administration of dopamine to increase the inotropic activity of the heart. Fluid overload may result in left-sided heart failure, right-sided failure, or both. Left-sided failure results in an increase in pulmonary interstitial and later alveolar fluid volume. Its early signs are a decrease in compliance and, if the patient is breathing spontaneously, tachypnea. The patient who has been extubated may develop a tracheal tug, intercostal and supraclavicular retractions, and an obvious increase in the work of breathing. In intubated patients, pulmonary edema fluid may present as "excess" secretions. In both intubated and extubated patients these secretions will cause coughing and the production of typical pulmonary edema fluid. A chest x-ray will confirm the diagnosis. If an endotracheal tube is in place it should be used to facilitate the administration of oxygen and positive end-expiratory pressure, and, if more conservative measures fail, controlled ventilation. The pharmacologic approach to fluid overload is to increase the size of the capacitance bed with morphine 0.05 to 0.1 mg/kg and administer a small dose of furosemide. With this therapy the pulmonary edema usually disappears within an hour or two, although the changes in compliance may be present for 12 to 24 hours. The extubated patient who is in severe distress should be given positive-pressure ventilation by bag and mask, and reintubated. If the patient is not in severe distress, oxygen must be administered while the pharmacologic treatment is begun. The pulse oximeter may provide additional information about the status of the patient's ability to ventilate. Patients with interstitial and alveolar edema will have a prolonged awakening time because of their decreased ability to remove inhalation agents through ventilation. Pulmonary edema from fluid overload is sometimes confused with postobstructive pulmonary edema. The airway management is the same, but with postobstructive pulmonary edema, there is no reason to administer diuretics.

REFERENCES

1. DuBois D, DuBois EF: Clinical colorimetry: Formula to estimate approximate surface area if height and weight be known. Arch Intern Med 17:863, 1916
2. Boyd E: Growth of Surface Area of Human Body. Institute of Child Welfare, Monograph Series 10. University of Minnesota Press, Minneapolis, 1935
3. Oliver WJ, Graham BD, Wilson JL: Lack of scientific validity of body surface as basis for parenteral fluid dosage. JAMA 167:1211, 1958

4. Berry FA: The renal system. In Gregory GA (ed): Pediatric Anesthesia. Vol. 1. Churchill Livingstone, New York, 1989

5. Arieff AI: Hyponatremia, convulsions, respiratory arrest, and permanent brain damage after elective surgery in healthy women. N Engl J Med 314:1529, 1986

6. Chung H, Kluge R, Schrier RW, Anderson RJ: Postoperative hyponatremia. Arch Intern Med 146:333, 1986

7. Sterns RH, Riggs JE, Schochet SS Jr: Osmotic demyelination syndrome following correction of hyponatremia. N Engl J Med 314:1535, 1986

8. Farrow-Gillespie A, Christensen S, Lerman J: Effect of the fasting interval on gastric fluid pH and volume in children. Anesth Analg 67:S59, 1988

9. Splinter WM, Stewart JA, Muir JG: The effect of preoperative apple juice on gastric contents, thirst, and hunger in children. Can J Anaesth 36:55, 1989

10. Sieber FE, Smith DS, Traystman RJ, Wollman H: Glucose: A reevaluation of its intraoperative use. Anesthesiology 67:72, 1987

11. Thomas DKM: Hypoglycemia in children before operation: Its incidence and prevention. Br J Anaesth 46:66, 1974

12. Welborn LG, McGill WA, Hannallah RS, et al: Perioperative blood glucose concentrations in pediatric outpatients. Anesthesiology 65:543, 1986

13. D'Alecy LG, Lundy EF, Barton KJ, Zelenock AB: Dextrose containing intravenous fluid repairs outcome and increases death after eight minutes of cardiac arrest and resuscitation in dogs. Surgery 100:505, 1986

14. Lundy EF, Kuhn JE, Kiwon JM, et al: Infusion of five percent glucose increases mortality and morbidity following six minutes of cardiac arrest in resuscitated dogs. J Crit Care 2:4, 1987

15. Lanier WL, Stangland KJ, Scheithauer BW, et al: The effects of dextrose infusion and head position on neurologic outcome after complete cerebral ischemia in primates: Examination of a model. Anesthesiology 66:39, 1987

16. Drummond JC, Moore SS: The influence of dextrose administration on neurologic outcome after temporary spinal cord ischemia in the rabbit. Anesthesiology 70:64, 1989

17. Steward DJ, Da Silva CA, Flegel T: Letter to the Editor: Elevated blood glucose levels may increase the danger of neurological deficit following profoundly hypothermic cardiac arrest. Anesthesiology 68:653, 1988

18. Burrows FA, Shutack JG, Crone RK: Inappropriate secretion of antidiuretic hormone in a postsurgical pediatric population. Crit Care Med 11:527, 1983

19. Randall HT: Fluid and electrolyte surgery. In Schwartz SI (ed): Principles of Surgery. McGraw-Hill, New York, 1969

20. Levens NR, Peach MJ, Carey RM: Role of intrarenal renin-angiotensin system in the control of renal function. Circ Res 48:158, 1981

21. Talbot NB, Richie RH, Crawford JD: Metabolic Homeostasis. Harvard University Press, Cambridge, MA 1969

5

PHYSIOLOGY AND SURGERY OF THE INFANT

Frederic A. Berry

The first year of life is characterized by an almost miraculous growth in size and maturity. The body weight alone changes by a factor of 3, and there is no other period in human life during which change occurs so rapidly. This chapter is divided into three main sections. The first deals with the transition from fetal to neonatal life and maturation (growth and development). The second section discusses the special physiologic and maturational problems of infants and their anesthetic implications. The third section discusses specific surgical problems and important considerations in their anesthetic management.

TRANSITION AND MATURATION
Transition

Transition, or adaptation of the infant, is that abrupt change which begins at birth, when the infant ceases to be a fetus and becomes a newborn, and then a neonate. The newborn period is the first 24 hours of life, and the neonatal period the first 30 days of life. The greatest part of transition occurs within the first 24 to 48 hours after birth, but it continues for approximately the first month of life. All systems of the body undergo transition, but the three that are of greatest interest to the anesthesiologist are (1) the circulatory system, (2) the pulmonary system, and (3) the renal system. The various systems are interdependent, and for purposes of discussion it will be assumed that each is normal. This interdependence is particularly true for the circulatory and pulmonary systems. The major changes that occur at birth are in the circulatory and pulmonary systems (Fig. 5-1A).

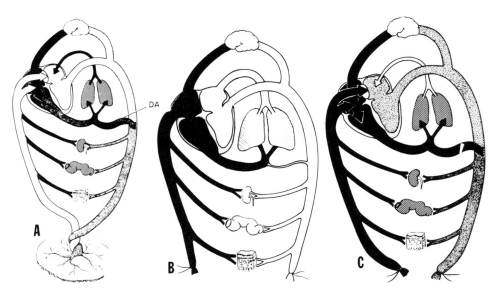

Fig. 5-1. **(A)** A schematic representation of the fetal circulation. Oxygenated blood leaves the placenta by way of the umbilical vein (vessel without stippling). It flows into the portal sinus in the liver (not shown), and a variable portion of it perfuses the liver. The remainder passes from the portal sinus through the ductus venosus into the inferior vena cava, where it joins blood from the viscera (represented by the kidney, gut, and skin). About half of the inferior vena cava flow passes through the foramen ovale to the left atrium, where it mixes with a small amount of pulmonary venous blood. This relatively well-oxygenated blood (light stippling) supplies the heart and brain by way of the ascending aorta. The other half of the inferior vena cava stream mixes with superior vena cava blood and enters the right ventricle (blood in the right atrium and ventricle has little oxygen, which is denoted by heavy stippling). Because the pulmonary arterioles are constricted, most of the blood in the main pulmonary artery flows through the ductus arteriosus *(DA)*, so that the blood in the descending aorta has less oxygen (heavy stippling) than blood in the ascending aorta (light stippling). **(B)** A schematic representation of the circulation in the normal newborn. After expansion of the lungs and ligation of the umbilical cord, pulmonary blood flow increases and the left atrial and systemic arterial pressures rise while the pulmonary arterial and right heart pressures fall. When the left atrial pressure exceeds the right atrial pressure, the foramen ovale closes, and all of the inferior and superior vena cava blood leaves the right atrium, enters the right ventricle, and is pumped through the pulmonary artery toward the lung. With the rise in systemic arterial pressure and fall in pulmonary artery pressure, flow through the ductus arteriosus becomes left-to-right, and the ductus constricts and closes. The course of the circulation is the same as in the adult. **(C)** A schematic representation of the circulation in an asphyxiated newborn with incomplete expansion of the lungs. The pulmonary vascular resistance is high, the pulmonary blood flow is low (note small caliber of pulmonary vein), and flow through the ductus arteriosus is large. With little pulmonary venous flow the left atrial pressure drops below right atrial pressure, the foramen ovale opens, and vena cava blood flows through the foramen into the left atrium. This partially venous blood goes to the brain by way of the ascending aorta. The blood in the descending aorta that goes to the viscera has less oxygen than that in the ascending aorta (heavy stippling) because of the right-to-left flow through the ductus arteriosus. The circulation is the same as in the fetus except that there is no oxygenated blood from the umbilical vein in the inferior vena cava. (From Phibbs,[37] with permission.)

Transition of the Circulatory System

The circulation of the fetus is characterized by the presence of three main shunts: the placenta, foramen ovale, and ductus arteriosus. The high pressure in the right atrium and the relatively low pressure in left atrium result in the foramen ovale being open, and a shunting of blood from the right to the left atrium, thereby bypassing the right heart and pulmonary vascular bed. In addition, the blood being pumped from the right ventricle to the lungs meets a rather high pulmonary vascular resistance, so that approximately 90 percent of this blood is shunted from the pulmonary artery through the ductus arteriosus to the descending aorta, and only about 10 percent perfuses the high-resistance pulmonary vascular bed. At birth, with the conversion of the pulmonary system from one of fluid-filled alveoli to air-filled alveoli, there is a sharp decrease in pulmonary vascular resistance, a marked increase in pulmonary blood flow, and an increase in systemic blood pressure (Fig. 5-1B). There is a reduction in mean pulmonary artery pressure to approximately 50 percent of mean aortic pressure by 24 hours of life.[1] The left atrial pressure exceeds the right atrial pressure and the foramen ovale is functionally closed. At the same time, there is an increase in the oxygenation of the blood.

The ductus arteriosus undergoes a two-stage closure during the newborn period. The first stage is a functional closure, which occurs during the first 10 to 15 hours after birth due to vasoconstriction of the medial smooth muscle of the ductal wall. This vasoconstriction is due to the effects primarily of oxygen. In the term infant, there is also a decreasing sensitivity to the vasodilating effects of prostaglandins and an increasing sensitivity to vasoconstriction from oxygen. The premature infant is more responsive to prostaglandins and, in addition, has less muscle in the ductus, which is part of the reason for the high incidence of patent ductus arteriosus. The second stage of ductal closure occurs by 2 to 3 weeks in the full-term infant and results in a permanent anatomic closure. This process involves infolding of the endothelium and hemorrhage, necrosis, and fibrosis of the connective tissue, which results in a band of fibrous connective tissue.

The neonatal pulmonary circulation remains sensitive to major alterations in PaO_2 and to acidosis for the first several weeks of life. Any pathophysiologic alterations that result in hypoxia and/or acidosis can cause an increase in pulmonary vascular resistance, a reopening of the ductus arteriosus, and a reopening of the foramen ovale (Fig. 5-1C). This is referred to as *persistent pulmonary hypertension*. It is evident that there are multiple causes of persistent pulmonary hypertension. Any process that causes respiratory failure with acidosis and hypoxia can cause persistent pulmonary hypertension. There are two other types of persistent pulmonary hypertension of interest to the anesthesiologist. One of these is found in infants who had chronic hypoxia in the last trimester of pregnancy, which results in meconium aspiration and a pathologic increase in the muscle content of the pulmonary vascular bed. Murphy et al. described a series of patients in whom this problem resulted in a fatal increase in pulmonary vascular resistance.[2] Their studies demonstrated that the amount of muscle found in the blood vessels of the terminal bronchiole, respiratory bronchiole, and in some cases the alveolar duct and alveolar wall was markedly increased over that found in the normal infant. There is no doubt that the muscular changes occurred in utero in 10 of the 11 infants reported, since all of them died within 4 days of birth.

The second type of persistent pulmonary hypertension occurs in infants with diaphragmatic hernia. It may be that the diaphragmatic hernia is a marker for abnormal embryologic growth (hypoplasia) of the lungs. The hypoplasia may be major or minor, and it may be unilateral or bilateral. At any rate, severity in infants born with a congenital diaphragmatic hernia may range from minimal interference with lung function and pulmonary vascular resistance and a good result from repair of the diaphragmatic hernia, to fatal hypoplasia of the lung, which is not remedial to any type of known therapy. This will be discussed more completely later in this chapter in the section, Congenital Diaphragmatic Hernia.

Transition of the Pulmonary System

The primary change that occurs in the transition of the pulmonary system is its transition from fluid-filled to air-filled alveoli. The first few minutes of life are characterized by the development of a residual lung volume and the establishment of normal tidal ventilation. The initial inflating pressures required are often in the range of 40 to 60 mmHg. However, by 5 to 10 minutes the normal ventilatory pressures as well as the normal tidal ventilation and residual volume, have been achieved. Table 5-1 lists the normal blood gas values for the first week of life.

Transition of the Renal System

The kidney in utero is a relatively passive organ. It serves mainly as a conduit for urine, since the placenta provides the necessary aspects of renal function. However, the fetal kidney does form urine, which, in contributing to the formation of amniotic fluid, is important for the normal development of the fetal lung, besides acting as a "shock absorber" for the fetus. The renal blood flow (RBF) and glomerular filtration rate (GFR) are low, owing to four factors: (1)

Table 5-1. Normal Blood Gas Values in the Newborn

Subject	Age	PO_2 (mmHg)	PCO_2 (mmHg)	pH	Base Excess (mEq/L)
Fetus (term)	Before labor	25	40	7.37	−2
Fetus (term)	End of labor	10–20	55	7.25	−5
Newborn (term)	10 minutes	50	48	7.20	−10
Newborn (term)	1 hour	70	35	7.35	−5
Newborn (term)	1 week	75	35	7.40	−2
Newborn (preterm, 1,500 g)	1 week	60	38	7.37	−3

a low systemic arterial pressure, (2) high renal vascular resistance, (3) low permeability of the glomerular capillaries, and (4) the small size and number of glomeruli. The first two factors—-a low systemic arterial pressure and a high renal vascular resistance-—are quite similar to the circulatory conditions found in the pulmonary system. These two factors change during the period of transition, whereas the last two factors change because of maturation. Immediately after birth there is a rapid increase in systemic arterial pressure and a rapid decrease in renal vascular resistance, so that over the first 24 to 48 hours the RBF and GFR increase markedly.

In summary, transition comprises the most rapid and greatest changes that occur in the human being in moving from the completely dependent fetal state to the newborn and neonatal states from which the individual begins the journey to complete independence. Thereafter, the major changes are due to maturation. These changes occur more slowly.

Maturation

Maturation refers to the growth and development of the various organ systems of the infant. The four organ systems that are discussed are the renal, respiratory, cardiovascular, and sympathetic and autonomic nervous systems. These organ systems are discussed in detail, but only insofar as their maturation directly affects their anesthetic management.

Maturation of the Renal System

The major changes that occur in the renal system are the rapid increase in the GFR and the maturation of the nephron.[3] Glomerulogenesis is completed at the 34th week of gestation, when the fetus weighs approximately 2,000 g. The renin-angiotensin-aldosterone system is intact in the newborn infant. As a matter of fact, there is a relative increase in aldosterone secretion, which is thought to be due to the need for sodium salts in the bone and the relative lack of maturation of renal feedback as a component of electrolyte balance. The infant in the first month of life is referred to as an *obligatory sodium loser*. This refers to the fact that the distal tubule, even with the increased secretion of aldosterone, cannot efficiently reabsorb essentially all of the sodium, even in the face of sodium loss. Therefore, there is an obligatory need to administer sodium in all intravenous solutions given to these infants. In the first 24 to 48 hours of life the infant has a limited ability to both concentrate and dilute the urine. However, over the next 3 or 4 days, there is, along with the increase in the RBF and GFR, an increased ability to concentrate and dilute the urine. Determining the rate of renal maturation is difficult because there is no agreement on the basis for comparing the renal function of the infant to the mature state. Two suggested methods of comparison of renal function between the infant and the adult involve using the body surface area or total body water. In the body surface area comparison, the 1-month-old infant has a renal system that is 40 to 50 percent mature; using total body water, the 1-month infant has a renal system that is

Table 5-2. Respiratory Handicaps
of Infants

Anatomy of the head and airway
Chest wall mechanics
Maturation of muscles
Higher closing volumes
High oxygen consumption (6–8 ml/kg/min)

approximately 70 to 80 percent mature. The latter comparison would appear to be more valid and agrees with the performance of the infant's renal system. From a practical standpoint, the kidney at 1 month of age is not the limiting factor in fluid and electrolyte balance and is capable of meeting almost any challenge from the surgeon or anesthesiologist.

Maturation of the Respiratory System

The infant has a number of respiratory handicaps that must be overcome by maturation of the respiratory system. These handicaps are of little consequence during periods of normal daily living, but when the infant is faced with the challenge of disease, anesthesia, and surgery, they may become life-threatening and in some situations life-limiting. The major respiratory handicaps are listed in Table 5-2.

Complicating Anatomic Factors in Infants

The infant is an obligate nose breather. The term *obligate nose breather* means that the infant can sustain life only through breathing through its nose. Even though they are able to cry and have intermittent breathing through their mouth, normal sustained breathing is through the nose. Relatively speaking, the infant's nose is narrow, and is thus easily obstructed by secretions and a nasogastric tube. Because infants are obligate nose breathers, anything that causes obstruction of the nasopharynx will greatly compromise their ventilation. This is why choanal atresia is a life-threatening illness in an infant. The infant is able to survive through crying and mouth breathing, but in time will fatigue unless the problem is solved. Another handicap of the infant is a large occiput (Fig. 5-2). The tongue is relatively large, and can also cause obstruction as well as interfere with laryngoscopy and intubation. The glottis is located at the C3 level in the premature infant, at the C3–C4 level in the newborn, and at the C5 level in the adult.

The larynx and trachea of an infant is funnel shaped rather than cylindrical, as in the child and adult (Fig. 5-3). The smallest diameter of the infant's airway is at the cricoid cartilage, whereas in the mature larynx, the opening of the vocal cords and the cricoid are the same. An endotracheal tube that passes through the vocal cords of an infant may not fit through the cricoid ring. Therefore, if an endotracheal tube does not easily pass beyond the cords, using a "Roto-Rooter" approach to insertion of the tube must be avoided. A smaller endotracheal tube must be used. Another factor that will obstruct an endotracheal tube after it passes through the cords is congenital subglottic stenosis. Some 20 percent

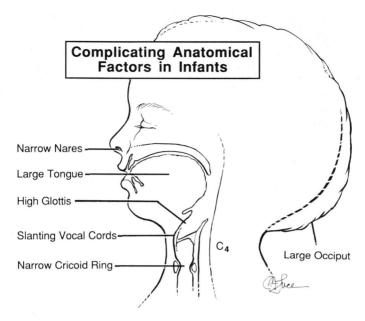

Fig. 5-2. Anatomic problems of infants.

of premature infants who have been ventilated have such a subglottic stenosis.[4] If the correct size endotracheal tube does not pass and even smaller endotracheal tubes do not pass easily, either the procedure should be cancelled or a pediatric endoscopist should be immediately summoned to endoscope the child and determine what the cause of obstruction is.

The combination of the relatively high location of the larynx and the large

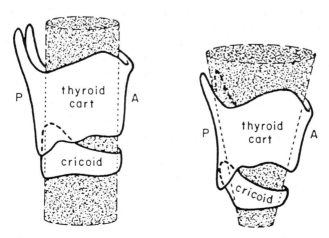

Fig. 5-3. Funnel-shaped larynx of infant on right compared to the cylindrical shape of the adult larynx on the left. (From Ryan et al.,[38] with permission).

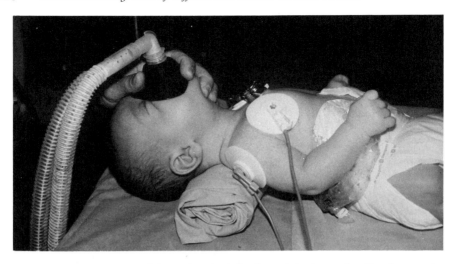

Fig. 5-4. Correct placement of the pad under infant's neck for improving the airway patency and for laryngoscopy.

tongue means that the tongue must be further displaced in order to visualize the larynx. The result is that the larynx would appear to be more anteriorly located in the infant than in the older child and adult.

These various anatomic factors suggest several practical techniques for improving airway patency and for laryngoscopy in infants. In an adult, a small pad placed under the occiput will improve the alignment of the airway axes and facilitate intubation (the sniffing position). By contrast, a similar pad placed under the head of the neonate will increase the already flexed position of the head and increase the problems. The correct place for the pad is under the neck, so that the head can be extended and the airway axes will come into better alignment (Fig. 5-4). Another practical point is to use slight cricoid pressure to depress the larynx. This will bring the larynx into better position for visualization and intubation. The pressure should be applied after the larynx or the arytenoids are visualized, so that the correct amount of pressure is applied. Too much pressure will distort the airway and make intubation more difficult. If the anesthesiologist's hand is large enough, the little finger can be used to apply the pressure (Fig. 5-5). At times, the insertion of a stylet will facilitate intubation, and one should therefore always be immediately available. The vocal cords slant anteriorly, which makes the insertion of an endotracheal tube slightly more difficult.

Chest Wall Mechanics

The chest wall mechanics of the infant normally undergo maturation. The ribs are relatively horizontal in the newborn and assume a more vertical angle with growth and development. This change is thought to improve the mechanical aspects of the action of the intercostal muscles. In addition, the ribs and cartilages

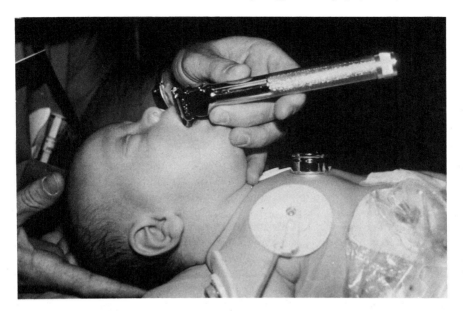

Fig. 5-5. Cricoid pressure applied with the little finger.

of the neonate are much more pliable than those in older infants, so that when negative pressure is developed within the thorax, the chest wall will collapse to a greater degree than it does in older infants and children, thereby reducing the amount of ventilation. This inefficient ventilation then becomes one of the factors in the development of fatigue and respiratory failure when the airway is compromised.

Maturation of Muscles

Not unexpectedly, the muscles of the infant have to mature along with everything else. There are two types of muscles within the body. Type I muscles compromise slow-twitch, high-oxidative fibers. These are the muscles that maintain prolonged activity, such as sustaining ventilation, and in the vernacular can be thought of as "marathon" muscles. Type II muscles comprise fast-twitch, low-oxidative fibers. These muscles are those that are active over a short period and can be thought of as the "sprinting" muscles and would be active in overcoming acute airway obstruction or coughing. Keens et al.[5] studied the pattern of the maturation of these muscle-fiber types in the human. They found that the premature infant had a very low amount of the Type I muscles that are important for sustaining activity. Table 5-3 gives the percentage of these muscles in both the premature and the newborn infant. In the diaphragm, the Type I muscles achieve the normal maturational levels at 2 months. It is evident from even a casual glance at the development of these Type I muscles that infants under 4 to 6 months of age are very susceptible to fatigue in the face of respiratory obstruction, chronic illness, and disease.

Table 5-3. Development of Type I (Marathon) Ventilatory Muscles: Percentage of Type I Muscles

	Premature	Newborn	Age at Maturity
Diaphragm	10	25	8 mos: 55
Intercostal	20	46	2 mos: 65

Closing Volumes

The closing volumes of infants are higher than those of adults but similar to those of the elderly; thus, there is overlap between the closing volume and the normal tidal volume (Fig. 5-6). The result is that atelectasis and hypoxia develop relatively more easily than in the older patient. When an infant coughs, breathholds, or has moderate degrees of laryngospasm in which they reduce their residual volume, they will rapidly develop shunting and desaturate. This is why an infant who is intubated and coughing on the endotracheal tube will often be desaturated and cyanotic. The high intrathoracic pressure will reduce venous return, which will in turn reduce cardiac output. Therefore, for a whole host of reasons, when the infant coughs and breathholds, they desaturate rapidly. One of the other respiratory handicaps of the infant is that hypoxia reduces the

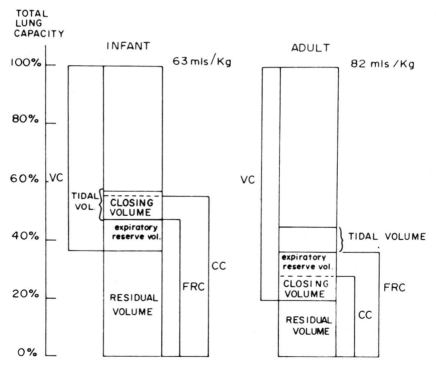

Fig. 5-6. Static lung volumes of the infant and adult. (From Smith and Nelson,[39] with permission.)

Table 5-4. Comparison of Normal Respiratory Values of Infants vs. Adults

	Infant	Adult
Respiratory frequency (breaths/min)	30–50	12–16
Tidal volume (ml/kg)	6–8	7
Dead space (ml/kg)	2–2.5	2.2
Alveolar ventilation (ml/kg/min)	100–150	60
Functional residual capacity (ml/kg)	27–30	30
Oxygen consumption (ml/kg/min)	6–8	3

respiratory rate and at times causes apnea, as opposed to the mature response of tachypnea in the face of hypoxia.

Respiratory Values of the Infant

Unquestionably, there exists a great deal of voluminous and difficult to remember physiologic data for the various respiratory values of the neonate as compared to the adult. The confusion is due to the enormous number of potential measurements that can be made versus the small number of measurements needed to determine the practical management of the infant. The most important difference is that the oxygen consumption is two to three times greater in infants.

Table 5-4 lists the respiratory values of the infant compared with those of the adult. The tidal volume is approximately the same. The functional residual capacity (FRC) is the same, as is the dead space and Vd/Vt. Since the tidal volume is the same and the oxygen consumption is two to three times higher in the infant, the major difference is that the respiratory frequency must be two to three times greater. The end result is that the resting alveolar ventilation is going to be two to three times greater and, when the alveolar ventilation is compared to the FRC, as in Figure 5-7, the ratio is seen to be approximately 5:1 for the neonate as compared to the adult ratio of 1.5:1. The same approximate ratio exists in the pregnant patient. The mechanisms, however, are different. The pregnant patient has an elevated diaphragm, a reduced FRC, and an increased alveolar ventilation. The practical aspects of a relatively low FRC compared to a high alveolar ventilation are the same. The advantage is a more rapid exchange of gases, with the result that the infant (or pregnant patient) will have anesthesia induced more rapidly and will awaken more rapidly. The disadvantage of this ratio is that it means the pregnant female has a relatively low oxygen reserve when the airway becomes obstructed. The practical result of the pregnant patient's reduced FRC and the infant's high oxygen requirement with a normal FRC is the same, a low oxygen reserve in the lungs. The neonate's high oxygen consumption is the reason why infants desaturate so rapidly when their airways become obstructed.

Maturation of the Cardiovascular System

Two areas within the cardiovascular system are mentioned: the baroresponse and the maturation of the heart. Murat et al. in a recent study demonstrated that the baroreflex is immature at birth and that volatile anesthetics and narcotics

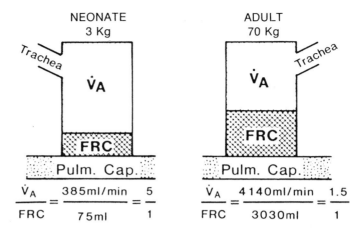

Fig. 5-7. Schematic representation of lung function showing the higher ratio of alveolar ventilation (V̇A) to FRC in the neonate compared to that of the adult. (From Graves and Kaplan,[40] with permission.)

further attenuate the baroreflex control.[6] The immaturity of this reflex would therefore limit the child's ability to compensate for hypotension by an increase in heart rate. This is discussed in detail in Chapter 3.

The second area of the cardiovascular system to be discussed is the maturation of the myocardium. Three main types of maturation have been described. They involve myocardial contractility, compliance of the ventricle, and sympathetic innervation. Friedman[7] studied the composition of cardiac muscle in the fetal and adult sheep and found that 30 percent of the fetal cardiac muscle mass is contractile mass, whereas 60 percent of the muscle in the adult is contractile mass. The implication is that the infant's myocardium will not be able to develop as great a degree of muscle contraction as the adult's. The other finding was that the smaller amount of contractile muscle mass of the infant resulted in a reduced compliance of the ventricle compared to the mature state. The clinical implication of this is that the infant has a limited ability to increase its stroke volume, and therefore depends mainly on changes in heart rate to increase its cardiac output. The other practical impact of these factors is that the newborn heart has a limited ability to increase its cardiac output in response to volume loading. The bottom line is that the neonate has a relatively limited ability to increase cardiac output[8] and, as one can see from Figure 5-8, the resting cardiac output of the neonate is relatively close to the maximum cardiac output. This means that the neonate has relatively little cardiac reserve compared to that of the more mature state of the cardiovascular system.

Maturation of the Autonomic and Sympathetic Nervous Systems

The infant is considered to have an increased vagal tone, resulting in bradycardia from vagal stimulation that in the mature state would have little effect.

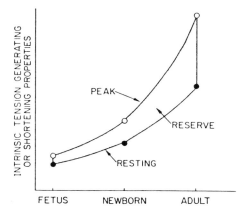

Fig. 5-8. Schema of reduced cardiac reserve in fetal and newborn animal hearts compared with adult hearts. **(A)** In newborn infant, resting cardiac muscle performance is close to peak of ventricular function because of limitations in diastolic, systolic, and heart rate reserve. **(B)** Similarly, pump reserve early in life is limited by these factors as well as by much higher resting cardiac output relative to body weight compared with the adult. (Data from Friedman and George.[8])

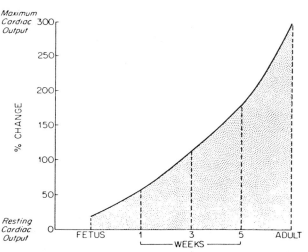

This appears to be especially true during periods of hypoxia. The normal heart rate in the newborn and in the small infant varies from 100 to 200 beats/min. As the child approaches 1 year of age, the normal rate varies from 90 to 120 beats/min. In the first month of life the definition of bradycardia is a heart rate below 120 beats/min. This may seem somewhat arbitrary and the number somewhat high, but changes occur very rapidly in an infant. If the heart rate starts at 120 beats/min and remains at 120 beats/min it can be considered normal for that infant. However, if the heart rate began at 180 beats/min and rapidly falls to 140 beats/min and then to 120 beats/min, the astute clinician would begin to respond to a rate of 120 beats/min rather than wait for the next possible decrement in rate. The major causes of bradycardia during anesthesia are hypoxia, vagal stimulation, and volatile anesthetics. The pulse oximeter has certainly been a great boon to the anesthesiologist in the differential diagnosis of what is causing bradycardia. As a matter of fact, the pulse oximeter has been

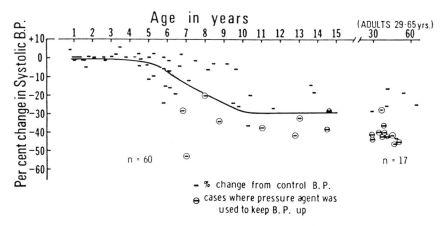

Fig. 5-9. Scattergram of percentage changes in systolic blood pressure from control plotted against age in years. −, maximal percentage change in systolic blood pressure following spinal anesthesia. 0, a case in which a pressor agent was given to prevent further decrease in blood pressure. (Data from Dohi et al.[9])

of great aid in preventing the development of bradycardia since early desaturation can be corrected before hypoxia develops. In the past hypoxia was one of the major causes of bradycardia. More and more we are finding that vagal stimulation and other unknown factors are quite prominent as causes of bradycardia. Hypoxia must always be considered as the cause of bradycardia until proven otherwise. The treatment of bradycardia is to ensure an adequate oxygen saturation, administer atropine or glycopyrrolate 0.02 mg/kg, and reduce the concentration of volatile anesthetic when applicable. If the bradycardia is accompanied by hypotension, after ensuring ventilation with oxygen the first step would be the administration of epinephrine 5 mg/kl as well as a fluid bolus of balanced salt solution. If the heart rate decreases further or if there is no appreciable response in the face of bradycardia and hypotension, cardiac massage should be begun.

The recent interest in regional anesthesia has brought about a new appreciation of the immaturity of the sympathetic nervous system in the infant and child. Dohi et al. (Fig. 5-9) have shown that infants and children less than 5 years of age have little or no change in blood pressure or heart rate following spinal anesthesia.[9] The immaturity of the sympathetic nervous system has two clinical implications: (1) a relative lack of response to adrenergic stimulation of the cardiovascular system in response to stress, and (2) a very low level of sympathetic tone, so that when a sympathectomy occurs with regional anesthesia there are no significant hemodynamic changes. For this reason, with high spinal anesthesic the blood pressure and pulse will remain normal. The symptomatology of a high spinal anesthetic will manifest itself with the onset of respiratory distress. The pulse oximeter has been shown to be invaluable for monitoring these infants with regional anesthesia.

PRACTICAL ANESTHETIC TECHNIQUES BASED ON FUNDAMENTAL CONSIDERATIONS

Should the Infant Be Routinely Intubated?

Most pediatric anesthesiologists routinely intubate most infants under the age of 1 year. In older patients the anesthesiologist determines a reason why the patient should be intubated, whereas in the patient under 1 year there should be reasons why the infant is not intubated. The reasons for not intubating infants include (1) the experience of the anesthesiologist, (2) the length of the procedure, and (3) the condition of the infant. This is a judgment call that requires careful consideration. If there is any doubt, the infant should be intubated. The infant's large occiput makes it difficult to maintain the head in reasonable alignment, and the large tongue makes the infant more prone to airway obstruction, which often results in the rapid development of hypoxia because of the ratio of alveolar ventilation to FRC and the high oxygen consumption. When there is any degree of obstruction, the infant must work harder to ventilate and the respiratory muscles are more likely to fatigue.

Should the Infant Be Ventilated?

One reason for ventilating or assisting the ventilation of these infants under 6 months is to rest their respiratory muscles during the operation, so that they will be fully ready to take over and maintain their own ventilation in the postoperative period. The infant may be able to ventilate spontaneously or with assistance for short periods, but as the procedure gets longer there is the danger of fatiguing the respiratory muscles. Therefore, if the procedure is short (i.e., up to 1 hour) and light levels of anesthesia are used, the infant can be allowed to ventilate spontaneously, whereas if there is any question, the ventilation should be assisted or controlled. If the operation is going to last for any longer period and require any relaxation, the ventilation will clearly have to be assisted or controlled. The pulse oximeter and stethoscope can also reflect the need for success in either assisting or controlling ventilation.

Should Anticholinergics Be Administered?

Anticholinergic administration is discussed in more detail in Chapter 2. Table 5-5 gives the dosages for anticholinergics. Because of secretions and the high degree of vagal tone, most anesthesiologists believe that infants under 6 to 8

Table 5-5. Dosage of Anticholinergics (mg)

	IV	IM	PO
Atropine	0.01	0.02	0.02
Glycopyrrolate	0.01	0.01	0.05

months of age should routinely receive an anticholinergic. I generally give anticholinergics to patients in this age group.

What Is the Best Technique of Intubation and Extubation?

There are always differences of opinion about every aspect of medicine, and intubation of the infant has not been spared this exercise. There has been a change in the issue of awake intubation in the neonate. Generally, the patients on whom I perform awake intubations are debilitated neonates and neonates with a full stomach. There has been recent concern in premature infants with fragile cerebral vessels and in infants who have undergone birth asphyxia and have impaired cerebral autoregulation because intubation with the infant awake might cause a period of hypertension, imposing the risk of an intraventricular hemorrhage. It has been suggested that infants who are to undergo intubation while awake be administered topical lidocaine to reduce the stimulation of the procedure, and that lidocaine 1 mg/kg IV be given just prior to intubation to minimize the hypertensive response. Other than in the situations referred to above, I prefer to anesthetize an infant before endotracheal intubation. Additionally, I prefer to paralyze the infant to facilitate the intubation. If an IV is in place, thiopental (Pentothal) 3 to 4 mg/kg should be administered as the infant is being oxygenated, and the halothane then begun. Most infants and children do not tolerate mask oxygen before induction so the technique is to blow a high flow of oxygen by the infants face. Succinylcholine 2 mg/kg IV is administered and the endotracheal tube is inserted. The doses for succinylcholine are higher for infants and young children. It is important to assure adequate oxygen saturation before the infant is intubated. If an IV is not in place, a nitrous oxide-halothane induction is accomplished. The halothane concentration is increased to 3 to 4 percent over 2 to 3 minutes. If adequate assistance is available, an intravenous infusion is started, the nitrous oxide is discontinued, and intravenous succinylcholine is administered. The other alternative is to discontinue the nitrous oxide for a period of 1 to 2 minutes as soon as the eyelid reflex is lost, and to then administer succinylcholine 4 mg/kg IM and intubate the infant. I prefer this technique if there is any question about the rapid starting of an IV. Prolonged attempts at starting an IV with a marginal airway is not as safe as securing the airway and then starting the IV. The halothane concentration should be immediately reduced after intubation until a dose-response effect on the blood pressure is determined, since controlled ventilation and high concentration of halothane can result in a very rapid halothane uptake. After intubation, the infant's chest movement must be carefully evaluated and the presence of breath sounds verified. Some clinicians prefer to use the volatile anesthetic for laryngoscopy and intubation. A recent study in infants and children demonstrated that it took approximately 1.4 MAC end-tidal halothane to accomplish laryngoscopy and intubation.[10] There is concern by some clinicians that, in the infant who has a decrease in cardiac reserve, the use of muscle relaxants to facilitate laryngoscopy and intubation is the preferred technique because there will be less potential depression of the cardiovascular system by the volatile anesthetic.

Timing of Extubation

The timing of extubation depends on three factors: (1) the reversal of neuromuscular blockade, (2) the level of anesthesia, and (3) the infant's temperature. There are differences of opinion about techniques for reversing the effects of nondepolarizing neuromuscular blocking agents. One view holds that it is necessary to determine the degree of neuromuscular blockade with a neuromuscular monitor and that the reversal depends on whether or not there is any residual paralysis. If there is no evidence of neuromuscular blockade, reversal agents are not given. The other view calls for reversal in any patient who has received nondepolarizing neuromuscular blocking agents regardless of the time of administration or the dose. There is no overwhelming consensus on this issue. Table 5-6 gives some of the criteria for the reversal of neuromuscular blocking agents. One useful test for use with infants is the reflex leg lift.[11] Mason and Betts report that a positive leg-lift sign is associated with a maximum inspiratory force of at least 32 cmH$_2$0.

Another difference of opinion concerns which agent to use for reversal of the effect of nondepolarizing blocking agents. Meakin et al.[12] reported a comparison of neostigmine and edrophonium as antagonists of pancuronium in infants and children. Figure 5-10 shows the difference in the reversal times with neostigmine and edrophonium, as well as the more rapid recovery that occurs in children as compared to adults. Reversal was attempted in all patients at the point of a 10 percent spontaneous recovery of muscle twitch. The impressive finding was that by 2 to 3 minutes the drug effects were 80 to 90 percent reversed with edrophonium, whereas with neostigmine approximately 8 to 9 minutes were required for 80 to 90 percent reversal. The other advantage of edrophonium is that it requires about only half as much atropine to block the adverse cardiac muscarinic effect.[13] The choice of which anticholinergic to use to prevent the cardiac muscarinic effects depends on which antagonist is used for neuromuscular reversal. Atropine has a rapid onset of action, whereas glycopyrrolate has a relatively slow onset, and edrophonium has a rapid onset of action, whereas

Table 5-6. Direct and Indirect Estimates of Respiratory Function With Partial Neuromuscular Blockade

	Moderate Weakness	Marked Weakness
Grip	25[a]	0–5
Twitch height	75	50
TOF	60	40–50
Inspiratory pressure	60–70	40
Vital capacity	75–80	60
Head lift (>5 sec)	Yes	No
Knee lift	Yes	No
Upper airway obstruction	Possible	Likely

[a] Numerical values are percent of control.

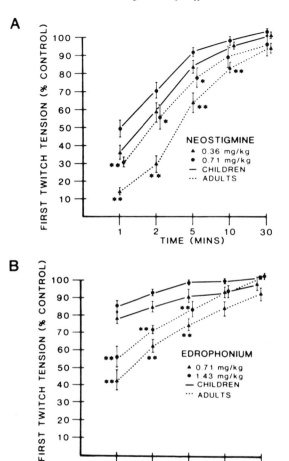

Fig. 5-10. Recovery of first-twitch tension as a percentage of control in pediatric patients (pooled data) compared with adults after neostigmine **(A)** and edrophonium **(B)**. Significant differences between adults and pediatric subjects are seen after the same dose of antagonist. *$P < 0.05$; **$P < 0.01$. (From Meakin et al.,[12] with permission.)

neostigmine has a relatively slow onset. A recent study in adults showed a significant decrease in heart rate with the combination of edrophonium and glycopyrrolate as compared to the combination of edrophonium and atropine.[14] If the glycopyrrolate is given 1 to 2 minutes before the edrophonium, the differences from atropine are minimized. In summary, the consensus is that if there is any question, nondepolarizing neuromuscular blocking agents should be reversed. I prefer to use edrophonium 1 mg/kg and atropine or glycopyrrolate 0.01 mg/kg. The reversal dose for neostigmine is 0.07 mg/kg, and the dose of atropine or glycopyrrolate is 0.01 mg/kg. The advantages of the rapid reversal of neuromuscular blockade are particularly advantageous in the small infant, since it shortens the period during which there is concern over inadequate reversal. In the older infant and child edrophonium may also have certain advantages in the situation where the child is lightly anesthetized, the surgery ends before expected and the neuromuscular reversal is given. The child's level of consciousness may return quickly and then one has the potential problem of a child who is awake and still intubated and/or weak. The use of edrophonium, which peaks in 2 minutes, would be much preferable in this situation since amnesia is difficult to predict or depend on.

The second criterion for the timing of extubation depends on whether or not the infant is awake. The reason for desiring the infant to be awake is that in the awake state the airway protective reflexes are active. At times, particularly with small infants, it is difficult to tell exactly when the patient is sufficiently awake to maintain their own protective airway reflexes. Infants often make nonspecific movements of the arms and legs, suggesting the ability to maintain the airway, but immediately go into laryngospasm when the tube is removed.

Therefore, if in doubt, the endotracheal tube should be left in position until the infant opens its eyes or makes meaningful movements. If there is any question, the infant should be taken to the recovery room while still intubated, and given an elevated FiO_2 until sufficiently awake to be extubated. If the infant is coughing with the endotracheal tube in place, lidocaine can be administered to increase tolerance until ready for extubation. The dose is 1 mg/kg in young infants and 1.5 mg/kg in older infants (1 year, arbitrary) and children. It can be repeated once in 5 minutes. Infants under 1 year of age do not develop traumatic croup very frequently, thus there are few contraindications to leaving the endotracheal tube in place in these patients.

The third criterion for the timing of extubation is the infant's temperature. It is well known that as the infant's temperature drops there is a decrease in respiratory drive. Although the temperature of 35°C is somewhat arbitrary, I use this as the temperature criterion of whether or not the infant is ready to be extubated. If the temperature is below 35°C, the endotracheal tube is left in. Heated, humidified air is given via the endotracheal tube, and heating lamps are placed on the infant until the infant's temperature reaches 35°C.

Monitoring of Pediatric Patients

Although we talk about "the basic monitors," we recognize that the concepts of monitoring don't refer only to the instruments used; the procedures require a vigilant physician.

The object of monitoring is to create an information interface between the patient and the anesthesiologist. The parameters monitored are the patient's response to the anesthetic agent and to the surgery. There has been an enormous improvement in monitoring technology in several areas.

The real excitement has come in the development of the pulse oximeter, and the end-tidal measurement of CO_2 and the anesthetic gases. These new monitors have certainly changed our appreciation of the uptake and distribution of anesthetic agents and cardiovascular and respiratory physiology, as well as the rapid change that can occur in patients. One of the most startling revelations from using these monitors has been the recognition of the occasional patient who, in spite of being 100 percent saturated and having a normal end-tidal CO_2 and appropriate end-tidal levels of anesthesia, has sudden cardiac dysrhythmias, resulting in significant alteration in blood pressure and an occasional cardiac arrest. In previous years we would have been concerned and the plaintiff's expert witness would have been positive that the patient had "unrecognized hypoxia." With this new generation of instruments it is becoming obvious that significant problems occur in the face of totally appropriate practice. We still do not completely understand the interactions of patients, drugs, and disease. There can be a bad outcome with no negligence and no explanation for its occurrence. We are gaining a new appreciation for this fact, but it will be questioned by certain plaintiffs' experts and especially by the plaintiffs' bar.

The routinely used monitors now are a pulse oximeter, stethoscope, blood pressure monitor, and electrocardiograph.

Temperature Monitoring

The question of when to monitor temperature is another matter of controversy, although the controversy is not too great. Certainly such monitoring is debatable for procedures that last from 5 to 15 minutes. The guidelines for temperature monitoring are somewhat arbitrary. The guidelines suggested by the ASA include that temperature monitoring be available for all patients. If surgery is to last longer than 15 minutes, then temperature monitoring can be quite helpful, particularly in the small infant, because they are especially susceptible to cooling. They have a large surface area:body weight ratio (2.3:1) and lose heat rapidly, either on the trip to the operating room or in the operating room itself, as their defense mechanisms are blunted by the anesthetic and the usually cool room temperature. I prefer an esophageal temperature if it can be conveniently obtained; my second choice is rectal temperature, and my last choice is axillary or skin temperature. The important factors in temperature monitoring are the absolute temperature and the temperature trend. For infants under 2 years of age there should be progressive warming of the operating room, with the room temperature 80 to 84°F for infants of approximately 2 to 3 kg. The other techniques for maintaining body temperature are humidification of the anesthetic gases, use of a warming mattress, warming of intravenous fluids, and use of heating lights. Another device for helping to maintain body temperature in the infant or child undergoing major thoracic or abdominal surgery is the plastic Steri-drape. This will prevent irrigation and other fluids from soaking and cooling the patient.

SURGICAL PROCEDURES IN NEONATES AND INFANTS UP TO 6 MONTHS OF AGE

For purposes of discussion, the surgical procedures for neonates and small infants can be divided into two groups: those that occur in the first week of life and those that occur within the first 6 months. The definition of a newborn is an infant in the first 24 hours of life; the definition of a neonate is an infant in the first month of life. The anesthetic considerations concern the transitional state of the infant, the specific surgical defect and its anesthetic implications, any associated congenital anomalies, and the maturation of the infant's organ systems.

General Philosophy of the Emergency Care of Infants

One of the most frightening problems to face the anesthesiologist is that of a newborn infant or neonate who needs surgery but because of the passage of time, lack of specific training, or lack of equipment, the anesthesiologist does not feel qualified to manage the anesthetic. An anesthesiologist who does not feel qualified to manage an emergency procedure has two options: calling in a colleague or transporting the infant to another medical center that is equipped to handle the emergency. In today's high-tech environment, very efficient methods for transporting critically ill infants have been developed and are almost nationally available. In addition, there are very few life-threatening emergencies in neonates that need immediate surgery. This latter type of problem would include airway obstruction or severe bleeding. Infants who have the congenital defects that are described in this chapter can be stabilized and transported. As a matter of fact, a period of stabilization is advantageous in these critically ill infants. There is no question that most anesthesiologists and surgeons, either during their training or immediately thereafter, were completely familiar with and able to perform safe and skillful anesthesia and surgery on these small infants. However, with the passage of time, the skills required to take care of these small infants are often lost, since the opportunities to maintain these skills are very infrequent. Another dimension in the care of the neonate is the availability of a support team with a neonatologist and dedicated nurses to help in the perioperative management. Therefore, except in immediate life-threatening emergencies, serious consideration should be given to transporting these infants to a hospital that has adequate facilities for treating them.

Surgical Procedures in Infants in the First Week of Life

This discussion does not attempt to cover the entire group of surgical emergencies that can occur in the first week of life, but covers the major conditions. The basic principles that are discussed here can then be applied to those procedures not covered. The most frequent surgical emergencies during the first week of life (not necessarily in order of occurrence) are (1) congenital diaphragmatic hernia, (2) tracheoesophageal fistula, (3) omphalocele and gastroschisis, and (4) intestinal obstruction.

Congenital Diaphragmatic Hernia

The concepts of the embryogenesis and medical and surgical management of the infant with congenital diaphragmatic hernia (CDH) have undergone considerable rethinking in the past decade. Initially, the problem was thought to be an embryologic defect in the diaphragm that resulted in the intestines compressing the lungs, thereby causing atelectasis or inhibiting development of the lung. It was believed that immediate surgery could save the patient. However, the mortality rate remained high, and this simplistic view did not explain the occasional child with CDH who also had severe hypoplasia of the contralateral lung. The basic pathology, a developmental arrest of the lung at various stages, resulted in a spectrum of lung development from a lung bud to what would appear to be a lung with minimal pathology. Therefore, there has been recent argument that the primary pathogenic mechanism in CDH is an inhibition of the growth of an embryonic lung, or perhaps both of them, and that the hernia in the diaphragm may be a secondary phenomenon.

Antenatal Diagnosis

The use of predelivery ultrasound has resulted in the fetal diagnosis of many congenital defects, and CDH is one of these. Mothers with polyhydramnios are highly suspect of a congenital anomaly and 30 percent of the cases of CDH are associated with polyhydramnios.

Clinical Presentation

Approximately 1 in 4,000 infants will have CDH. It is evident that the degree and severity of CDH can be enormous. At one end of the spectrum is an infant who has only lung buds and no effective pulmonary system; at the other end of the spectrum is the infant with what is referred to as *eventration of the diaphragm*, in which the major problem is incomplete muscularization of the diaphragm. In the latter situation, the abdominal pressure will elevate the diaphragm into the thoracic cavity, although it takes days or weeks for symptoms to occur. In the case of an infant with very abnormal lungs, the symptomatology will begin at birth, as the infant is unable to oxygenate. The Apgar score may be normal or slightly low initially, but will continue to remain in the 3 to 7 range. Immediate intubation and stabilization is needed in that infant. Approximately 80 to 90 percent of diaphragmatic hernias appearing in the first week of life occur on the left side in the foramen of Bochdalek. There are several other potential hernias through the diaphragm, such as that which may occur through the anterior foramen of Morgagni, but these are usually not symptomatic early and present later in life. Hernias may also occur through the esophageal hiatus, but these hernias are also quite small and are not usually detected in the neonatal period.

The chest cavity may contain varying amounts of the gut, depending on the size of the hernia and the lung. The chest may contain the stomach, spleen, small and large bowels, and liver, and the abdomen may not be able to contain its contents, thereby requiring some form of prosthetic material for closure. The classic physical findings are usually present at birth in severe cases of CDH. The newborn will have a scaphoid abdomen secondary to the herniation of the intestinal contents into the chest and the breath sounds on the affected side will be diminished. The radiograph is confirmatory (Fig. 5-11). The immediate therapy is stabilization with endotracheal intubation, ventilation, and nasogastric intubation to decompress the gastrointestinal tract. At this point a determination

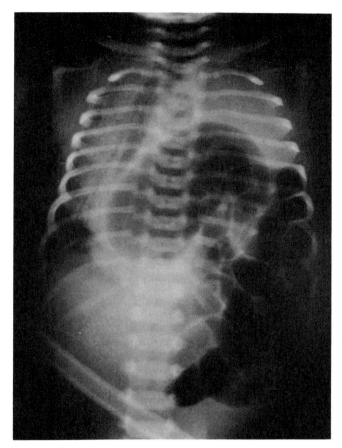

Fig. 5-11. Radiograph of an infant with CDH, with intestinal contents herniated into the left chest.

needs to be made about the degree of pulmonary hypoplasia. The mortality of congenital diaphragmatic hernia remains very high (50 percent) because of the fact that these infants have effectively no lung tissue. There is a spectrum between the infant who has only a lung bud and often only a lung bud on both sides, to the infant who may be minimally affected or have normal lungs bilaterally. The outcome for these infants is directly related to the degree of pulmonary hypoplasia, the gestational age, and other congenital defects. However, there is no question but that the prime determinant of mortality and morbidity is the degree of pulmonary hypoplasia.

Prediction of Pulmonary Hypoplasia

The first step after the immediate emergency stabilization of the infant is to determine the amount of pulmonary tissue that the infant has, because this will affect survival. There are various techniques used to predict the amount of pulmonary hypoplasia that is related to outcome. Bohn et al. have suggested several criteria to predict pulmonary hypoplasia.[15] They used the preoperative $PaCO_2$ and correlated this with an index of ventilation (VI), which is determined by multiplying the mean airway pressure by the respiratory rate. In a study of 66 infants with CDH, they found that preoperatively if an infant had a $PaCO_2$ above 40 the infant had a 77 percent mortality. Even when the $PaCO_2$ could be reduced below 40 with high respiratory rates and pressures the mortality rate still remained greater than 50 percent. They then correlated the $PaCO_2$ with a VI. They found that when the VI was greater than 1,000 even though the $PaCO_2$ may have been reduced, the mortality rate was still greater than 50 percent. The $PaCO_2$ was also used in the postoperative period to predict pulmonary hypoplasia. If the $PaCO_2$ could be reduced to less than 40, 30 of 31 infants in this group survived. However, when the $PaCO_2$ was greater than 40, only 2 of the 27 infants survived.

Effect of Surgical Repair on Respiratory Mechanics

Sakai et al. measured compliance of the respiratory system in nine patients (five survivors and four nonsurvivors) before and after operation.[16] All of the infants were diagnosed within 6 hours of birth, and after a period of stabilization an abdominal approach was used to repair the CDH. In one infant the compliance improved immediately after surgical repair and in another it showed no change; both of these infants had an uneventful postoperative course. Postoperative compliance immediately decreased from 10 to 77 percent in the remaining seven infants, and the four infants with more than a 50 percent decrease died. It was their conclusion that immediate repair of the hernia resulted in a reduction in pulmonary compliance and rather than improving outcome, frequently resulted in a deterioration of the infant. Therefore, they believed that a period of stabilization and resuscitation with a period of cardiorespiratory stability are indicated before the repair is undertaken. It has been suggested that infants who remain hypoxic and iso- or hypercarbic following this bridge of stabilization should be placed on extracorporeal membrane oxygenation (ECMO) to allow a degree of development of the lung before surgery is undertaken. This has not yet proved to be of much benefit. The reason is that the severely hypoplastic lung is not likely to improve in the short time (1 to 2 weeks) that ECMO can be used. ECMO is discussed further in the section on postoperative care.

Associated Cardiac Anomalies

Infants with CDH have a high incidence (23 percent) of associated cardiac anomalies. As part of the initial stabilization and resuscitation, evaluation for possible congenital cardiac anomalies needs to be conducted.

Anesthetic Considerations for CDH

The majority of the infants with this condition will undergo postoperative ventilation for a period of time. Those infants who are thought to have minimal pulmonary hypoplasia and in whom early extubation is anticipated, with little if any postoperative ventilation, should have an anesthetic tailored to this plan. Narcotics should be minimized. Postoperative analgesia can be accomplished with caudal bupivacaine (see Ch. 11). One of the considerations in infants with CDH is that because they may have air in the gastrointestinal tract, nitrous oxide should be avoided because of the possibility of further compromising the thoracic contents and increasing the difficulty of returning the intestinal system to the abdominal cavity. At times the abdominal peritoneal cavity is not capable of accepting the migratory intestinal system, resulting in the need for a Dacron or Marlex closure of the abdomen; under these circumstances the surgeon will need superb muscle relaxation and the infant will need postoperative ventilation.

After the abdominal contents have been returned to the abdomen, the lung is evaluated. The lungs should be gently re-expanded under direct vision using a ventilatory pressure of no greater than 30 to 40 cmH$_2$O. The lung that has little hypoplasia will respond quickly to these inflation pressures, whereas the hypoplastic lung will have moderate or at times no response to these inflation pressures. Further efforts to expand the hypoplastic lung should not be attempted, as they may result in a pneumothorax on the contralateral side. Any sudden deterioration in the clinical condition of the infant, as manifested by a decrease in heart rate or blood pressure or change in oxygen saturation suggests that such a catastrophe has occurred. In such cases a chest tube must be inserted expeditiously. There is a difference of opinion among surgeons about the prophylactic insertion of a contralateral chest tube in order to avoid that possibility.

Postoperative Care

The postoperative care of the infant who has minimal hypoplasia of the lung will be relatively straightforward. This type of infant needs either minimal or no postoperative ventilation. On the other hand, the infant who has moderate to severe degrees of pulmonary hypoplasia, or who may be premature, or who may also have an associated congenital cardiac anomaly may require the full spectrum of postoperative care, including ECMO. Infants who have little pulmonary tissue will remain desaturated, and in spite of a high VI will have a normal or slightly elevated CO$_2$. These infants rarely survive. Other infants will have varying degrees of hypoplasia and reactive pulmonary vasculature, which may respond in time to varying degrees of supportive care. This disease remains very frustrating for the anesthesiologist and surgeon. However, with a realization of the embryogenesis of the defect a more realistic view of outcome should be taken.

Extra Corporeal Membrane Oxygenation

Several centers have been using ECMO in neonatal respiratory failure. The procedure involves cannulating the right carotid and internal jugular vein and placing the infant on a pump oxygenator to oxygenate the blood and thereby rest the lung. The lung is kept inflated with low pressures to reduce barotrauma and a F$_{I}$O$_2$ of 40 percent to reduce oxygen trauma. The results for some forms of respiratory failure have been quite good, although those for CDH have been disappointing, but in view of the embryology of the defect, it is not surprising. ECMO is not without complications. Campbell et al. reported that in a group of 35 infants undergoing ECMO, 11 developed focal seizures.[17] In addition, Patrias et al. reported retinal vascular changes in infants undergoing ECMO.[18]

Long-term Pulmonary Function

Long-term follow-up studies of children who survive surgery reveal normal lung volumes in most patients. In one study, there was equal distribution of lung volumes on the two sides and ventilation to the hernia side was reduced in only 2 of 19 patients.[19] Xenon 133 radiospirometry was performed in nine patients and in all nine patients blood flow was reduced to the hernia side. This would be consistent with a reduction of the vascularity of that lung. In spite of this small reduction in blood flow there was little effect on airway resistance or the distribution of ventilation.

Esophageal Atresia and Tracheoesophageal Fistula

Esophageal atresia is a relatively frequent congenital defect, occurring in approximately 1 in 3,000 births. Approximately 10 percent of patients with esophageal atresia have a blind proximal esophageal pouch and no tracheoesophageal fistula (TEF). Approximately 85 percent of infants with esophageal atresia will have a blind esophageal pouch and a fistula between the membranous portion of the distal trachea and the distal esophagus. The fistula is usually located in the distal third of the trachea but may be at the carina or a main stem bronchus. The embryologic defect in the development of TEF occurs between the fourth and sixth week of intrauterine life, and the associated congenital anomalies develop at approximately the same time. The basic defect is the imperfect division of the foregut into the anteriorly positioned larynx and trachea and the posteriorly positioned esophagus. Fifty percent of affected infants have associated congenital anomalies, which are categorized in Table 5-7. The two major causes

Table 5-7. Incidence of Associated Anomalies by Organ System

Organ System	Incidence (%)
Musculoskeletal	24.0
Cardiovascular	22.8
Gastrointestinal	20.3
Genitourinary	12.2
Craniofacial	9.7
CNS	7.2
Pulmonary	2.1
Chromosome	1.7

Total patients: 102 with 237 associated anomalies; 82% survived, 18% expired.

(Modified from German,[36] with permission.)

of death in TEF are (1) the associated cardiac anomalies, which account for over 50 percent of the mortality, and (2) prematurity.

Clinical Presentation

Atresia of the esophagus in the fetus leads to an inability to swallow amniotic fluid and the subsequent development of polyhydramnios. This is not the only reason why polyhydramnios develops, but atresia of the esophagus should be ruled out in infants of mothers with this condition. Esophageal atresia may be diagnosed in the delivery room, when an attempt is made to pass a catheter into the stomach. Sometimes the diagnosis is not suspected, and becomes apparent only with the early feedings of the infant, which result in coughing and cyanosis. At this point, a nasogastric tube is passed and a radiograph taken.

The two major complications of esophageal atresia and a distal fistula between the trachea and upper gastrointestinal system are dehydration and pulmonary aspiration. Two types of pulmonary aspiration may occur: aspiration of saliva and feedings from the blind upper esophageal pouch and regurgitation of gastric secretions retrograde through the fistula and their aspiration into the lungs (Fig. 5-12). There are two approaches to the management of these infants: primary repair and staged repair. If the TEF is discovered early and the infant is well hydrated, a primary repair is undertaken. This involves a direct approach to ligate the fistula and then a primary repair of the esophagus if the two ends can be approximated. If the anastomosis is tenuous, some surgeons would do a gastrostomy at the end of the case. If an anastomosis is not possible, an esophagostomy and feeding gastrostomy are done, and a colon interposition performed at a much later date. The other approach to the treatment of a TEF is referred to as the staged repair. If the infant has pneumonia, is premature, or has respiratory distress syndrome (RDS), or if there are other congenital anomalies that result in the overall condition of the infant being poor, a gastrostomy is done under either local or general anesthesia and the infant is given several days of supportive care. When the infant responds to the supportive care and its condition improves, it is returned to the operating room for ligation of the fistula and repair of the esophagus as outlined above.

Some premature infants have the challenging combination of a TEF and RDS. Often these infants need intubation and ventilation. Their high gastrointestinal compliance coupled with their relatively poor pulmonary compliance may result in inadequate ventilation, the possibility of regurgitation and aspiration, and the potential for gastric dilatation with rupture. The solution to this problem is not easy. Various approaches have been used. Bloch proposed doing bronchoscopy on such infants, placing a Fogarty balloon catheter in the fistula and leaving it in place for several days while the RDS abated.[20]

Anesthetic Considerations

There is a difference of opinion about the best technique for the intubation of infants with TEF. There are those who prefer awake intubation, whereas my preference is for the infant to be anesthetized and then intubated. As noted above,

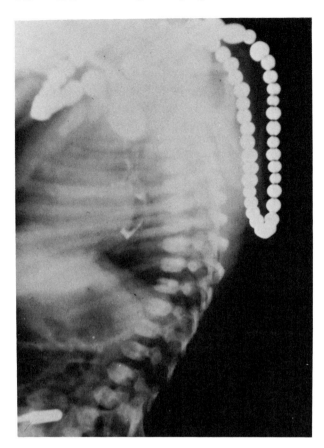

Fig. 5-12. TEF with contrast medium in blind upper esophageal pouch and spillage of contrast medium into the tracheobronchial system.

regurgitation with the aspiration of gastric secretions is one of the feared complications of TEF. The danger of intubation with the infant awake is that it will cry and struggle, thereby increasing the intra-abdominal pressure, which may lead to regurgitation and aspiration. If the infant has a gastrostomy tube in place, it should be left open in order to minimize the danger of regurgitation and aspiration. The technique used for intubation makes no difference. A gentle induction of anesthesia with halothane and nitrous oxide is my preferred technique. The reason for this is to minimize the chance of regurgitation and aspiration. The infant is allowed to breathe spontaneously and is given gentle assisted ventilation with monitoring by a stethoscope on the chest. When the abdomen becomes soft the infant is laryngoscoped and 1 percent lidocaine 3 mg/kg is sprayed on the larynx and vocal cords and the trachea intubated. Lidocaine 1 percent is used because it allows easy, accurate determination of the dose in these small infants.

In premature infants with decreased compliance who are over the main problem of RDS, after the above induction of anesthesia a Fogarty catheter is passed down the trachea into the esophageal fistula to block the esophagus to prevent the stomach from filling with anesthetic gas and avoid the dangers of aspiration during surgery. This is accomplished after the induction and topicalization with lidocaine. A rigid bronchoscope is used to identify the fistula, which is usually in the posterior membranous part of the distal trachea. The Fogarty catheter is passed into the fistula, the bronchoscope is removed, and then the patient is gently intubated.

One of the problems with the introduction of a Fogarty catheter into the esophageal fistula is that during the surgical procedure the Fogarty catheter may back into the trachea. The sign that this has happened is that the patient will be difficult to ventilate. However, often during this time period there is manipulation of the lung or of the surgical field, so it may be difficult to determine exactly why ventilation is difficult. For that reason, if ventilation becomes difficult or impossible, the differential diagnosis is (1) the endotracheal tube has been compressed or distorted by the surgeon, (2) the Fogarty catheter has slipped retrograde into the trachea, or (3) the tip of the tube may have entered into the fistula. This latter event may happen in the case of a large fistula or if the endotracheal tube is pushed further down into the trachea. The immediate measures to be taken include notifying the surgeon and unpacking the lung to see if this solves the problem. The surgeon will be able to palpate the tip of the endotracheal tube and determine if it is in the trachea or in the fistula. If not, the air should be taken out of the Fogarty catheter. If this is not successful, the Fogarty catheter should be removed entirely. If this doesn't work, then the endotracheal tube should be backed up 1 cm.

Other techniques have been used to prevent the ventilation of the stomach with anesthetic gas. It has been suggested that the tip of the endotracheal tube should be placed beyond the fistula to minimize the chances of inflating the stomach. If the tip of the endotracheal tube is past the fistula, ventilation will also be easier to control. At least two techniques have been described for placing the tube in the desired location. If the infant has a gastrostomy, the tip of the gastrostomy tube is placed under a water seal. After intubation, gentle pressure is placed on the anesthesia bag so that the gas will flow into the fistula and bubble out through the gastrostomy tube (Fig. 5-13). The endotracheal tube is then advanced down the trachea until the bubbling stops. At this point the distal end of the tube should be past the fistula. The other technique that has been described is to advance the endotracheal tube down the trachea, past the carina, into one of the mainstem bronchi.[21] The infant has the same angles between trachea and mainstem bronchi as the adult, therefore the most frequent course for the endotracheal tube to take would be into the right mainstem bronchus. The tube is then slowly withdrawn while listening to the chest, and when bilateral breath sounds appear and bilateral chest movement is verified, the endotracheal tube should be located just above the carina (Fig. 5-14).

At present, the immediate outcome for most infants with TEF depends on the associated congenital anomalies and whether or not the infant was premature. One of the congenital anomalies reported in 5 percent of infants with TEF is a right aortic arch, which greatly complicates the repair. Therefore, it is suggested that infants with esophageal atresia be screened preoperatively for the presence

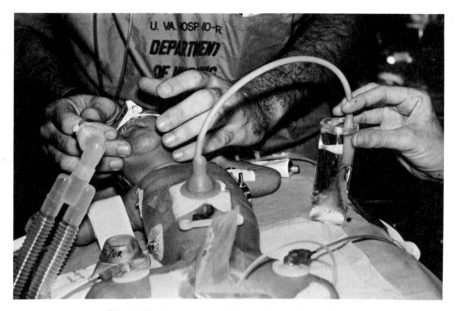

Fig. 5-13. Gastrostomy tube under water seal.

of a right aortic arch. This will allow a surgical approach through the left chest. Should the right aortic arch not be discovered preoperatively and the right chest be opened, several management alternatives are available. The management is certainly a matter of surgical judgment. Harrison et al. suggest that it is safest to close the thoracotomy without further dissection or after simple ligation of the TEF, and to later perform the definitive esophageal repair through a left thoracotomy.[22]

Anesthetic Technique and Postoperative Care

Full-term or near full-term infants without other congenital anomalies or respiratory problems can be anticipated to have a very smooth postoperative period. In general, extubation is planned for the end of surgery and the anesthetic technique tailored accordingly. A short-acting muscle relaxant such as atracurium is used. Medium- to high-dose narcotics should be avoided (see Ch. 3). Postoperative analgesia can be accomplished by using caudal marcaine (0.25 percent marcaine 1 ml/kg with epinephrine 1:200,000). This will provide analgesia for approximately 12 hours. If the infant has a severe congenital anomaly or is premature with the residual of RDS, the postoperative period can be complicated by the need for postoperative ventilation. In this case the anesthetic should be planned accordingly.

A significant percentage of infants with TEF have residual symptomatology of the esophagus or tracheobronchial tree for several years.[23] Some of these infants may develop esophageal stricture and need dilatation. Others have vary-

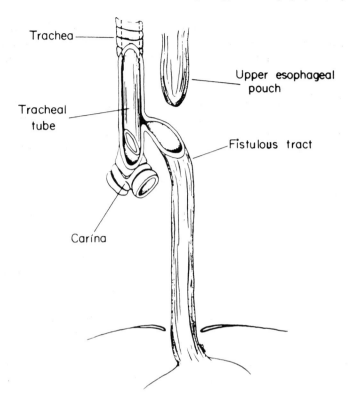

Fig. 5-14. In a patient with a TEF of the commonest type, distal placement of the tip of the tracheal tube blocks the fistulous opening in the trachea and prevents gastric distention during intermittent positive-pressure ventilation. (From Salem et al.,[21] with permission.)

ing degrees of tracheomalacia, which can be a recurrent problem for the first several years of life. Jolly et al.[24] report a 68 percent incidence of gastroesophageal reflux following the repair of esophageal atresia and distal TEF. Milligan and Levison reported a long-term follow-up (7 to 18 years) of patients with these abnormalities.[25] Clinically, the patients appeared normal. The investigators studied varying parameters of pulmonary function and bronchial reactivity. The pulmonary function studies demonstrated obstructive airway disease in 54 percent and restrictive lung disease in 20 percent of the patients.

Omphalocele and Gastroschisis

Some clinicians have difficulty remembering the differences between an omphalocele and gastroschisis. Even though these two conditions resemble each other, they have entirely different etiologies and are entirely different in terms of the associated congenital anomalies.[26] An *omphalocele* is a congenital anomaly secondary to an embryologic defect, whereas gastroschisis is the result of a developmental defect. Early in fetal development the pleuroperitoneal cavity is a single compartment. During the fifth to tenth weeks of fetal life, the gut is herniated into the extraembryonic coelom. During this time period the diaphragm develops to separate the thoracic and abdominal cavities. The diaphragm is developed from the (1) septum transversum, (2) the pleuroperitoneal membranes, (3) the dorsal mesentery of the esophagus, and (4) muscular components of the body wall. The development of the diaphragm is usually completed by the eighth fetal week. In the ninth to tenth week, the developing gut returns to the peritoneal cavity. An omphalocele occurs because of the failure of the gut to return to the abdominal cavity. The resulting omphalocele is covered with a fine membrane called the *amnion*, which protects the intestine and abdominal contents from infection and the loss of fluid. The umbilical cord is found at the apex of this large sac (Fig. 5-15).

In gastroschisis the pathologic process is thought to be due to the intrauterine interruption of the omphalomesenteric artery.[27] This leads to an interruption of the abdominal wall next to the base of the umbilical cord, with herniation of the gut through the abdominal wall. The umbilical cord is found on the side of the herniated viscera (Fig. 5-16). There is usually no involvement of the muscles of the abdominal wall. The intestinal contents, which may include the liver, are not covered by any membrane and are therefore at risk for the development of infection and for the loss of enormous amounts of protein-rich extracellular fluid. An omphalocele may occur in various malformation syndromes, such as the Beckwith-Wiedemann syndrome, which comprises mental retardation, congenital heart disease, and a large tongue. Approximately 20 percent of infants with an omphalocele will have a congenital heart lesion. The frequency of associated

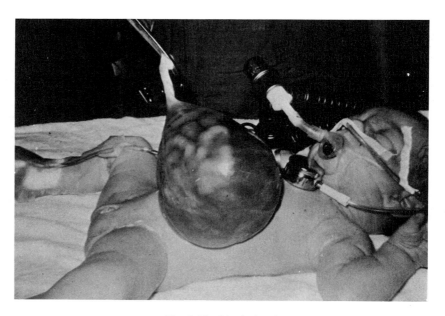

Fig. 5-15. Omphalocele.

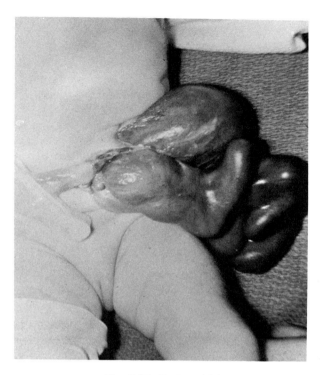

Fig. 5-16. Gastroschisis.

defects is twice as great in omphalocele as in gastroschisis. Approximately 70 percent of the associated defects in gastroschisis involve the gastrointestinal tract, and consist primarily of intestinal atresia or stenosis, most often in the jejunum and ilium, and malrotation.

Antenatal Diagnosis

α-Fetoprotein (AFP) is a protein present in tissues during fetal development. Closure of the abdominal wall and the neural tube prevents a release of large quantities of this protein into the amniotic fluid. On the other hand, an open neural tube, such as in meningomyelocele, or an open abdominal wall, such as with omphalocele and gastroschisis, will result in an increased amount of AFP in the amniotic fluid. High levels of AFP in the amniotic fluid can cross the placenta and be detected in maternal blood. Thus, abnormal levels of AFP in the mother or from amniotic fluid raises concern over the possibility of either an abdominal wall or a neural tube defect in the fetus. Ultrasonography is reliable in helping to diagnose either condition.

Preanesthetic Considerations

The two major differences in the apparently similar conditions of omphalocele and gastroschisis are that the associated defects with omphalocele are of much greater clinical significance, and that the potential for fluid loss and infection in gastroschisis is much more significant. Preoperative preparation of the infant with an omphalocele mainly involves the identification of other congenital defects (e.g., cardiac defect) that may complicate the anesthetic management. The infant with gastroschisis needs careful attention to the prevention and treatment of infection as well as extracellular fluid replacement. These infants often need large quantities of full-strength balanced salt solution for adequate volume resuscitation. During surgery, as soon as the amnion is removed from an omphalocele, the same potential exists for the loss of extracellular fluid.

The surgical approach to the defect will be directly related to the magnitude of the defect. At times all of the abdominal contents can be returned to the peritoneal cavity and a primary closure of peritoneum and skin can be accomplished. This occurs with small defects and small amounts of extraperitoneal viscera. At times there is not enough peritoneum to cover the abdominal contents but there is enough skin so that skin closure can be done. In the worst case scenario the large amount of extraperitoneal abdominal viscera results in inadequate stretching of the peritoneal cavity, and the abdominal viscera cannot be contained within the abdomen without undue pressure. This high intra-abdominal pressure will cause circulatory and ventilatory problems. In this situation a Dacron silo is incorporated into the abdominal wall to contain and cover the abdominal viscera (Fig. 5-17). The repair is then staged with the size of the silo being reduced every 2 or 3 days, thereby allowing the abdominal contents to slowly stretch the peritoneum, with the final result being a complete closure of the abdominal wall. It would be desirable to have some objective criteria by which to judge whether the complete operative reduction of the her-

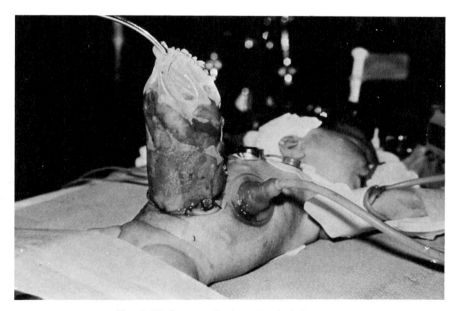

Fig. 5-17. Dacron silo for extruded viscera.

niated viscera would be successful and not result in the above-mentioned ventilatory and circulatory problems. A recent study looked at intragastric pressure, cardiac index, and central venous pressure following complete primary closure.[28] In this study a complete closure was accomplished in eight infants. However, four of these infants required reoperation and placement of a silo within 24 hours because of poor peripheral perfusion and oliguria. It is of interest that the infants who required reoperation had intragastric pressures of 20 mmHg or more and a decrease in cardiac output. Other intraoperative changes of blood pressure, heart rate, and systemic vascular resistance were not predictive of outcome. This study strongly suggests that intragastric pressure should be monitored during attempted complete closure of omphalocele or gastroschisis and that if the intragastric pressure is greater than 20 mmHg a compromise of blood flow to the abdominal organs will result. A pressure less than 20 mmHg would appear to be predictive that the complete closure will be successful. It would seem that these criteria could also be applied to the predictive criteria when the final closure is done after the removal of a Dacron silo. There is a recent report of a dog model in which there was a close correlation between bladder pressure measurements and intra-abdominal pressure. This would provide an alternative measure of intra-abdominal pressure.

If the defect is small and closure is simple, routine monitoring and intravenous access are sufficient. However, if there is any question about the ability to close the defect and the liver is involved in the process, several potentially complicating factors must be considered. The first of these relates to monitoring. Often, there is malrotation of the abdominal viscera, so there may be torsion of the vascular pedicle of the liver as well as pressure on the vena cavae. This can cause quite rapid and severe fluctuations of venous return and cardiac output, resulting in a vacillating blood pressure. It is helpful to have a direct arterial readout of these pressure changes to assist the surgeon in the approach to replacement of the viscera.

A central line is quite useful in these patients for the administration of crystalloid, blood, and antibiotics, and as a good source for following the hematocrit, blood chemistries, and venous blood gases intra- and postoperatively. These infants can lose enormous amounts of fluid, and vigorous fluid therapy must therefore be anticipated. Another major anesthetic problem with these infants is that the heat loss from their bodies can be enormous when a large amount of their abdominal viscera is exposed. Measures must be taken to warm the room, warm and humidify the anesthetic gases, and warm all intravenous fluids.

Several problems should be anticipated in the postoperative period, particularly if the abdomen is tight as the result of a tight closure. The latter will increase the intra-abdominal pressure, with possible circulatory and ventilatory consequences. The increased intra-abdominal pressure will elevate the diaphragm and encroach upon the ventilatory ability of the infant. If there is any question, the patient should remain intubated and ventilated until the effects of the anesthetic have been completely dissipated and the infant can be carefully monitored in an intensive care unit. The circulatory problems of a tight closure are threefold: (1) renal parenchymal blood flow is reduced and there is an outpouring of renin, which may result in a low urine output, (2) venous return from the lower extremities is obstructed, which may result in significant edema following surgery, and (3) the bowel becomes ischemic.[28]

If a silo is needed to allow the peritoneum and skin to stretch so that they can comfortably contain the abdominal contents, the surgical approach after the placement of the silo involves a staged reduction in the size of the silo, and when all of the abdominal contents are able to be returned to the peritoneal cavity without undo pressure, final closure of the defect. The silo is usually reduced in size every other day. There is some urgency to closure of the abdomen and removal of the silo, since the presence of a foreign body encourages infection. The operation to reduce the silo does not involve major, painful stimulation, but as the silo is reduced (in a fashion similar to squeezing a tube of toothpaste), the infant may feel some degree of discomfort as the peritoneum and abdominal skin are stretched and the diaphragm is elevated. If the infant is already intubated and ventilated, the anesthetic technique is moot. However, if the infant is breathing spontaneously, our anesthetic technique has been to administer ketamine 0.5 mg/kg IV while the silo is tightened down. This blunts the discomfort while at the same time allowing the anesthesiologist and surgeon to determine the appropriate silo reduction commensurate with the maintenance of adequate ventilation and circulation. The infant's pulse, blood pressure, skin color, and oxygen saturation are all followed. The dose of ketamine is titrated to prevent excessive crying and movement by the infant. This is a technique that requires clinical judgment. Small decreases in arterial pressure and increases in pulse rate are frequent with this procedure, but these two parameters return to normal while the silo is being resutured. The oxygen saturation is followed, and if it drops below 90 while breathing room air, then the size of the silo is enlarged accordingly. We have not used intragastric or bladder pressures to monitor the silo reduction but it certainly would seem to be a reasonable technique to assist in this procedure. The procedure takes approximately 20 to 25 minutes. The usual total dose of ketamine is between 1 and 2 mg/kg. The final closure of the abdominal wall defect requires a full anesthetic with intubation, controlled ventilation, and excellent muscle relaxation. The infant is left intubated after the surgery, and is weaned by following its clinical condition and blood gas values.

Intestinal Obstruction

Intestinal obstruction occurs in two major anatomic locations in the neonate, the upper intestinal tract and lower intestinal tract. The most frequent is duodenal obstruction. The others involve the lower gastrointestinal tract, either at the terminal ileum or in the rectum (megacolon or Hirshsprung's disease) or anus (imperforate anus). Infants who have duodenal atresia have a high incidence of associated congenital anomalies, including a 20 percent incidence of congenital heart disease and a frequent association with trisomy 21 (Down syndrome). If the lesion is located in the terminal ileum or colon, the incidence of associated congenital anomalies is much lower. Imperforate anus is associated with a high incidence of associated anomalies. The major potential problem of infants with obstruction is fluid and electrolyte balance. The anesthesiologist should not initiate anesthesia until the fluid deficits have been repaired.

Upper Gastrointestinal Tract Obstruction

Obstruction of the upper gastrointestinal tract will usually present within 12 to 24 hours because the infant cannot tolerate oral feeding. The diagnosis in these infants is usually made fairly rapidly with only mild to moderate disturbances of fluid and electrolyte balance.

The preoperative preparation of these patients depends on how long it took for the defect to be recognized. Upper gastrointestinal tract fluid losses are high in sodium content and should be replaced with balanced salt solution. One of the major anesthetic concerns with upper gastrointestinal tract obstruction is aspiration. Gastric decompression cannot be guaranteed with a nasogastric tube but it will result in a reduction in the quantity of fluid in the upper gastrointestinal tract. In addition, the fluid can be buffered with bicarbonate in order to reduce the dangers of an acid aspiration. The usual airway management of these infants is awake intubation facilitated with topical anesthesia to reduce the pain and discomfort. There has been concern by some that in the premature infant with immature cerebral blood vessels, the hypertension from an awake intubation might increase the chances of an intracerebral bleed. Therefore topical anesthesia for the oropharynx with lidocaine is appropriate. In addition, lidocaine 1 mg/kg IV can be administered 1 minute before attempts at intubation. The major issue in the anesthetic technique for these infants is ensuring adequate relaxation, and if the infant is robust with no other medical problems a technique should be chosen that will allow extubation at the end of the procedure. Caudal anesthesia (0.25 percent marcaine 1 ml/kg with epinephrine 1:200,000) can be administered shortly after the infant is intubated or at the end of surgery. If the caudal anesthesia is administered before surgery begins it will provide some of the muscle relaxation and anesthesia necessary for surgery. This will allow the infant to awaken more rapidly at the termination of surgery and to recover its protective airway reflexes. If it is administered at the end of surgery it will provide excellent postoperative analgesia for 12 hours, thereby reducing or eliminating the immediate postoperative need for narcotic analgesia. The muscle relaxant of choice at the present time in these infants is atracurium. If at the end of surgery the infant is awake with intact protective airway reflexes and the effects of the muscle relaxant either reversed or dissipated, consideration should be given to extubating the infant. However, if there is any question, the endotracheal tube should be left in place and the infant taken to the recovery room and extubated there. If the infant has other congenital defects or if the incision is long and the operation involved considerable intra-abdominal trauma, consideration should be given to leaving the endotracheal tube in place with positive end-expiratory pressure for a period of time immediately after surgery until the situation is stabilized.

Lower Gastrointestinal Tract Obstruction

Lesions in this area take longer to become evident. However, an imperforate anus should be recognized shortly after birth. Most infants with lower gastrointestinal tract obstruction present with abdominal distention, little or no meconium passage, and vomiting. There is a potential for an enormous amount of sequestration of fluid within a dilated intestinal tract. The weight of the infant will not reflect the reduction of extracellular fluid volume since the majority of fluid loss is within the intestinal lumen. In infants with upper gastrointestinal tract losses, vomiting may result in a loss of weight and this can be used as a guidelines to adequate fluid resuscitation. These infants often have greater derangements of fluid and electrolyte balance than those infants with an upper gastrointestinal tract obstruction, and therefore it may take longer to prepare them for surgery. Premature surgery should be avoided. Skin turgor, urine output, and serum electrolytes are the best guides to adequate fluid resuscitation in these infants. Before surgery is undertaken, the serum sodium should be greater than 130 mEq/L and the urine output 1 to 2 ml/kg/hr. The presence of a nasogastric tube does not guarantee emptying of the stomach, and consideration should be given to doing an awake intubation in these infants if they have been vomiting. The same procedure needs to be followed as described above. If the infant has had minimal or no vomiting consideration can be given to doing a rapid-sequence induction. Preoxygenation for 1 to 2 minutes with oxygen blown over the infant's face will increase the oxygen reserve in the lungs. However, persistent attempts to place a mask on the face of an uncooperative infant may be counterproductive and result in desaturation as the infant cries and breathholds. Thiopental 3 to 4 mg/kg followed by succinylcholine 2 mg/kg or atracurium 0.8 mg/kg along with cricoid pressure as tolerated represents a reasonable approach to the rapid-sequence intubation of these infants. The presence of air within the intestine discourages the use of nitrous oxide and therefore the technique is usually that of either a volatile agent (which I prefer) or a narcotic technique. Usually the amount of narcotic that would be required to do the anesthetic without the use of a volatile agent would result in a dose of narcotic that would require postoperative ventilation. The other possibility is to administer caudal anesthesia after the induction and intubation. This would reduce the amount of anesthetic and muscle relaxant required and provide excellent postoperative analgesia.

These infants can be more difficult than those with upper gastrointestinal tract obstruction since their disease involves considerably more of the intestinal tract, the incision may be longer, and they may not have been in as good condition because they have been obstructed for periods of up to a week. The question of extubation at the end of surgery arises. If the infant is in good condition with no other congenital defects and is ready for extubation at the end of surgery or shortly thereafter, then they should be extubated. If there is any question these infants should be left intubated with positive end-expiratory pressure in the postoperative period until it is determined that they are ready for extubation.

Surgical Procedures in Infants 1 Week to 6 Months of Age

The major surgical procedures done on infants 1 week to 6 months of age are both diagnostic and therapeutic. It is this period that infants who have been intubated and ventilated for varying periods begin to develop subglottic stenosis, and infants who have undergone repair of TEF may have problems with aspiration and stridor. The major diagnostic procedures done on infants other than laryngoscopy and bronchoscopy, which are discussed in another chapter, are eye examinations, computed tomographic (CT) scans, and arthrograms for congenital dislocation of the hip. This discussion is primarily concerned with anesthetic considerations in therapy for necrotizing enterocolitis, retinopathy of prematurity, hernias, gastrointestinal tract obstruction, and diagnostic procedures.

Necrotizing Enterocolitis

Necrotizing enterocolitis (NEC) is a disease of premature infants that fortunately has decreased in frequency in the last several years. The exact cause of NEC has yet to be determined. Milner et al. proposed that the risk factors for developing NEC include an overwhelming hypotensive and ischemic injury to the intestines in association with sepsis.[29] Other predisposing factors in this condition were believed to be intestinal immaturity and oral feedings. Leung et al. described the association of NEC with infants with symptomatic congenital heart disease who were receiving prostaglandins.[30] It was believed that the prostaglandins caused apnea and hypotension, and that this predisposed some infants to NEC. A retrospective study of infants with myelomeningocele by Costello et al. showed an association with NEC, and the investigators recommended that there should be a more cautious approach to the introduction of feeding in infants with myelomeningocele.[31] Rotbart et al. have recently reported a strong association between rotavirus infection and NEC.[32] Kosloske proposed that NEC occurs by the coincidence of two or three pathologic events: intestinal immaturity, colonization by pathogenic bacteria, and excess protein substrate in the intestinal lumen.[33] NEC is the result of a cascade of pathologic events. The immature intestine has a decreased ability to absorb substrate, which leads to stasis. The consequence of stasis is bacterial proliferation, which leads to focal infection. Further pooling of fluid, ischemia, and infection may lead to necrosis of the intestinal mucosa, which may be followed by perforation. The picture is complicated by severe fluid loss, peritonitis, septicemia, and disseminated intravascular coagulation. The first signs that NEC may be developing are distension, irritability, and the development of metabolic acidosis. The first line of treatment for NEC is medical: stopping oral intake and administering antibiotics, fluids, and blood products. However, the anesthesiologist will become involved after conservative medical management has failed and the infant continues a downhill course. These infants are than brought to the operating room to remove the gangrenous bowel and for an ileostomy.

These infants need an enormous amount of supportive care before they arrive in the operating room because of the severe degree of septicemia, metabolic acidosis, fluid loss, and disseminated intravascular coagulation. They often require a period of intubation and ventilation in the nursery along with correction of the circulatory, metabolic, and clotting derangements. These infants may be so critically ill that they will only tolerate small amounts of anesthesia, such as ketamine 0.5 to 1 mg/kg. Small doses of fentanyl (i.e., 1 to 3 μg/kg) can be administered if the ketamine is tolerated. As resuscitation and surgery continues and the infant's condition improves, more narcotics or small doses of volatile anesthetics can be added as tolerated.

Usually, these infants are well monitored with an arterial line and a central line when they arrive. They represent some of the most challenging cases in anesthesia. The peritonitis and necrosis of the intestine result in enormous losses of extracellular fluid, which needs to be replaced with large quantities of balanced salt solution. The hematocrit in these infants should be maintained somewhere between 30 and 35. Postoperatively, they are returned to the newborn intensive care for continued medical management.

Retinopathy of Prematurity

Premature infants are at risk for developing the retinopathy of prematurity (ROP). The exact causes and relationship to the inspired oxygen concentration has not been well defined. There has been an increase in ROP in low-birthweight infants, but this is due to an increased survival in infants at risk. The major risk group is premature infants weighing less than 1,500 g. However, in all circumstances in which an infant is at risk for ROP, it should be remembered that they are also at risk for hypoxia of the central nervous system. When there is any doubt, the central nervous system has priority over the retina. The pulse oximeter will assist in determining the appropriate FiO_2 in the premature infants at risk. In infants more than 1,500 g, however, there is little risk in developing ROP, and my choice of anesthetic is a volatile agent plus oxygen. If there is a concern about ROP, the oxygen saturation should be maintained somewhere between 95 and 98 percent. If attempts at maintaining this oxygen saturation are accompanied by large swings in saturation that result in desaturation to levels below 90, a higher FiO_2 should be used and attempts to adjust the FiO_2 to such a fine line abandoned.

Hernia

The incidence and complications of hernia are quite different in infants under 1 year of age compared to those of the older child and adult. Premature infants have a much higher incidence of inguinal hernia. The major complication of a hernia is incarceration with the potential for intestinal obstruction, necrosis, and gonadal infarction. Two studies of infants with hernias under a year of age report an incidence of incarceration of 31 percent.[34,35] Rescorla and Grosfeld reported a series of 100 infants less than 2 months of age.[34] Thirty-one percent presented with incarceration, 9 percent presented with intestinal obstruction, and 2 percent presented with gonadal infarction. Therefore, this puts hernia repair in the urgent category rather than the elective. Those who would suggest that hernia repair should be delayed until the infant is 6 months to 1 year of age must carefully weigh this against the problems of incarceration.

Incarcerated hernias fall into two categories: reducible and irreducible. If the hernia is reducible most surgeons wait for 24 to 48 hours after reduction to allow the swelling to go down before performing surgery. If the hernia is irreducible it needs to be operated on relatively quickly. If a gonad is involved in an irreducible hernia the rate of gonadal infarction is high (20 to 30 percent). The complication rate in the above study was 4.5 percent for reducible incarcerated hernias and 33 percent for irreducible incarcerated hernias. In Rescorla and Grosfeld's study 30 percent were premature, 42 percent had a history of the respiratory distress syndrome (16 percent had been ventilated), and 19 percent had congenital heart disease. Therefore, in the premature infant and in the premature nursery graduate, we may be presented with a surgical condition that has a high rate of complications and a group of infants that may have a high rate of complications. Refer to Chapter 16 for a further discussion of problems of premature infants.

Anesthetic Techniques

There has been a great deal of discussion about whether the anesthetic technique has anything to do with the incidence of postoperative apnea in premature nursery graduates. Most clinicians think that the occurrence of apnea in premature infants is a maturation problem and that after they achieve a conceptual age of 44 to 46 weeks that apnea will no longer be a problem. However, the debate continues whether or not regional anesthesia for these infants is preferred over general anesthesia. There are risks and complications with all anesthetic techniques. Regional anesthesia in the form of a caudal or spinal technique has been supported by many. However, it is becoming evident that not all infants will tolerate lying quietly, even with an anesthetic, for the purposes of a hernia repair. Therefore, in some of these infants it is necessary to use sedation, but when sedation is used this greatly increases the incidence of apnea.

It may be difficult for clinicians who only occasionally work with premature nursery graduates to maintain their skills in doing spinal or caudal anesthesia. Therefore, most often general anesthesia will be the technique of choice. However, regional anesthesia can be added to the general anesthesia to minimize the depth of anesthesia and provide postoperative analgesia. Techniques for regional anesthesia include caudal and ilioinguinal and iliohypogastric block. These blocks can be performed after the induction of anesthesia or at the termination of surgery. There would appear to be more advantages to performing them after induction to reduce the amount of general anesthesia and muscle relaxants that are needed. Ilioinguinal and iliohypogastric nerve blocks have about the same degree of postoperative analgesia as caudal analgesia, and are less invasive procedures. Details of the technique for regional anesthesia are given in Chapter 11.

Another question in infants undergoing general anesthesia is whether or not they should be intubated. There are surgeons who can repair hernias in 15 minutes. In that situation, if the infant is otherwise normal and has no significant respiratory problems, mask anesthesia would be acceptable. On the other hand, if the infant is a premature nursery graduate who may have some degree of residual lung disease and a reactive airway, the risk and benefits of intubation need to be carefully evaluated. Sometimes after the decision is made to use mask anesthesia it may turn out that it is difficult to maintain oxygen saturations of 95 percent. Then consideration should be given to stopping the procedure and intubating the infant. The figure of 95 percent saturation is somewhat arbitrary, but inability to accomplish so high an oxygen saturation is a tipoff that there may be difficulty ahead.

Pyloric Stenosis

One of the most frequent pediatric surgical emergencies is the infant with pyloric stenosis. The pathology is hypertrophy of the pyloric smooth muscle. There is edema of the pyloric mucosa and submucosa. The obstruction leads to progressive episodes of vomiting, which becomes projectile. Although pyloric stenosis usually presents between 2 and 10 weeks of life, the symptoms may occur as early as the second day and as late as the fifth month of life. The primary fluid and electrolyte losses are of water, sodium, potassium, chloride, and hydrogen ion. If the vomiting becomes protracted, varying degrees of hyponatremic, hypochloremic, and hypokalemic metabolic alkalosis will develop. It should be remembered that these infants represent a medical emergency, for fluid and electrolyte replacement, and not a surgical emergency. Time must be taken to restore the fluid and electrolyte deficits. If the diagnosis is made early and the deficit is minimal, these infants may be prepared for surgery in as little as 2 to 3 hours. On the other hand, if the deficits and electrolyte derangements are great, it may take as long as 12 to 24 hours to repair them. See Chapter 4 for a discussion of this issue.

Techniques of Intubation

There are differences of opinion about the techniques of intubation for infants with pyloric stenosis. There are a great number of proponents of intubation with the infant awake. I prefer to intubate infants with pyloric stenosis after the induction of anesthesia, usually in a rapid-sequence fashion. However, there are certain maneuvers that must be accomplished before the induction. First, if the infant doesn't have a nasogastric tube in place, a large well-lubricated (No. 14) suction catheter is passed orally into the stomach. The tube is then suctioned while the abdomen is gently massaged. Five milliliters of standard sodium bicarbonate solution are injected down the orogastric tube. The tube is then suctioned and removed and the infant gently agitated to distribute the bicarbonate. I use one of two techniques for the induction and intubation of the infant. If an

IV is in place, a rapid-sequence induction with oxygenation, thiopental 3 to 4 mg/kg, cricoid pressure, succinylcholine 2 mg/kg, and intubation of the infant is performed. If the infant has no IV and it doesn't appear as if one could be started easily, an inhalation induction is accomplished with halothane nitrous oxide and then either succinylcholine 4 mg/kg IM is administered, followed by intubation or an IV is started and then the patient is intubated.

The surgery for pyloric stenosis requires two periods of relaxation: one when the pylorus is delivered into the wound and the other when the peritoneum is being closed. The basic anesthetic technique involves a volatile agent (halothane 1 to 1.5 percent with 70 percent nitrous oxide) with small doses of succinylcholine at the appropriate time if needed. The dose of succinylcholine is 0.5 to 1 mg/kg. The endotracheal tube is left in place until the infant is completely awake and can protect its own airway. If atracurium is used for the rapid-sequence intubation this will usually provide sufficient muscle relaxation for the surgery, which usually takes 20 to 30 minutes.

Postoperative analgesia can be provided in two ways. One is to infiltrate the skin, subcutaneous tissue, muscle, and peritoneum with marcaine at the outset of surgery or at the time of closure. The other technique is to perform a caudal block with marcaine.

Associated Congenital Anomalies

Infants born with one congenital anomaly have a higher incidence of a second congenital anomaly than does the overall infant population. As an example, infants with an omphalocele have a 60 percent chance of having another anomaly. The location of the omphalocele may determine the type of anomaly (i.e., a hypogastric omphalocele is more frequently associated with exstrophy of the bladder, and an epigastric omphalocele is more frequently associated with an increased incidence of cardiothoracic anomalies). The most frequent life-threatening associated congenital anomalies are those of the cardiovascular system.

The presence of another congenital anomaly has serious implications for the infant, the family, and the surgical team. First, the associated anomaly may delay surgery for the primary anomaly because of the need for evaluation and possible treatment. An example of this is a congenital heart defect. Second, the associated defect may impact on the anesthetic management of the patient. If the infant has a symptomatic congenital heart defect it may well need extensive perioperative monitoring and supportive care. Third, the associated anomaly often determines the survival of the infant. For example, in trisomy 21 (Down syndrome) with duodenal atresia and a congenital heart defect, the long-term survival of the infant depends on the associated congenital heart defect.

REFERENCES

1. Clyman R: Ontogeny of the ductus arteriosus response to prostaglandins and inhibitors of their synthesis. Semin Perinatol 4:115, 1980
2. Murphy JD, Vawter GF, Reid LM: Pulmonary vascular disease in fatal meconium aspiration. J Pediatr 104:758, 1984

3. Berry FA: The renal system. In Gregory GA (ed): Pediatric Anesthesia Vol. I. Churchill Livingstone, New York, 1989

4. Jones R, Bodnar A, Roan Y, et al: Subglottic stenosis in newborn intensive care unit graduates. Am J Dis Child 135:367, 1981

5. Keens TG, Bryan AC, Levison H, et al: Developmental pattern of muscle fiber types in human ventilatory muscles. J Appl Physiol 44:909, 1978

6. Murat I, Lapeyre G, Saint-Maurice C: Isoflurane attenuates baroreflex control of heart rate in human neonates. Anesthesiology 70:395, 1989

7. Friedman WF: The intrinsic physiologic properties of the developing heart. Prog Cardiovasc Dis 15:87, 1972

8. Friedman WF, George BL: Medical progress: Treatment of congestive heart failure by altering loading conditions of the heart. J Pediatr 106:697, 1985

9. Dohi S, Naito H, Takahashi T: Age-related changes in blood pressure and duration of motor block in spinal anesthesia. Anesthesiology 50:319, 1979

10. Watcha MF, Forestner JE, Connor MT, et al: Minimum alveolar concentration of halothane for tracheal intubation in children. Anesthesiology 69:412, 1988

11. Mason LJ, Betts EK: Leg lift and maximum inspiratory force, clinical signs of neuromuscular blockade reversal in neonates and infants. Anesthesiology 52:441, 1980

12. Meakin G, Sweet PT, Bevan JC, et al: Neostigmine and edrophonium as antagonists of pancuronium in infants and children. Anesthesiology 59:316, 1983

13. Cronnelly R, Morris RB, Miller RD: Edrophonium: Duration of action and atropine requirement in humans during halothane anesthesia. Anesthesiology 57:261, 1982

14. Azar I, Pham AN, Karambelkar DJ, et al: The heart rate following edrophonium-atropine and edrophonium-glycopyrrolate mixtures. Anesthesiology 59:316, 1983

15. Bohn D, Tamura M, Perrin D, et al: Ventilatory predictors of pulmonary hypoplasia in congenital diaphragmatic hernia, confirmed by morphologic assessment. J Pediatr 111:423, 1987

16. Sakai H, Tamura M, Hosokawa Y, et al: Effect of surgical repair on respiratory mechanics in congenital diaphragmatic hernia. J Pediatr 111:432, 1987

17. Campbell LR, Bunyapen C, Holmes GL, et al: Right common carotid artery ligation in extracorporeal membrane oxygenation. J Peds 113:110, 1988

18. Patrias, Rabinowicz IM, Klein MD: Ocular findings in infants treated with extracorporeal support. Pediatrics 82:560, 1988

19. Reid JS, Hutcherson RJ: Long term follow-up of patients with congenital diaphragmatic hernia. J Pediatr Surg 11:939, 1976

20. Bloch EC, Filston HC: A thin fiberoptic bronchoscope as an aid to occlusion of the fistula in infants with tracheoesophageal fistula. Anesth Analg 67:791, 1988

21. Salem MR, Wong AY, Lin YH, et al: Prevention of gastric distention during anesthesia for newborns with tracheoesophageal fistulas. Anesthesiology 38:82, 1973

22. Harrison MR, Hanson BA, Mahour GH, et al: The significance of right aortic arch in repair of esophageal atresia and tracheoesophageal fistula. J Pediatr Surg 12:861, 1977

23. Davies MRO, Cywes S: The flaccid trachea and tracheoesophageal congenital anomalies. J Pediatr Surg 13:363, 1978

24. Jolley SG, Johnson DG, Roberts CC, et al: Patterns of gastroesophageal reflux in children following repair of esophageal atresia and distal tracheoesophageal fistula. J Pediatr Surg 15:857, 1980

25. Milligan DWA, Levison H: Lung function in children following repair of tracheoesophageal fistula. Pediatrics 95:24, 1979

26. Grosfeld JL, Weber TR: Congenital abdominal wall defects: Gastroschisis and omphalocele. Curr Prob Surg 19:158, 1982

27. Hoyme HE, Higginbottom MC, Jones JL: The vascular pathogenesis of gastroschisis: Intrauterine interruption of the omphalomesenteric artery. Pediatrics 98:228, 1981
28. Yaster, Buck JR, Dudgeon DL, et al: Hemodynamic effects of primary closure of omphalocele/gastroschisis in human newborns. Anesthesiology 69:84, 1988
29. Milner ME, de la Monte SM, Moore GW, Hutchins GM: Risk factors for developing and dying from necrotizing enterocolitis. J Pediatr Gastroenterol Nutr 5:359, 1986
30. Leung MP, Chau K, Hui P, et al: Necrotizing enterocolitis in neonates with symptomatic congenital heart disease. J Pediatr 113:1044, 1988
31. Costello S, Hellmann J, Lui K: Myelomeningocele: A risk factor for necrotizing enterocolitis in term infants. J Pediatr 113:1041, 1988
32. Rotbart HA, Nelson WL, Glode MP, et al: Neonatal rotavirus-associated necrotizing enterocolitis: Case control study and prospective surveillance during an outbreak. J Pediatr 112:87, 1988
33. Kosloske AM: Pathogenesis and prevention of necrotizing enterocolitis: A hypothesis based on personal observation and a review of the literature. Pediatrics 74:1086, 1984
34. Rescorla FJ, Grosfeld JL: Inguinal hernia repair in the perinatal period and early infancy: Clinical considerations. J Pediatr Surg 19:832, 1984
35. Puri P, Guiney EJ, O'Donnell B: Inguinal hernia in infants: The fate of the testis following incarceration. J Pediatr Surg 19:44, 1984
36. German JC, Mahour FH, Woolley MM: Esophageal atresia and associated anomalies. J Pediatr Surg 11:299, 1976
37. Phibbs R: Delivery room management of the newborn. In Avery GB (ed): Neonatology, Pathology and Management of the Newborn. JB Lippincott, Philadelphia, 1981
38. Ryan FJ, Lodris ID, Coté CJ, Goudsouzian N (eds): A Practice of Anesthesia for Infants and Children. Grune & Stratton, Orlando, FL, 1986
39. Smith CA, Nelson NM: Physiology of the Newborn Infant. 4th Ed. Charles C Thomas, Springfield, IL 1976
40. Kaplan RF, Graven SA: Anatomic and physiologic differences of neonates, infants, and children. Semin Anesth 3:4, 1984

6

ANESTHESIA FOR THE CHILD WITH A DIFFICULT AIRWAY

Frederic A. Berry

The presentation of the patient with a difficult airway covers a spectrum of possibilities that depends on the severity of the airway obstruction. At the most intimidating end of the spectrum is the infant with Pierre Robin syndrome or cystic hygroma (Fig. 6-1) who has an obvious airway obstruction causing varying degrees of alarm not only in the infant and parents but in the anesthesiologist as well. Children at the other end of the spectrum, such as those with Goldenhar syndrome (Fig. 6-2), may not be recognized because they do not have airway problems in the unanesthetized state. These children may present for elective correction of the anatomic defect that is associated with the airway problem, for elective correction of associated congenital abnormalities, or for the emergency treatment of an acquired injury (i.e., broken bones, acute abdomen, or open-eye injury).

Usually, the infant or child with a difficult airway is easily recognized, either by symptomatology or anatomic features. However, in a small but significant number of cases a difficult airway is unrecognized during the preanesthetic assessment, and becomes recognized only upon the induction of anesthesia. The problem usually begins with difficulty in the basic management of the airway, resulting in episodes of desaturation, and progresses to varying degrees of difficulty with intubation. Because the anesthesiologist may not be psychologically prepared or have the necessary equipment or game plan to manage the airway problem, these unrecognized cases may represent a greater management challenge than that of the patient whose difficult airway is recognized preoperatively. Such was the case with the patient with Goldenhar syndrome in Figure 6-2, who had two anesthetics without any surgery because he could not be intubated. Various reasons may be perceived for these problems, such as "old" succinylcholine, an inadequate concentration of anesthetic agent, an incorrectly shaped laryngoscope blade, or a physician who is simply having a bad day. The anes-

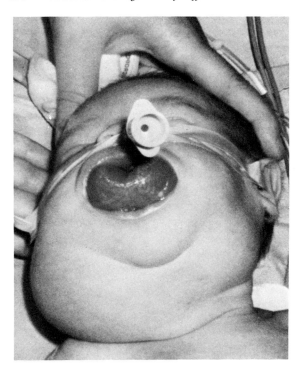

Fig. 6-1. Infant with massive cystic hygroma and severe upper airway obstruction after nasotracheal intubation.

thesiologist's most frequent thought in the situation of a difficult intubation is that the patient is not adequately relaxed. The skilled anesthesiologist must acquire the expertise and confidence to recognize the clinical situation for what it is (i.e., an anatomic anomaly) and then activate his or her contingency plan for a difficult airway. One of the goals of this chapter is to assist the anesthesiologist in identifying patients with such anomalies preoperatively, before struggling through inelegant attempts at airway management and intubation. The second goal of this chapter is to help the anesthesiologist identify the reason or reasons why a patient cannot be intubated and to develop contingency plans for the managed airway. The problem may be insufficient muscle relaxation, but it may also be an anatomic abnormality. The skillful anesthesiologist must learn to discriminate between a technically inadequate intubation and an anatomic problem. A rapid alternative can then be taken before the patient becomes hypoxic, receives an ''industrial dose of succinylcholine, or has his upper airway demolished. The course of action open to the anesthesiologist depends on the clinical situation. If the patient is hypoxic, in and out of laryngospasm, or having runs of various frightening cardiac dysrhythmias, it may be time to turn off the anesthetic, awaken the patient, and return another day. If the airway is manageable, the patient is well oxygenated and the anesthesiologist is not in tatters, various options for establishing the airway are available. These options are discussed in this chapter.

One of the most rewarding aspects of anesthesia practice is the development

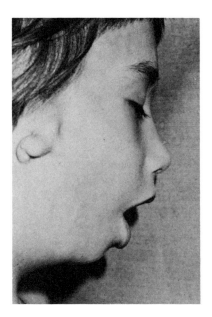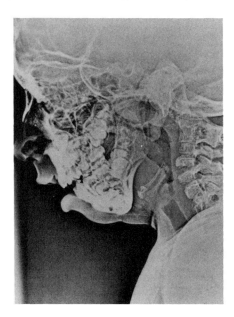

Fig. 6-2. Photo and lateral radiograph of a boy with Goldenhar syndrome. Note the fused cervical vertebrae, malformed mandible, and proximity of the hyoid bone to the mandible.

of skills in the art and science of managing the difficult airway. Planning is 90 percent of winning any battle. This is a well-recognized phenomenon of war, athletic contests, and most of life's endeavors. The same can be said about the management of the difficult airway, which at times truly appears to be a battle. The approach to the difficult airway is discussed under three main headings: (1) the anatomy of the airway and of intubation, (2) the physiology and pharmacology of the protective airway reflexes, and (3) the clinical management, which is based on points 1 and 2.

ANATOMY OF THE DIFFICULT AIRWAY AND OF INTUBATION

The difficult airway is a relatively rarely encountered phenomenon unless the anesthesiologist works in a center that specializes in such cases. Most anesthesiologists experience a high rate of success with the day-to-day airway management and intubation of patients, with the result that intubation techniques become so automatic and routine that, over time, an understanding of the anatomy of the airway and of intubation becomes less clear. It is therefore important to be aware of the basic anatomic factors involved in intubation so that in the preanesthetic evaluation of the patient and the clinical application of techniques for laryngoscopy and intubation, these factors are well understood. The skillful anesthesiologist must be able to quickly discern when there is an anatomic problem, and to know how to apply this knowledge to techniques of intubation. This discussion therefore begins with the preanesthetic evaluation of the patient and the development of an anesthetic plan, with special emphasis on the recognition of anatomic problems and a discussion of the techniques of intubation and their anatomic basis.

Preanesthetic Evaluation

The foundation of all anesthesia begins with the preoperative visit. Difficult airways are encountered very infrequently, and many can be overcome by inelegant, traumatic, but eventually successful techniques of intubation that unfortunately often leave the anesthesiologist no wiser but fortunately leave the patient with an intact central nervous system. It may be difficult to detect a difficult airway unless there is an obvious anomaly or the parents of the child recount a difficult anesthetic experience. The parents may describe a host of difficulties, such as the intubation taking an inordinate amount of time, that the operation was terminated because the child could not be intubated, or that airway difficulties resulted in a tracheotomy or an unexpected visit to the pediatric intensive care unit. The history of a difficult anesthetic experience should never be ignored, regardless of what the anesthesiologist considers his or her level of skill to be; there are skilled anesthesiologists everywhere. Thus, when the history of a difficult anesthetic experience is elicited, the anesthesiologist should be prepared for the worst. The history may reveal other problems as well, including problems with respiratory infections and problems with feeding that led to severe coughing and cyanosis. Any infant or child who has airway problems associated with either respiratory infections or feedings will probably have the same problems with induction and awakening from anesthesia. These problems include the early development of airway obstruction, coughing, laryngospasm, and regurgitation.

Anatomic Features of the Difficult Airway

The physical examination may reveal gross abnormalities, such as a massive cystic hygroma, or abnormalities that may be much more subtle. An example of the latter is the small (micrognathic) or deformed mandible (Fig. 6-2). The child shown in this figure has Goldenhar syndrome; the lateral radiograph demonstrates the enormous malformation of the mandible that results in a decreased potential displacement space for laryngoscopy. This will be discussed later in greater detail. There are various maneuvers used to evaluate the airway in such cases. The infant or child can be asked to open the mouth and extend the neck. This provides the anesthesiologist with a great deal of information about the mobility of the neck and mandible. If the child will not cooperate with the examiner, the parent should be asked to have the child follow these simple requests.

There are other anatomic features to look for. These include the size of the tongue, the faucial pillars, uvula, soft palate, the shape and size of the mandible,

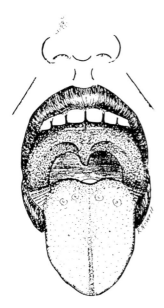

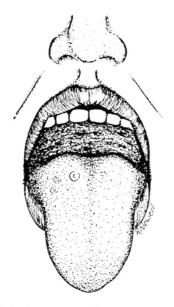

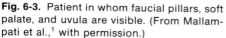

Fig. 6-3. Patient in whom faucial pillars, soft palate, and uvula are visible. (From Mallampati et al.,[1] with permission.)

Fig. 6-4. Patient in whom none of the three pharyngeal structures are visible. (From Mallampati et al.,[1] with permission.)

and the distance from the underside of the middle of the body of the mandible to the hyoid bone. A narrow, highly arched palate also increases the difficulty of intubation. Mallampati et al. described a technique to predict the degree of difficulty in laryngeal exposure in a group of adult patients based on the ability to visualize the faucial pillars, soft palate, and uvula.[1] The patients were divided into three classes, depending on the ability to visualize the oral airway with the patient sitting, open mouth, and protruding the tongue maximally. Then the patients were anesthetized and laryngoscoped following administration of succinylcholine. They were graded according to visualization of the glottis. There was a strong correlation between the ability to visualize the faucial pillars, soft palate, and uvula and the ability to successfully laryngoscope the patient (Fig. 6-3). In patients in whom there was no visualization of any of these airway structures, there was a high degree of difficulty experienced in visualizing the airway structures with a laryngoscope (Fig. 6-4).

Anatomy of Intubation

A quick analysis of the mechanics of laryngoscopy will illustrate the importance of the above-described factors. The first step in laryngoscopy is the alignment of the oral, pharyngeal, and laryngeal axes (Fig. 6-5). It is evident that increasing degrees of impairment in opening the mouth and extending the neck will increase the difficulty of direct laryngoscopy. Laryngoscopy involves dis-

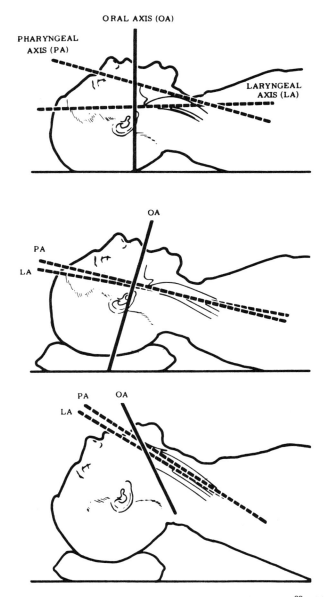

Fig. 6-5. Alignment of the airway axes for intubation. (From Stoelting,[20] with permission.)

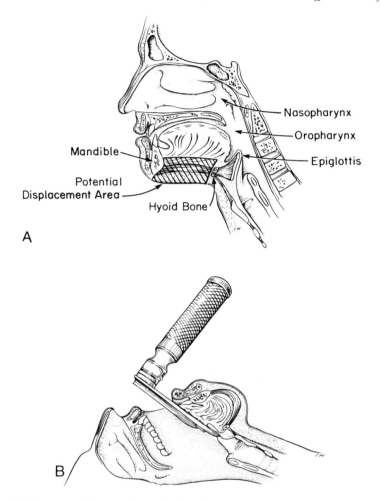

Fig. 6-6. (A) Diagram of airway, demonstrating "potential displacement area" for intubation. **(B)** Laryngoscopy with displacement of the tongue and soft tissue into the "potential displacement area."

placement of the soft tissue of the oropharynx, allowing a line of vision to be developed from the teeth or mandibular alveolar ridge to the epiglottis and larynx. The soft tissue is displaced into a potential space that is encompassed, and therefore potentially restricted, by an incomplete bony ring bound posteriorly by the hyoid bone, laterally by the rami of the mandible, and anteriorly by the mentum of the mandible (Fig. 6-6). An alteration in the shape or size of the bony structures in this area results in a decrease in the space in which the soft tissue can be displaced with the laryngoscope. This occurs in the Pierre Robin syndrome and in the syndromes that include mandibular dysplasia as part of their pathology, such as Treacher Collins syndrome, Goldenhar syndrome, and some of the hemifacial microsomias. An increased amount of soft tissue in the area of the tongue will have the same effect. This may occur in various tumors of the tongue and oropharynx, such as cystic hygroma or hemangioma. The degree of interference with laryngoscopy depends on the disproportion between the size of the potential space and the amount of soft tissue to be displaced. The use of muscle relaxants will maximize the potential displacement space. However, the disproportion may be so great that laryngoscopy is unsuccessful even with maximal relaxation. The problem is the bony ring, albeit incomplete, that restricts and confines the displacement of the tongue and soft tissue, and that cannot be relaxed by any dose of neuromuscular blocking agent. Preoperative assessment of this region allows the anesthesiologist to anticipate the degree of tissue displacement that might be possible.

Measurement of the anteroposterior distance from the middle of the inside of the mentum of the mandible to the hyoid bone is one method for assessing the potential space for laryngoscopy. This is referred to as the *Schwartz hyoid maneuver*. The distance can easily be measured by gently placing the examining fingers in the space, as shown in Figure 6-7. In adults, the minimum distance for a normal airway is about 3 cm (two fingers). The distance in infants and children is proportionately smaller, approximately 1.5 cm in newborn infants. Often, when the anteroposterior diameter is reduced, the lateral distance is also reduced. The result of an increased soft tissue mass or a decreased potential space is a reduction in the ability to successfully laryngoscope the patient. This

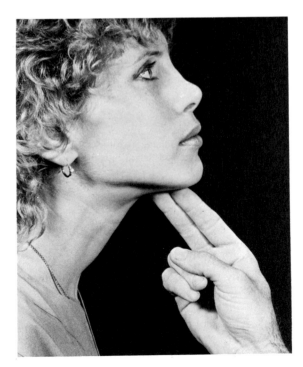

Fig. 6-7. The Schwartz hyoid maneuver to determine the adequacy of the "potential displacement area."

leads to varying degrees of difficulty with endotracheal intubation, ranging from minimal difficulty in visualization to total inability to visualize the epiglottis or any part of the larynx. This is referred to as an *anterior larynx*. Anatomically, the larynx is not any more anterior in these patients than in a patient who can easily be laryngoscoped; it is, however, "anterior" to the line of vision. The problem is that the laryngoscope remains in a posterior position, since the soft tissue cannot be displaced anteriorly. If the patient's neck cannot be extended or the mouth opened to align the airway axes, this will add to the difficulties of laryngoscopy and intubation. The inability to extend the neck is found in patients with fused cervical vertebrae, such as in Goldenhar syndrome, and also occurs in patients with cervical arthritis.

THE PHYSIOLOGY AND PHARMACOLOGY OF THE DEPRESSION OF THE PROTECTIVE AIRWAY REFLEXES

Physiology of the Protective Airway Reflexes

The patient with a difficult airway experiences early and frequent obstruction that is difficult to overcome. The two main causes of problems in patients with a difficult airway are the altered anatomy of the airway and the protective reflexes of the airway. These reflexes are coughing, apnea, swallowing, and laryngospasm. Under normal circumstances, the protective reflexes and other physiologic mechanisms of the oropharynx and hypopharynx allow a remarkable coordination of vocalization, ventilation, and alimentation, while the protective reflexes prevent any trespass by a foreign body, including an endotracheal tube, into the tracheobronchial tree. The activation of these reflexes will lead to laryngospasm, which is accompanied by coughing, apnea, and varying degrees of airway obstruction. The apnea and airway obstruction leads to hypoxia as the oxygen reserve of the functional residual capacity (FRC) is utilized. Positive pressure is often used to ventilate the obstructed patient. Positive pressure greater than 5 to 10 cmH_2O will cause barotrauma to the larynx, which may well intensify and contribute to the laryngospasm and airway obstruction. I have seen many instances in which partial laryngospasm that could have been managed with gentle positive end-expiratory pressure (PEEP) of 5 to 10 cmH_2O converted into total laryngospasm by the application of 20 to 30 cmH_2O of pressure in an attempt to "break" the laryngospasm. Positive pressure cannot break complete laryngospasm. Excessive positive pressure also may result in inflation of the stomach and the danger of regurgitation and aspiration. On the other hand, obstruction of the airway associated with hypoxia may lead to negative postobstructive pulmonary edema (see Ch. 13). Inflation of the stomach may also reduce ventilation owing to elevation of the diaphragm secondary to the increased intra-abdominal pressure. In order to ventilate the patient and intubate the trachea, the protective reflexes of the airway must be overcome.

Pharmacology of the Depression of the Protective Airway Reflexes

Control of the airway can be accomplished by the pharmacologic depression of the neurogenic control of the protective reflexes, by the pharmacologic depression or paralysis of the muscles that execute these reflexes, or by a combination of the two. The depression of the reflexes can be accomplished by topical anesthesia, general anesthesia, or a combination of the two. Muscle relaxants can be given to paralyze the muscles that execute the protective reflexes. However, the use of muscle relaxants to paralyze the muscles of the protective airway reflexes in order to "facilitate" intubation may be fraught with danger. Muscle relaxants should be given only after very careful evaluation of the patient. On the other hand, administering small doses of succinylcholine to a patient with complete laryngospasm who is developing severe desaturation may relax the laryngospasm and allow the patient to be ventilated. This is discussed later in this chapter.

CLINICAL MANAGEMENT OF THE DIFFICULT AIRWAY

Informed Consent

After the potentially difficult airway is identified, the anesthesiologist must share this information with the parents and the surgeon. The parents must be informed that there is an increased risk in anesthetizing their infant or child, including the rare but nonetheless ever-present danger of a fatal airway problem. They must answer two questions: (1) Are they willing to take the increased anesthetic risk associated with the difficult airway, including the potential for an emergency cricothyrotomy, in order to have whatever surgical procedure is planned for their child? (2) If an airway cannot be established by nonsurgical means, should an elective tracheotomy be done to permit the surgery, or should the procedure be cancelled and replanned for another day? The surgical team as well as the parents must answer this second question. If the airway problem is severe or the postoperative course potentially protracted, consideration should be given to performing an elective tracheotomy at the beginning of the procedure. This is an infrequent occurrence, but the need for it occasionally arises. Although this can be a very difficult question to answer preoperatively, it is even more difficult to answer during prolonged attempts at intubation, when a decision must be made and the possibilities have not been discussed with the parents.

Elective Tracheotomy

There are two approaches to management of the airway for tracheotomy: following placement of an endotracheal tube and without an endotracheal tube. The preferred technique is after placement of an endotracheal tube. However, intubation may be quite difficult, and in lieu of repeated unsuccessful attempts at intubation that may cause hypoxia and dysrhythmias, elective tracheotomy can be done without intubation if management of the airway is adequate. The technique combines general anesthesia with a volatile agent such as halothane with local anesthesia of the upper airway and trachea. If the child is cooperative, topical lidocaine should be applied to the oropharynx before induction. This allows early placement of an oral airway should obstruction occur. If the child is not cooperative, attempts at oral topicalization should be abandoned until after general anesthesia is induced. Small amounts of lidocaine can then be applied to the tongue and hypopharynx. Care must be taken not to evoke laryngospasm, however. Nitrous oxide is often used for the initial induction, but is discontinued after adequate levels of halothane have been tolerated so that the FRC will contain the highest possible concentration of oxygen should obstruction occur. After adequate general anesthesia is obtained, the area of the tracheotomy is infiltrated with 0.5 percent lidocaine with 1:200,000 epinephrine. The tracheotomy should proceed in an expeditious but controlled manner. If the patient is coughing and otherwise indicating inadequate anesthesia, the procedure should be interrupted until control is obtained. This can be done by increasing the concentration of halothane, by giving lidocaine 1.5 mg/kg IV, or by infiltrating more local anesthetic. After stabilization, the procedure continues. When the trachea is ready for the incision, lidocaine 1 to 2 mg/kg can be injected into the trachea to minimize coughing.

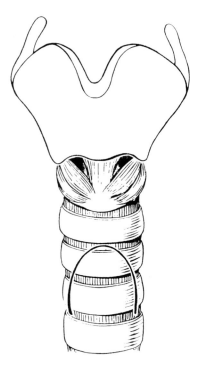

Fig. 6-8. Inverted U incision for tracheotomy.

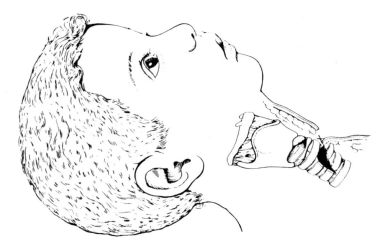

Fig. 6-9. Suture of tracheal wall to skin to maintain an open airway even if the tracheotomy tube is displaced.

Many techniques have been described for performing tracheotomies. One technique, known as the inverted U tracheotomy, has certain advantages that make it particularly appealing (Fig. 6-8). The two major features of this technique are the inverted U-shaped incision it employs and the suturing of the tracheal flap to the skin edge. The advantage of the inverted U-shaped incision is that there is less damage to the tracheal cartilage, resulting in a more favorable reconstitution of the trachea when the trachea is closed. The advantage of suturing the tracheal flap to the skin is that if the tracheotomy tube is accidentally dislodged, the airway remains patent (Fig. 6-9). This advantage is extremely important for the anesthesiologist in the operative and postoperative periods. When the tracheotomy is no longer needed, the trachea is released from the skin by cutting the sutures. An infrequent potential disadvantage of the technique is that a reapproximation of the edges of the tracheal incision may have to be done.

Emergency Management of the Difficult Airway

Airway obstruction and hypoxia can occur with such alarming speed that the surgeon and emergency airway equipment must be in the operating room before the induction of anesthesia. In unusual circumstances, control of the airway may be lost and not re-established. In the face of an impossible airway, the anesthesiologist cannot remain frozen performing unsuccessful techniques, but must initiate a different approach. This requires an emergency surgical opening of the airway. Three approaches are mentioned in the literature: (1) emergency tracheotomy, (2) emergency cricothyrotomy, and (3) emergency transtracheal ventilation.[2] In my experience, emergency tracheotomy cannot be performed rapidly enough. Therefore, the most rapid method for oxygenating the patient is by cricothyrotomy. This technique is the method of choice for management of the

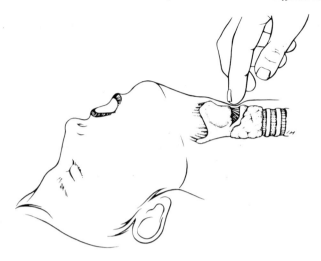

Fig. 6-10. Palpation of the cricothyroid membrane.

obstructed airway when endotracheal intubation cannot be accomplished. The cricothyroid membrane is identified and a transverse incision is made down to the cricothyroid membrane (Fig. 6-10). The cricothyroid membrane is then incised (Fig. 6-11). A tracheal dilator is inserted to enlarge the opening in the membrane, and a tracheotomy tube or endotracheal tube is inserted. After stabilization of the patient, either a permanent tracheotomy is done and the surgery is performed or the cricothyrotomy is used for the operation and immediate postoperative period and then allowed to close. If the patient is not stable, the operation is terminated and performed another day. Several mechanical devices for performing a cricothyrotomy have been introduced but there have been

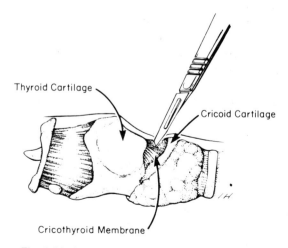

Thyroid Cartilage

Cricoid Cartilage

Cricothyroid Membrane

Fig. 6-11. Incision of the cricothyroid membrane.

problems with these devices. It is my opinion that the surgical approach described above is the technique of choice at this time.

Preoperative Preparation

After identification of the difficult airway or once it is suspected that one may be lurking just inside the oropharynx, the anesthesiologist must prepare a game plan. This includes consultation with colleagues, a perusal of the medical literature, and preparation of the anesthesia equipment for the various contingencies that might arise. This equipment includes: (1) endotracheal tubes of several sizes, (2) straight and curved laryngoscope blades, and (3) functioning fiberoptic equipment, if the anesthesiologist is appropriately trained in its use.[3–6] The fiberoptic laryngoscope or bronchoscope can potentially facilitate intubation in patients with a difficult airway. However, skillful use of these instruments must be acquired in the normal airway, where intubation can easily be accomplished if airway problems arise. The period of ongoing management of the difficult airway is not the time to learn how to use unfamiliar equipment.

Premedication

The ordinary pediatric patient may be premedicated for two reasons: sedation and the drying of secretions. In the patient with a potentially difficult airway, a third possible reason arises: increasing the gastric pH and reducing the gastric volume in order to minimize the problems of acid aspiration.[7–9] If the patient has a documented or suspected difficult airway, sedation should be avoided because of the possibility of airway obstruction on the ward, in the elevator, or while awaiting the induction of anesthesia. The best rule to follow is that if there is any question that sedation might lead to airway obstruction, it should be avoided. Drying agents are useful since many patients with a difficult airway appear to have excessive secretions. In addition, instrumentation of the airway during attempts at intubation increases the flow of secretions. Atropine 0.02 mg/kg PO or glycopyrrolate 0.05 mg/kg PO is recommended for reducing these secretions. A potential problem that is rare in the pediatric patient but more frequent in the one with a difficult airway is the aspiration of gastric contents. This occurs more frequently in patients with a difficult airway because of the problem of airway obstruction, which often leads to the use of excessive positive pressure in order to either break a ''laryngospasm'' or increase ventilation. At any rate, the stomach is often distended, which may increase the possibility of regurgitation and aspiration. To minimize this danger, cimetidine and/or metoclopramide have been recommended by some.[7–9] The use of cimetidine and metoclopramide have not achieved full acceptance in routine practice, and perhaps with the longer use of these drugs, we may find that their disadvantages outweigh their advantages. This subject is discussed in more detail in Chapter 2.

The Induction and Maintenance of Anesthesia

There has been an increasing appreciation for the psychological trauma that occurs with the separation of the parent and child at the time of anesthesia and surgery. This has led to techniques of induction that allow the parents to be with the child during the early phases of induction. These techniques may still be used for the child with a difficult airway, but careful screening must be done beforehand. If there is a history of obstruction with induction, the child should have anesthesia induced in the operating room, with the surgical team ready. Whether or not the parent should be allowed in the operating room with the child is a very difficult issue. The anesthesiologist who is very experienced with parents in the induction area might be able to manage the airway and the parents. On the other hand, the inexperienced anesthesiologist may decide that it would be better if the parents not accompany the child. Otherwise, induction may be accomplished in the induction area, but with the recognition that the patient may have to be rapidly moved to the operating room. The major danger during the induction of anesthesia is obstruction of the airway. Early in the induction phase of anesthesia, the muscles of the oropharynx begin to relax, and the airway may become either partially or fully obstructed. Attempts at correcting this with an oral airway often result in activation of the protective airway reflexes, such as coughing, apnea, and laryngospasm, because of the very light level of anesthesia. A technique used to minimize this problem is topicalization of the oropharynx with lidocaine before induction. Lidocaine paste (5 percent) can be placed on the tongue, and as it melts will be distributed into the oropharynx of the small infant or child. If the child will not allow the anesthesiologist to do this, it may be able to be accomplished by the parent. This will topicalize the supraglottic airway either partially or completely, and allow the early introduction of an oral airway without activation of the protective reflexes.

An induction technique for infants and children from 1 to 4 years of age is the use of rectal methohexital. (Chapter 2 discusses this in more detail.) The technique allows an induction with a minimum of hassle for the child. The parents appreciate it, since the separation from their child is peaceful. The dose is 30 mg/kg, and the drug is administered as a 5 percent solution. Approximately 95 percent of patients will be induced within 5 to 10 minutes and the anesthetic lasts approximately 60 to 90 minutes, depending on the anesthetic technique used. After induction, the child is put on the abdomen or side, with its head turned. This will help maintain the airway while the child is being transported to the operating room. If there is any question about the ability to manage the airway with this type of induction, it should not be used. There are several other methods for inducing anesthesia in infants and children with difficult airways. These include inhalation, ketamine, and intravenous barbiturates. Regardless of the technique employed, I favor the preinduction use of topical anesthesia whenever it is easily tolerated. If an IV is in place, glycopyrrolate is administered, and small doses of a barbiturate are given to sedate the child, who is then moved to the operating room, where the induction can be completed with further doses of sodium thiopental or an inhalation induction. The dose of sodium thiopental in this situation is 1 to 2 mg/kg. The usual induction dose of this drug in children is from 4 to 6 mg/kg, which may relax the muscles of the oropharynx, leading to a rapid obstruction of the airway. If the child is cooperative but does not have an IV in place, an inhalation induction is accomplished. This is begun with a 70/30 mixture of nitrous oxide/oxygen, using a high flow. After the child adjusts to the smell of the nitrous oxide and the anesthetic system, halothane is slowly introduced in 0.5 percent increments. As the child tolerates each increment of halothane, the concentration is increased. It usually takes about 30 seconds for each increment to be tolerated. If the child coughs, holds its breath, or shows any other signs of intolerance of the halothane, the level of halothane is maintained for a longer period or turned back for a short period before the next incremental increase. The usual dialed induction concentrations of halothane are 3 to 5 percent. After the lid reflex is lost, the nitrous oxide is decreased to 50 percent. If this is tolerated, the nitrous oxide is decreased to 25 percent and then finally turned off. The nitrous oxide is discontinued as soon as possible so that the lungs contain the highest possible F_IO_2, thereby increasing the margin of safety should obstruction occur. The patient is allowed to breathe spontaneously throughout the entire induction. As the anesthetic level deepens, the patient's ventilation is gently assisted. Spontaneous ventilation offers a margin of safety: if the patient experiences an obstruction, the continued redistribution of the halothane will result in a lowering of the concentration of halothane. The anesthetic will lighten and the patient will, it is hoped, regain control of the airway.

The Uncooperative Child With a Difficult Airway

The uncooperative child with a difficult airway presents a real challenge for the induction of anesthesia. Crying increases the amount of secretions and often leads to a very unpleasant induction experience. In this situation the anesthesiologist may elect any of several techniques. At times a gentle inhalation induction can be performed on a crying child. However, "gorilla inductions," in which the patient is forcefully restrained on the operating table with an anesthetic mask clamped tightly over the face have no place in pediatric anesthesia. Two other methods for inducing anesthesia in uncooperative children are preferable: the use of rectal methohexital or ketamine. In an uncooperative child who is already upset, administration of rectal methohexital may prove even more upsetting and difficult to accomplish. Therefore, in this situation ketamine 3 mg/kg IM is given. Following the ketamine, an inhalation anesthetic is begun as tolerated. If the child experiences intermittent obstruction at the beginning of the induction, the F_IO_2 is begun at 50 percent rather than 30 percent because of the concern for obstruction and the difficulty of oxygenation. The halothane is introduced as tolerated. An IV should be started as soon as possible after the induction, regardless of the technique used.

Laryngospasm

Problems may occur during the induction of anesthesia. Patients with a difficult airway usually experience obstruction at very light levels of anesthesia. They do this for a number of reasons, which include excessive secretions, abnormal airway, and relaxation of the oropharynx. The placement of an oral airway often activates the protective reflexes unless topical anesthesia has been applied. Varying degrees of laryngospasm may occur, leading to varying degrees of obstruction and ventilation.[10] Part of the reflex of laryngospasm is apnea and coughing, which further complicates the management of the airway. All of these factors culminate in the inability to properly oxygenate and anesthetize the patient. Positive pressure of 5 to 10 cmH$_2$0 gently applied will increase the pressure gradient from the anesthetic circuit to the lungs and increase the ventilation and thereby the oxygenation and anesthetization of the patient if the obstruction and laryngospasm are partial. Cricoid pressure should be applied to minimize gastric distension. On occasion, the inexperienced anesthesiologist, feeling quite uncomfortable at this point, will apply excessive positive pressure in an attempt to "break" the laryngospasm. Positive pressure cannot "break" laryngospasm. As a matter of fact, positive pressure of greater than 10 cmH$_2$0 can and of itself lead to laryngospasm, coughing, and apnea. Usually, the unsettled anesthesiologist will keep using the flush valve to fill the anesthetic bag because the excessive pressures and poor fit of the anesthetic mask lead to an empty breathing bag. This greatly prolongs the induction, since the anesthetic is continually flushed from the system and diluted. The patient in this circumstance may become more lightly anesthetized and be more of a problem. In addition, the high pressure that is applied to the airway may result in the passage of the gases down the esophagus and into the stomach. The resulting scenario is all too familiar: the stomach will distend, elevating the diaphragm and reducing the ventilation even more. The anesthetic level will lighten and the patient may begin to struggle. The pharmacologic maneuvers necessary to control the difficult airway depress the protective reflexes of the airway. This is the reason for the use of topical anesthesia before the induction of anesthesia; for the gentle induction with varying combinations of nitrous oxide and halothane; and for the small amounts of PEEP and cricoid pressure to improve ventilation should obstruction occur. Another problem of complete airway obstruction with resulting large negative intrathoracic pressures and hypoxia is the occurrence of postobstructive pulmonary edema. Chapter 13 carries a discussion of this problem.

After the induction of anesthesia is accomplished, an IV should be begun as quickly as possible. The advantage of this is to facilitate airway management. If secretions are a problem, glycopyrrolate 0.01 mg/kg IV should be given. A newly rediscovered technique for easing an induction is the use of lidocaine in a dose of 1 to 1.5 mg/kg IV. This may be repeated in 5 minutes. Lidocaine will deepen anesthesia, depress the protective airway reflexes, and enable the anesthesiologist to proceed with a smoother inhalation induction. No more than 3 mg/kg of lidocaine should be given intravenously in a 5-minute period and no more than 6 mg/kg in 30 minutes. The goal of all of these pharmacologic maneuvers is to achieve a high-enough concentration of anesthetic to depress the protective reflexes and facilitate ventilation and intubation. At times, laryngospasm and airway obstruction may be irreversible, and ventilation of the patient will be impossible despite turning off of the anesthetic. Serious ventricular dysrhythmias may also occur. This is a very difficult clinical situation. As the airway obstruction increases, it is often difficult to determine if the cause is laryngospasm, anatomic obstruction of the upper airway, or a combination of these factors. As ventilation and oxygen saturation diminish, so do the possibilities for solving the problem through inhalation techniques. Most would consider the use of succinylcholine controversial for elective intubation in a patient with a difficult airway. However, in the condition of progressive obstruction as described, succinylcholine 1 mg/kg IV will produce muscle relaxation, enabling the patient to be ventilated if the problem is laryngospasm. However, it must be recognized that if the problem is an anatomic airway obstruction, muscle relaxants may increase this obstruction. Giving muscle relaxants has been referred to as "burning bridges." However, if the airway cannot be managed and the patient cannot be ventilated, the bridges are already burning, and succinylcholine may be an appropriate emergency drug in an attempt to oxygenate the patient. If laryngospasm is the problem, ventilation of the patient should be possible within 30 to 45 seconds. After ventilation is accomplished and the airway controlled, then attempts can be made at laryngoscopy and intubation. If ventilation cannot be accomplished, the problem is due to factors other than laryngospasm and a cricothyrotomy must be performed immediately. If there is any doubt, the choice is immediate cricothyrotomy.

Topicalization of the Airway

At times, the lack of cooperation of the child makes topical anesthesia before induction difficult or impossible. In this case, two options are open to the anesthesiologist after the initial induction of anesthesia. The best of the two is a translaryngeal or transtracheal block with lidocaine 3 mg/kg. This technique is quite useful early in the scenario of an obstructed airway or even before it becomes obstructed, and will reduce the risk of laryngospasm. This block is technically difficult to preform in infants under 1 year of age because of the small anatomy involved and the danger of penetration of undesired tissue by the needle. For this reason, the technique is infrequently used in infants less than 1 year old. The second option is to coat the oral airway with lidocaine paste or to use 10 percent lidocaine spray into the hypopharynx after induction. Usually this will anesthetize the area, but it may induce a period of coughing and apnea or laryngospasm if the child is very lightly anesthetized. Lidocaine spray is not recommended for children under 6 months of age because of the potential for large doses being administered, with resulting cardiovascular and/or central nervous system toxicity.

Ketamine for Intubation of Infants

The last technique described for induction and intubation is that which is used in small infants under 1 year of age, such as the patient in Figure 6-12. Glycopyrrolate is administered preoperatively in an oral dose of 0.05 mg/kg. After

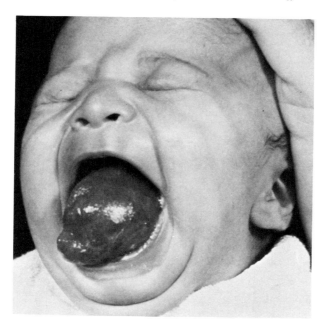

Fig. 6-12. Infant with a large hemangioma of the tongue that partially obstructed the airway and interfered with alimentation.

adequate oral topicalization of the infant's airway, a 3-mg/kg dose of ketamine is administered intramuscularly. An IV is begun. Laryngoscopy is attempted while oxygen is insufflated (Fig. 6-13). If the child moves and this interferes with laryngoscopy, small doses of ketamine (0.5 mg/kg) are given to facilitate the laryngoscopy. There are several methods for insufflating oxygen. A laryngoscope with an oxygen source at the tip has been described. An assistant can hold the anesthesia mask to the side of the face, and using a high flow of oxygen, can increase the FiO_2 during the laryngoscopy. A nasal or hypopharyngeal catheter can be used to provide a high oxygen concentration in the oro- and hypopharynx. Frequent episodes of apnea, coughing, and movement indicate a need for more topical anesthesia and more ketamine. If an IV is in place initially, the ketamine can be given intravenously. The initial dose is 1 mg/kg, followed by titrated doses of 0.5 mg/kg. The key to the technique is good topical anesthesia.

Laryngoscopy and Intubation

After the patient has been adequately anesthetized by whatever technique is chosen, the time for laryngoscopy has arrived. If the patient coughs, swallows, or shows any other evidence of inadequate anesthesia that interferes with laryngoscopy, the depth of the anesthesia is inadequate, and deeper anesthesia or more topical anesthetic is needed. Laryngoscopy can be considered successful if any part of the larynx or epiglottis is visualized. If only the arytenoids or epiglottis

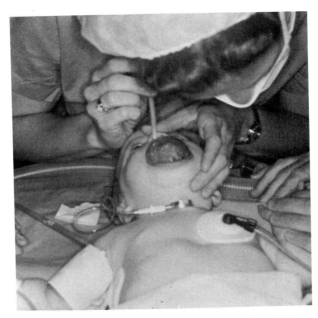

Fig. 6-13. Ketamine and topical anesthesia for intubation.

is visualized, a stylet may be needed to direct the tip of the endotracheal tube. A moderate angle of approximately 70 to 90 degrees is needed. The end of the stylet should remain within the tip of the endotracheal tube to avoid damage to the larynx or trachea. The endotracheal tube is advanced slowly in the midline toward the laryngeal opening, and is placed under the laryngeal side of the epiglottis. Two maneuvers can be used for intubation: (1) the epiglottis can be lifted with the tip of the endotracheal tube, allowing better visualization of the larynx and visual direction of the endotracheal tube; or (2) the tube can be advanced in a blind fashion underneath the epiglottis, listening for breath sounds or watching for condensation of moisture in the endotracheal tube with exhalation. When it is thought that the tip of the tube is in the opening of the larynx, the endotracheal tube is advanced off the stylet. The tube and stylet should never be forced into the larynx.

When difficulty exposing the glottis occurs, two people may be able to successfully complete the procedure. The laryngoscopist uses his or her left hand to apply posterior pressure over the larynx, thereby exposing the glottis. This may require considerable pressure. The second person passes the endotracheal tube while the laryngoscopist holds position and visualization. This is referred to as the "two-handed" laryngoscopy technique (Fig. 6-14) (Creighton RE, personal communication).

If laryngoscopy is unsuccessful (which is defined as the inability to visualize any part of the airway), several options are available: (1) blind oral or blind nasal intubation, (2) retrograde intubation, (3) fiberoptic intubation, (4) tracheotomy, or (5) aborting the surgery if the anesthesiologist does not feel con-

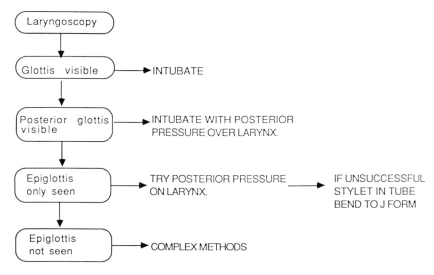

Fig. 6-14. Approach to difficult airway. (Courtesy of R.E. Creighton, M.D.)

fident to proceed or if the patient has dysrhythmias that cannot be corrected or persistent episodes of desaturation that are difficult to reverse. It should be stressed that this last option should be followed when in doubt.

Techniques of Blind Oral and Blind Nasal Intubation

The major requirements for "blind" intubation techniques are (1) an anatomic appreciation of the path that the endotracheal tube must take to enter the larynx, (2) adequate anesthesia to prevent the airway reflexes from defeating attempts to intubate the patient, and (3) spontaneous ventilation.

Blind Oral Intubation

For blind oral intubation, a stylet shaped to conform to the anticipated anatomy of the patient's airway is used. This configuration is usually the J or hockey-stick shape. The bent end of the tube must be relatively short in an infant in order to enter the larynx. The stylet should be lubricated and should be removable from the endotracheal tube in vitro. The ultimate frustration is the successful introduction of an endotracheal tube followed by the inability to extract the stylet. A MAC blade is used to open the airway. Laryngoscopy per se (i.e., visualization of the airway) should not be attempted further. The inability to visualize the airway has already been established, and further attempts may lead to trauma and may distort the airway. The purpose of the laryngoscope is to maintain and open the airway. The blade is placed in the vallecula and lifted until the breath sounds are their loudest. The endotracheal tube is advanced in the midline in the anticipated path for intubation. Increasing breath sounds indicate that the tip of the tube is approaching the larynx. The connector to the precordial stethoscope can be placed in the tip of the endotracheal tube in order to better appreciate breath sounds. A decrease in breath sounds indicates that the tip is too far to the right, too far to the left, or has slipped under the larynx into the esophagus. The endotracheal tube must be withdrawn a short distance and redirected. The tube should be advanced short distances with inspiration, since the laryngeal opening is maximal at that time. After breath sounds are heard maximally and condensation appears rhythmically with exhalation, the endotracheal tube is slipped off the stylet and, it is hoped, into the trachea. If at any time during the procedure the patient bites the laryngoscope, coughs, or exhibits other difficult behavior, attempts at intubation should be suspended temporarily and the anesthetic level deepened and/or topical anesthesia administered. Transtracheal or translaryngeal techniques are often quite useful at this point if they have not already been used. The major reason for failure to intubate the patient with the blind technique is inadequate anesthetic depression of the protective airway reflexes.

Blind Nasal Intubation

The technique for blind nasal intubation requires a sound understanding of the anatomy of the area as well as proper preparation of the patient. The nasopharynx should be topicalized with a local anesthetic and a vasoconstrictor even if general anesthesia is used. Topicalization accomplishes two goals: it provides anesthesia of the nasopharynx and it produces vasoconstriction to decrease trauma and bleeding. The drugs used for topicalization are a combination of equal parts of 0.25 percent phenylephrine and 4 percent lidocaine. If the need for a nasal intubation is anticipated before the induction of anesthesia, the solution is applied before induction. This can only be accomplished in cooperative patients. The reason for early topicalization is that should airway obstruction occur at extremely light levels of anesthesia, the nasotracheal tube can be used as a nasopharyngeal airway. This technique was used in the patient in Figure 6-15. The topical anesthesia will diminish the likelihood of activation of the protective airway reflexes at these light levels of anesthesia. One difficulty encountered in nasotracheal intubation is the relatively anterior position of the larynx. In practical terms, the nasotracheal tube has to angle upward into the larynx. One way to achieve a slight anterior deflection of the nasotracheal tube is to curl it within its package prior to the time of intubation. During prolonged attempts at nasotracheal intubation the tube may become warm and quite pliable, and will not curve anteriorly into the larynx. Another way to create an anterior angulation of the tube is to place a stylet in the tube and then remove it immediately before intubation. Currently, there is a commercially available endotracheal tube with a controllable tip. However, this tube is not made in pediatric sizes.

As the nasotracheal tube is blindly advanced, the anesthesiologist must continually mentally picture the position of the tip of the tube. The first major obstruction is the adenoid tissue of the nasopharynx. This tissue is friable and

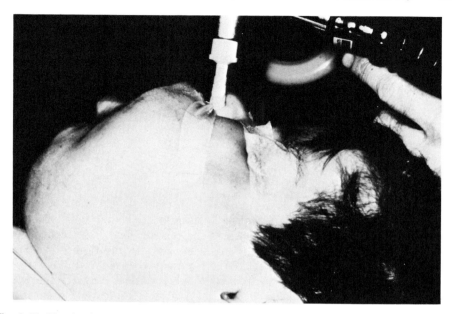

Fig. 6-15. Nasal tube used as a nasal airway in a child with massive lymphangiomas. Obstruction had occurred immediately after induction in this case. Topical anesthesia applied before induction allowed the insertion of the nasal tube into the hypopharynx, immediately restoring ventilation and allowing a smooth completion of the induction and nasotracheal intubation.

bleeds quite easily despite gentle manipulation. At times a small core of adenoid tissue may remain within the nasotracheal tube. After the tube passes this area, a quick look into the hypopharynx with the laryngoscope at the tip of the tube will reveal whether or not any tissue has been cored by the tube. If so, this tissue should be suctioned out of the tube. The next obstruction to passing the tube is the area of the epiglottis. Often the nasotracheal tube will course into the vallecula. Several maneuvers can be performed in an attempt to pass the tube under the epiglottis. These various maneuvers include turning the patient's head from side to side or gently pushing the larynx to one side with the anesthesiologist's free hand. The signal that the nasotracheal tube has passed the epiglottis is that the breath sounds will become louder. At this point the anesthesiologist should note the length of nasotracheal tube that has been inserted. A relatively short distance now remains between the tip of the tube and the larynx. With each inspiration the tube is moved forward approximately 1 to 2 cm, and if intubation is unsuccessful, as revealed by a decrease or absence of breath sounds, the tube need only be withdrawn 2 to 3 cm, to the point previously noted on the nasotracheal tube, and not back into the hypopharynx. Successful intubation is indicated by breath sounds, coughing, the condensation of moisture with exhalation, bilateral chest movement and breath sounds after attaching the anesthesia circuit and inflating the lungs, visualizing with a fiberoptic bronchoscope, and where available, end-tidal CO_2. Surgery should not begin if there is any doubt about placement of the tube. If there is doubt about the length of nasotracheal tube that is in the trachea, the position of the tube can be confirmed by taking a chest x-ray or through the use of a fiberoptic bronchoscope. If the nasotracheal tube is barely within the larynx, changing the position of the head during the surgical procedure might well result in extubation. Also, changes in head position may result in endobronchial intubation if the tip of the tube is at the carina. Coughing, changes in oxygen saturation, and premature ventricular contractions are signs that the endotracheal tube has irritated the carina or is endobronchial.

Use of a Stylet in Nasotracheal Intubations

Occasionally, all maneuvers, whether visual or blind, to advance a nasotracheal tube into the larynx fail, as the tube continuously courses posteriorly into the esophagus. This is easy to visualize in the case of blind nasotracheal intubations, as the nasotracheal tube remains in a posterior position in the hypopharynx under the epiglottis, as depicted in Figure 6-16. In some children during the visual placement of a nasotracheal tube, advancement of the nasotracheal tube into the larynx may not be successful because of inadequate room in the hypopharynx for McGill forceps to guide the tube into the larynx. In these situations, a stylet can be used.[11] The nasotracheal tube is introduced as in Figure 6-16.[11] The stylet is premeasured before the nasotracheal tube is introduced since introducing the nasotracheal tube with a stylet can cause considerable damage to the nasopharynx. The stylet should be bent according to the anatomic path of the nasotracheal tube, with a short 30-degree angle on the distal end. The stylet should be well lubricated and introduced gently down the nasotracheal tube. If the stylet has not been premeasured before the introduction of the nasotracheal tube, another tube of the same length can be used to measure the

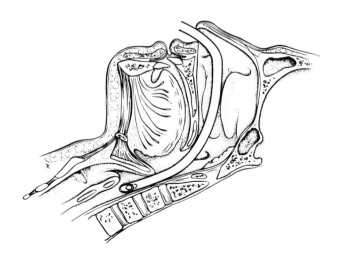

Fig. 6-16. Nasotracheal tube passing into the esophagus.

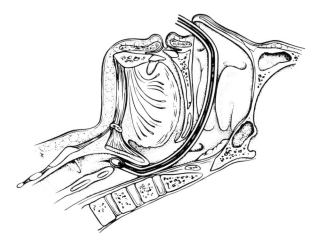

Fig. 6-17. Stylet with a slight anterior angle passed into the nasotracheal tube to redirect the tip of the tube.

appropriate length of the tube. After the nasotracheal tube is in place and the stylet has been introduced, the proximal end of the tube and stylet can be gently levered posteriorly, as in Figure 6-17, resulting in an anterior movement of the distal stylet and tube. As the tube is maneuvered and approaches the larynx, breath sounds will get louder and condensation may appear with exhalation in the tube. At this point, the endotracheal tube can be slipped off the stylet (Fig. 6-18). The nasotracheal tube will follow the direction in which the stylet has been curved. If the stylet is too soft, it will lose its anterior angulation. At times, the tip of the nasotracheal tube will become lodged in the anterior commissure

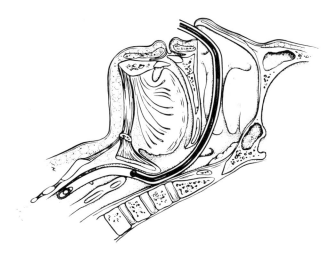

Fig. 6-18. Nasotracheal tube advanced off the stylet and into the trachea.

of the cords and will not easily advance. In this case, the nasotracheal tube should be backed out a short distance until the patient's breath sounds become louder, and should then be advanced. The other maneuver that is sometimes successful in this situation after the stylet has been completely removed is to rotate the tube 360 degrees so that the bevel will rotate and redirect the tube through the larynx. This technique of a stylet in the nasotracheal tube has been used mainly in the operating room for blind nasotracheal intubations when, for one reason or another, laryngoscopy and direct visualization are impossible. Another application of this technique has been in the emergency room or intensive care unit when the same situation has prevailed.

Retrograde Intubation

The principle of retrograde intubation is the passage of a stylet (either a wire stylet in a plastic catheter or a "J" wire) in a retrograde direction, through a needle in the cricothyroid membrane, into the oropharynx or nasopharynx.[12] The stylet will pass out through the mouth or nose of the patient, or become obstructed in the hypo- or nasopharynx, in which case it can be visualized in the hypopharynx by laryngoscopy and pulled out with McGill forceps or a Kelly clamp. The endotracheal tube is slid over the wire and into the trachea. The risk:benefit ratio of this procedure must be carefully evaluated. The cricothyroid membrane develops at approximately 2 to 3 years of age. The use of the retrograde technique in children under this age not only may be technically difficult, but there is also concern about the normal development of these immature structures.

Either orotracheal or nasotracheal intubation can be accomplished through the technique of retrograde intubation. In the case of orotracheal intubation the stylet is extracted through the mouth. In the case of nasotracheal intubation a small suction catheter is introduced through the nose into the hypopharynx. The retrograde stylet and the suction catheter are then pulled out through the mouth and tied together, and the suction catheter that was introduced through the nose is withdrawn back through the nose, thereby pulling the stylet back through the oropharynx and out through the nasopharynx.

Various combinations of needles and stylets have been described, including an epidural needle and a disposable epidural catheter, a No. 20 Angiocath with a "J" wire, and a No. 14 Intracath with a long catheter. There are basically two techniques for accomplishing retrograde intubation: (1) with the patient awake but topicalized and sedated and (2) with the patient anesthetized and topicalized. The first technique requires a very cooperative patient; very few teenagers will tolerate this type of an anesthetic, and the vast majority under age 15 will need general anesthesia to accomplish retrograde intubation. In these patients the retrograde technique is accomplished with the patient anesthetized and breathing spontaneously. A local anesthetic is infiltrated into the skin and cricothyroid membrane, and a translaryngeal block is done. For the latter, a small syringe containing topical lidocaine 3 mg/kg is placed on the needle selected. The needle is introduced in a slightly cephalad direction. The syringe serves three purposes:

(1) it acts as a firm handle to help pass the needle through the cricothyroid membrane, (2) it determines when the tip of the needle is within the larynx, and (3) it permits a translaryngeal block to be accomplished. The position of the needle is confirmed by aspiration of air with the syringe. At this point, a translaryngeal block is done with lidocaine if it was not done earlier in the induction. After the intralaryngeal position of the needle is verified by air aspiration, the stylet is inserted through the needle and advanced gently into the hypopharynx. If it does not pass smoothly it should not be forced. The patient's mouth is opened and the hypopharynx visualized. The stylet is then brought out through the mouth. Sometimes the stylet will spontaneously come out through the mouth or the nose. For oral intubation, the endotracheal tube is then threaded over the stylet. It takes two people to do a retrograde intubation, one to secure the stylet and the other to advance the endotracheal tube. The stylet is placed under mild tension by having the assistant holding both of its ends, and the endotracheal tube is then advanced into the larynx. Since the end of the stylet is anterior in the larynx, the tip of the endotracheal tube may catch on the anterior commissure of the vocal cords and be difficult to pass. In this case, tension on the stylet should be relaxed and the endotracheal tube withdrawn slightly and then readvanced into the larynx while listening to the patient's breath sounds. When the breath sounds are loud the wire stylet is pulled out of the endotracheal tube and the endotracheal tube is advanced down the trachea.

Sometimes the distal angle that the endotracheal tube must traverse may be so sharp that the tube will not bend sufficiently anteriorly and will therefore advance posteriorly below the larynx. In order to angulate the tube anteriorly into the larynx, a standard, firm metal stylet with a 70- to 90-degree bend at the tip can be introduced into the endotracheal tube beside the wire stylet ("J" wire or catheter) already present, and the patient's breath sounds followed to determine the location of the tip of the endotracheal tube. When the breath sounds are maximal the endotracheal tube is advanced over the metal stylet, the wire stylet is pulled out of the endotracheal tube, and the endotracheal tube is advanced down the trachea.

If the older child or teenager is cooperative, retrograde intubation using a neurolept technique can be accomplished. In this situation, the skin and the cricothyroid membrane, as well as the oro- and hypopharynx, have to be well anesthetized. A transtracheal or transcricothyroid block should be performed with lidocaine 3 mg/kg. If a nasotracheal intubation is to be used, the nasopharynx should be topicalized as previously described. Any amount of coughing, swallowing, or movement will make this technique extremely difficult, and indicates the need for further topical anesthesia, sedation, or both.

The Unsuspected Difficult Airway

As the anesthesiologist fine-tunes his or her practice and becomes more familiar with the various congenital and acquired airway problems, there will be fewer and fewer unsuspected difficult airways encountered.[3] However, there are children who appear to be almost normal yet have very difficult airways. Many of these children also have other anatomic abnormalities that should suggest the potential presence of a difficult airway. An example of this association is found in the Treacher Collins and Goldenhar syndromes. These patients may have microstomia or a dermoid cyst of the eye, which may be the reason why such a patient is having surgery. Children with abnormal ears should have a careful evaluation of the airway.

The unsuspected difficult airway presents just as its name suggests. It may manifest itself early in the induction of anesthesia, with an obstruction developing and becoming difficult to reverse. It may become manifest at the time of laryngoscopy, with difficulty in visualizing the larynx or any other part of the airway. Various explanations for the difficulty enter the anesthesiologist's mind, but the first of these is usually inadequate relaxation or an inappropriate laryngoscope blade. Often, several doses of succinylcholine and multiple changes of the laryngoscope blade bring no improvement in the ability to visualize the airway. At this point two other possibilities enter the differential diagnosis: (1) an anatomic deformity of the airway and (2) masseter spasm. The latter is an active clenching of the jaw, and in some patients it is an early sign of the malignant hyperthermia syndrome. Chapter 15 discusses this subject in detail.

The last but most frequent possibility is that there is an anatomic deformity of the airway. One of the goals of an anesthesiologist must be a recognition of his or her level of technical expertise and experience, so that when a difficult laryngoscopy occurs, a rapid evaluation of the situation should quickly pinpoint the difficulty. A nerve stimulator will determine if the relaxation is sufficient. Attention should then be directed to reevaluating the anatomy of laryngoscopy and the airway. The airway axis should be reevaluated and realigned. The soft tissue under the mandible should be reevaluated by the Schwartz hyoid maneuver. Difficult intubations and laryngoscopies do not occur very frequently in the practice of anesthesia and, as previously suggested, can usually be overcome with rather inelegant techniques. However, today's increasing sophistication and expectation of high-quality anesthesia care require the early recognition of difficulty and a decision about the clinical management of the situation. When an unexpected difficulty is encountered, the possibilities are (1) termination of the procedure, (2) a blind or retrograde intubation, (3) fiberoptic or "light wand" intubation, and (4) a tracheotomy followed by the planned surgery. When possible, a colleague should be called in for a quick consultation while the situation is being tidied up. If in doubt or if there have been major problems with airway management resulting in hypoxia, frequent episodes of laryngospasm, cyanosis, or cardiac dysrhythmias, it is probably in the best interest of all concerned to discontinue the anesthesia, awaken the patient, and have the patient return another day with an intact central nervous system.

MISCELLANEOUS CONSIDERATIONS
Fiberoptic Intubation

Advances in technology have made fiberoptic instruments useful adjuncts in airway management.[6] Not only do these instruments have superior optics, but they are equipped with a suction apparatus that allows the clearing of secretions, thus enabling the operator to better visualize the airway. Unfortunately, these instruments also carry a price tag that is beyond reach for the majority of anesthesiologists in today's era of cost containment and diagnosis-related groups (DRGs). The major point to be remembered about fiberoptic laryngoscopic techniques is that they should be mastered before the difficult airway is encountered.

The "Light Wand"

The difficult airway has on some occasion or another tempted every anesthesiologist to become creative, and has therefore led to a limitless number of anesthetic techniques and equipment. To facilitate tracheal intubation, one technique is to use the "lighted" stylet seen in Figure 6-17 (hence the name "light wand").[13–15] The principles of the technique are (1) adequate anesthesia of the airway, (2) assuring that the curvature of the stylet simulates the curvature of the airway, and (3) illumination of the airway. The tip of the light wand will illuminate the area of the hypopharynx, the epiglottis, and the larynx in a diffuse manner as the instrument is advanced. When the light is directed through the vocal cords, the upper trachea will be brightly illuminated for a distance of several centimeters. The room must be darkened to accentuate the change from the diffuse illumination of the area above the vocal cords to the bright illumination of the trachea. The endotracheal tube is advanced into the larynx in the standard fashion. The most frequent reason for the failure of light wand-directed intubation is inadequate anesthesia of the larynx. The technique is limited to children who are at least 6 to 7 years of age, since the smallest endotracheal tube that will fit over the light wand is 5.5 mm. One danger of this technique is that the bulb may break off and lodge in a bronchus.[16]

Steroids

Multiple attempts at intubation will result in varying degrees of trauma to the airway, with the subsequent development of secretions and varying amounts of edema. This, of course, will add to the problems already presented by the difficult airway. The question often arises as to whether or not steroids will prevent or reduce the development of edema. Recent evidence in the treatment of infectious croup with steroids in relatively high doses has documented the benefit of this therapy.[17] It has been suggested that the use of high-dose steroids in cases of traumatic croup might likewise be beneficial. Therefore, the use of dexamethasone 0.5 to 1.0 mg/kg after or during a difficult intubation is justified empirically, since traumatic croup in the child with a difficult airway is a potentially dangerous situation. A discussion of traumatic croup is found in Chapter 16.

Techniques of Ventilation

Usually, a smaller than normal endotracheal tube is used with a difficult airway in order to facilitate intubation. This may increase the airway resistance to spontaneous ventilation during surgery. The question arises as to whether or not it would be wiser to mechanically ventilate the patient in order to avoid the potentially elevated negative intrathoracic pressures that may be generated with spontaneous ventilation in the presence of a small endotracheal tube. These pressures, in conjunction with hypoxia that may accompany a difficult intubation, may in some circumstances lead to postobstructive pulmonary edema. One such case is described in Chapter 13. Some clinicians favor spontaneous ventilation in patients who have a difficult airway, because they believe that should extubation occur, the patient will be able to ventilate spontaneously and maintain the airway. If the intubation was accomplished relatively smoothly with minimal desaturation, spontaneous ventilation using end-tidal gas measurements is acceptable. However, if the patient has undergone multiple episodes of obstruction leading to severe desaturation, my preference is to ventilate the patient intraoperatively. It is obvious that this is an area of clinical judgment in which the risk of accidental extubation must be balanced against the problems of a difficult intubation. For short procedures the question is probably moot. However, if there has been difficulty with intubation, the preference is for controlled ventilation. If the patient's oxygen saturation does not achieve the levels that are expected at that FiO_2 then in addition to controlled ventilation, the application of 5 to 8 cmH_2O of PEEP should be administered.

Timing of Extubation

Unfortunately, the problems presented by the difficult airway do not end with the end of surgery; the last major hurdle is how and when to extubate the patient. Simply stated, the extubation should be accomplished when the patient is awake, when the protective reflexes are intact, and with airway expertise standing by in case of difficulty. One major clinical problem is awakening the patient before he reacts to the presence of an endotracheal tube. Suctioning should be performed while the patient is still relatively deeply anesthetized. The anesthetic should then be gradually or rapidly discontinued, according to the situation. One anesthetic technique for rapidly returning the patient to a greater state of awareness and airway reflex control is to use muscle relaxants monitored by a nerve stimulator, a low concentration of halothane, or isoflurane in 70 percent nitrous oxide. The muscle relaxants can rapidly be reversed with edrophonium 1 mg/kg and atropine 0.02 mg/kg.[18] There is a 90 percent reversal in 2 minutes with this regimen, whereas with neostigmine 0.06 mg/kg and atropine 0.02 mg/kg, 90 percent reversal requires approximately 10 minutes. Some children will react to the endotracheal tube before the anesthesiologist thinks they are ready for extubation. This may result in coughing, apnea, desaturation, and dysrhythmias. In this situation, lidocaine 1 to 1.5 mg/kg IV will depress the reflexes sufficiently to allow the child to reawaken and tolerate the endotracheal tube until conditions are appropriate for extubation. The dose of lidocaine may be repeated in 5 minutes. The child can remain in the operating room for extubation or be taken to the recovery room. All monitors should be left on the patient until extubation is successfully completed. While the child is awakening from anesthesia there should be as little stimulation as possible. This refers to the suctioning of secretions, turning of the patient, and premature, unnecessary attempts to awaken the patient. If it is evident that the endotracheal tube is obstructed by secretions, it is obvious that adequate suctioning must be accomplished. However, in our anxiety to achieve supposed perfection, we often cause more difficulty than we prevent. An example of this is a child who has awakened quietly with an endotracheal tube in place but who has a small amount of secretions either in the endotracheal tube or the mouth. Small amounts of insignificant secretions can make a lot of noise and not interfere with ventilation. Secretions of this nature should be left alone. On the other hand, some secretions will obstruct endotracheal tubes, and signs of obstruction such as decreased air movement and retraction of the ribs indicate the need for suctioning. However, in the case of noisy secretions, suctioning at this point may well stimulate the protective reflexes, resulting in a child who is coughing and breathholding, and what was going to be a relatively smooth awakening and extubation can turn into a nightmare by these well-intentioned but inappropriate attempts to completely clear the airway before extubation. These are difficult judgment calls. The child who is awake and ready for extubation is perfectly capable of swallowing secretions and is capable of coughing up secretions.

Indications that the child is ready to be extubated include opening of the eyes in response to a command, nodding appropriately, or in the infant, reaching up and pulling at the endotracheal tube. At times the child is disoriented and out of control, and the extubation becomes more of a judgment call. The small child or infant should be placed in the prone position for extubation so that secretions can run out of the oropharynx during the extubation process. At this point the child would have been breathing 100 percent oxygen for several minutes and when the signs for extubation are present, the child should be extubated. When the child is in the prone position, coughing up any secretions will immediately clear the airway. If the child is on his back and coughs, the secretions may not clear the airway and may be aspirated down the trachea with a deep breath. The child should be monitored with a pulse oximeter during this extubation period and a bag and mask should be available for administration of 100 percent oxygen after the extubation. Clinicians with airway expertise and appropriate equipment must be at the bedside at the time of extubation. If after extubation the patient becomes obstructed and difficult to manage, and narcotics have been administered, it should be rapidly reversed. The initial dosage of naloxone for this purpose is 0.01 mg/kg, and it should be administered intravenously. This dose can be repeated several times. If effective, the same total intravenous dose should be given intramuscularly, since the duration of action of intravenous naloxone is shorter than the duration of action of narcotics.[19] If the child remains obstructed in spite of all attempts at airway management and reintubation cannot be rapidly accomplished, it is important to be prepared to immediately go forward with an emergency cricothyrotomy.

Postcase Analysis

Several things must be done after the difficult airway is encountered and, hopefully, successfully managed. An accurate, legible, and complete note must be included in the anesthetic record, in the progress notes, or in both. The parents must be told of the problem, and a letter describing the problem and method of its management should be given to the parents.

REFERENCES

1. Mallampati SR, Gatt SP, Gugino LD, et al: A clinical sign to predict difficult tracheal intubation: A prospective study. Can Anaesth Soc J 32:429, 1985
2. DeLisser EA, Muravchick S: Emergency transtracheal ventilation. Anesthesiology 55:605, 1981
3. McIntyre JWR: The difficult tracheal intubation. Can J Anaesth 34:204, 1987
4. Childres WF: New method for fiberoptic endotracheal intubation of anesthetized patients. Anesthesiology 55:595, 1981
5. Davidson AJ, Reynolds AC, Stewart ET: Use of a flexible, radiopaque directable catheter for difficult tracheal intubations. Anesthesiology 55:605, 1981
6. Patil BU, Stehling LC, Zauder HL: Fiberoptic Endoscopy In Anesthesia. Year Book Medical Publishers, Chicago, 1983
7. Goudsouzian N, Cote CJ, Liu LMP, et al: The dose-response effects of oral cimetidine on gastric pH and volume in children. Anesthesiology 55:533, 1981
8. Solanki DR, Suresh M, Ethridge HC: The effects of intravenous cimetidine and metoclopramide on gastric volume and pH. Anesth Analg 63:599, 1984
9. Rao TLK, Madhavareddy S, Chinthagada M, et al: Metoclopramide and cimetidine to reduce gastric fluid pH and volume. Anesth Analg 63:1014, 1984
10. Roy WL, Lerman J: Laryngospasm in paediatric anesthesia. Can Anaesth Soc J 35:93, 1988
11. Berry FA: The use of a stylet in blind nasotracheal intubation. Anesthesiology 61:469, 1984
12. Borland LM, Swan DM, Leff S: Difficult pediatric endotracheal intubation: A new approach to the retrograde technique. Anesthesiology 55:577, 1981
13. Macintosh R, Richards H: Illuminated introducer for endotracheal tubes. Anaesthesiology 12:233, 1957
14. Berman RA: Lighted stylet. Anesthesiology 20:382, 1959
15. Holzman RS, Nargozian CD, Florence FB: Lightwand intubation in children with abnormal upper airways. Anesthesiology 69:784, 1988
16. Stone DJ, Stirt JA, Kaplan MJ, McLean WC: A complication of light-wand-guided nasotracheal intubation. Anesthesiology 61:780, 1984
17. Kairys SW, Olmstead EM, O'Connor GT: Steroid treatment of laryngotracheitis: A meta-analysis of the evidence from randomized trials. Pediatrics 83:683, 1989
18. Meakin G, Sweet PT, Bevan JC, et al: Neostigmine and edrophonium as antagonists of pancuronium in infants and children. Anesthesiology 59:316, 1983
19. Longnecker DE, Grazis PA, Eggers GWN Jr: Naloxone for antagonism of morphine-induced respiratory depression. Anesth Analg 52:447, 1973
20. Stoelting RK: Endotracheal intubation. In Miller RM (ed): Anesthesia. Churchill Livingstone, New York, 1981

7

PEDIATRIC ENDOSCOPY

Andrew M. Woods

BRONCHOSCOPY

During the first half of the twentieth century, pediatric bronchoscopy was an art practiced by a limited number of skilled practitioners. The dominant anesthetic technique was topical anesthesia of the airway and intramuscular narcotics. The pioneers in endoscopy railed against the dangers of general anesthesia for pediatric bronchoscopy, and with some justification. Imagine, if you will, providing an ether anesthetic to a toddler undergoing bronchoscopy for removal of an endobronchial foreign body. The room is dark to enable the endoscopist to view the airway through a long metal tube illuminated only by light reflected off a reflector attached to the forehead of the endoscopist. The endoscopist struggles to grasp the dimly lit foreign body, a peanut, which is far down the right mainstem bronchus. The bronchoscope is occluding the bronchus to the right upper lobe as well as the entire left mainstem bronchus. The lung distal to the foreign body is atelectatic. You detect a slowing of the child's heart rate and a weakening of the pulse. Turning on the lights in the operating room you find a deeply cyanotic child who may or may not recover when the bronchoscope is withdrawn into the trachea and ventilation with oxygen provided.

Faced with this not uncommon scenario, endoscopists usually opted for topical anesthesia and narcotic sedation, assisted by several strong assistants to restrain the child during the procedure. There was some assurance that a struggling child was at least still alive. Regardless of anesthetic technique, pediatric bronchoscopy during this era still carried an excessively high mortality rate.

Contrast this with pediatric bronchoscopy during the closing decades of the same century. Inhalation anesthesia with assisted ventilation is maintained through a semiclosed system that connects directly into the lumen of the bronchoscope. This same lumen also provides space for the passage of special airway instruments and a telescope that provides a clear image of the airway. The view of the endoscopist is shared by the operating room staff via a color television camera and monitor. The operating room is well lit, and monitors document the adequacy of oxygenation and carbon dioxide removal in the child.

Although the skills of the anesthesiologist and the endoscopist are important, the safety of modern pediatric bronchoscopy is equally related to advances in equipment. Optimum anesthetic care for children undergoing airway endoscopy requires a thorough understanding of this equipment and how it interacts with physiologic functions, both normal and pathologic, and various anesthetic techniques.

Bronchoscopes

Bronchoscopes are of two main types: rigid and flexible. Rigid bronchoscopes provide a higher-quality image and larger channels for instrumentation compared to flexible bronchoscopes, whereas flexible bronchoscopes provide access to distal airways inaccessible to rigid instruments and allow for endoscopy in awake patients with only surface anesthesia.

Rigid Bronchoscopes

The modern rigid bronchoscope consists of two main components: a hollow metal tube, referred to as a sheath (Fig. 7-1), and a narrow telescope of similar length that may be inserted into the sheath (Fig. 7-2). A high-intensity halogen bulb in a separate cabinet provides a common light source for both the sheath and the telescope, with linkage via flexible fiberoptic cables. The light cable attaches at the proximal end of the sheath, and a movable prismatic deflector can be partially advanced into the lumen to project light to the distal end of the sheath. This illumination, however, is markedly inferior to that provided by the telescope that is inserted through the sheath. The light is transmitted through tiny flexible fibers in the telescope casing and emerges at the distal end, delivering high-intensity illumination anywhere the endoscopist directs the distal end of the instrument.

The space between the sheath and the telescope is critical since this is the lumen through which gas exchange must occur. Thus, especially for the smaller

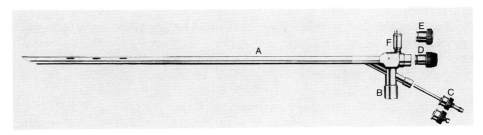

Fig. 7-1. Rigid bronchoscope. A, Sheath. B, 15-mm connector. C, Injection cannula for jet ventilation. D, Rubber-capped telescope guide. E, Proximal window. F, Prismatic light deflector and connector for fiberoptic light cable. (Courtesy of Karl Storz Endoscopy-America, Inc., Culver City, CA.)

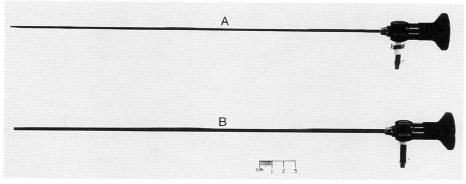

Fig. 7-2. Hopkins telescopes. **(A)** 2.8-mm diameter, 30-cm length. **(B)** 4.0-mm, 30-cm length.

sheaths required in infants, it is imperative to have a telescope with a small diameter. The Hopkins rod lens telescope represents a great advance in telescope miniaturization, as the traditional arrangement of a series of small lenses separated by large air spaces is replaced with a series of glass rods separated by small air spaces. This ingenious system allows for a much smaller diameter telescope with a much larger viewing angle, greatly increased light transmission, and excellent resolution.

At the time of its introduction, the most important consequence of this brighter illumination system for the anesthesiologist was that it allowed endoscopists to work in well lighted operating rooms with no compromise of viewing. No longer was the anesthesiologist forced to assess cyanosis in a darkened room using a flashlight aimed at the child's feet. Now, pulse oximetry is more reliable than visual observation in detecting oxygen desaturation. Another benefit of the brighter illumination system is that it allows the use of miniature television cameras, which can provide all operating room personnel with visual access to the patient's airway.

Pediatric bronchoscope sheaths are classified as either infant or child sizes based upon length. For the Storz instruments, the infant sheaths are 20 cm in length; the child sheaths are 30 cm long. There is a range of diameters provided for both lengths, and different-size instruments are identified by a nominal size, which is imprinted on the sheath. The infant sheaths are identified as 2.5, 3.0, and 3.5, and the child sheaths are labeled 3.5, 4.0, 5.0, and 6.0. The nominal sizes do not correspond exactly with the actual internal diameters of the sheaths, as seen in Table 7-1. Reference to Table 7-2 shows that the external diameters of the Storz sheaths are slightly larger than the corresponding-size endotracheal tubes. The greatest difference is in the 4.0 size, in which the sheath is 1.3 mm larger in diameter than a 4.0-mm endotracheal tube.

Table 7-3 is a guide to sheath size for use in various age groups. However, airway pathology will often necessitate a smaller instrument than that suggested by this guide. In cases in which a sheath of maximum size is required to facilitate instrumentation, a tight fit in the airway may result. If tested, there will be no air leak between the sheath and the trachea, even at tracheal pressures above

Table 7-1. Storz Bronchoscope Dimensions

Nominal Size	Measured Internal Diameter (mm)	Measured External Diameter (mm)
2.5	3.2	4.0
3.0	4.2	5.0
3.5	4.9	5.7
4.0	5.9	6.7
5.0	7.0	7.8
6.0	7.4	8.2

(Data from Karl Storz Endoscopy-America Inc., Culver City, CA.)

50 cmH$_2$0. Although this will result in mucosal ischemia in the trachea, it is usually of minimal consequence if the sheath is in the trachea for only a short period of time, except in cases of pathologic airway narrowing, such as subglottic stenosis. When longer procedures are anticipated, and there is a tight fit between the sheath and the trachea, preoperative administration of steroids may be warranted to lessen the degree of postoperative airway edema.

Another reason for the attention given to the sheath size is concern for airflow during bronchoscopy, particularly when the telescope is in place.[1,2] The lumen

Table 7-2. National Catheter Endotracheal Tube Dimensions

Nominal Size	Measured Internal Diameter (mm)	Measured External Diameter (mm)
2.5	2.4	3.5
3.0	3.0	4.0
3.5	3.5	4.9
4.0	4.0	5.4
5.0	5.0	6.9
6.0	5.8	7.9

(From Lockhart and Elliot,[2] with permission.)

Table 7-3. Suggested Endotracheal Tube and Bronchoscope Sizes for Children (by Age)

Age	Cricoid Airway Diameter (mm)	Endotracheal Tube Size (internal diameter, mm)	Bronchoscope Size
Premature	4.0	2.5–3.0	2.5
Term newborn	4.5	3.0–3.5	3.0
6 months	5.0	3.5–4.0	3.0
1 year	5.5	4.0–4.5	3.5
2 years	6.0	4.5–5.0	3.5
3 years	7.0	5.0–5.5	4.0
5 years	8.0	5.5–6.0	5.0
10 years	9.0	6.5 cuffed	6.0[a]
14 years	11.0	7.0 cuffed	6.0[a]

[a] A larger adult-size bronchoscope may be helpful if there is a large air leak and positive-pressure ventilation is being used.

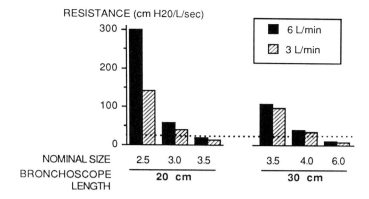

RESISTANCE (cm H20/L/sec)

■ 6 L/min

▨ 3 L/min

NOMINAL SIZE

BRONCHOSCOPE LENGTH

Fig. 7-3. Resistance to airflow through pediatric ventilating bronchoscopes. Resistance to airflow at two different flow rates was measured through three infant bronchoscopes, nominal-size 2.5, 3.0, and 3.5 and three child bronchoscopes, nominal-size 3.5, 4.0, 6.0. The infant bronchoscopes were evaluated with a 2.8-mm diameter, 20-cm telescope in the lumen; the child bronchoscopes had a 4.0-mm diameter, 30-cm telescope in place. The dotted line represents the upper limit of normal respiratory resistance for an infant.

for gas exchange is the space between the wall of the sheath and telescope. The standard telescope for the infant sheaths has a diameter of 2.8 mm. The actual internal diameter of the 2.5 sheath is 3.2 mm (see Table 7-1). The circumferential 0.2 mm space between the telescope and the sheath is inadequate for gas exchange. Figure 7-3 depicts the resistance associated with various sizes of Storz sheaths at clinically relevant flow rates. Note the drastic decrease in resistance associated with very small increases in the diameter of the sheath. This reflects the fact the resistance is inversely related to the fourth power of the radius. Figure 7-3 also illustrates another important concept that relates to airway pathology. For the 2.5 sheath there is a much higher resistance associated with a 6-L/min flow rate compared to the resistance measured at 3 L/min. This difference is due to the turbulent flow associated with this small sheath. Contrast this with the resistances measured across the 6.0 sheath. Regardless of flow rate, 3 or 6 L/min, the resistance is the same. This indicates that the flow through this system is essentially laminar. The important point is that, under conditions of turbulent flow, resistance increases with increases in flow rates. This does not happen when flow is laminar.

With the 3.0 infant sheath/telescope, the resistance is comparable to a 3.0-mm endotracheal tube, and should be adequate for most infants. Referring again to Figure 7-3, there is a seeming paradox in that the resistance associated with the 3.5 child sheath/telescope is higher than that measured in the 3.5 infant sheath/telescope. This is because the telescope used in the child sheath has a diameter of 4.0 mm, so that the actual cross-sectional area available for gas exchange is less than in a similar-diameter infant sheath with a 2.8-mm telescope. Also, the child sheath is 50 percent longer than the infant sheath, and length and resistance are linearly related. Problems using the 3.5 child sheath with a 4.0-mm telescope are most likely to arise in paralyzed patients.[3] While the resistance to gas flow through this instrument is easily overcome by the pressure generated using a 1-L breathing bag, the passive recoil of the infant lung and chest wall may be insufficient to allow adequate emptying before the next breath. Air trapping and stacking of respirations may occur, and this can result in hemodynamic compromise as well as barotrauma.

There are several approaches to managing this problem. The simplest solution is to allow longer expiratory times, often greater than 5 seconds. Significant air trapping can also be avoided by periodically removing the telescope for a few seconds. If paralysis is not essential, allowing spontaneous ventilation will improve gas egress. Exhalation under anesthesia is an active process, and much higher pressures are generated compared to those resulting from passive recoil. Studies in paralyzed patients have shown that abdominal compressions can restore adequate gas exchange in situations of airflow resistance caused by the bronchoscope.[3] Alternatively, Storz manufactures a 2.8-mm telescope that is 30 cm in length and fits all child sheaths (Fig. 7-2). While the optics are slightly inferior to the 4.0-mm telescope, the difference is significant only if photography is involved. Use of this smaller-diameter telescope in the 3.5 child sheath decreases resistance to a range that should allow adequate lung emptying, even during anesthetic techniques utilizing muscular paralysis (Fig. 7-4).

It should be emphasized that problems related to the telescope interfering with gas exchange are usually of major consequence only for the smallest infant sheath, the 2.5, when the telescope is in place. When this instrument is used, one must deliver low flows of oxygen (1 L/min) through the sheath with the pop-off valve left open, provide only an occasional positive pressure breath, and remove the telescope frequently to allow lung emptying. Failure to do so may lead to increases in intrathoracic pressure with adverse hemodynamic consequences as well as increased risk for pneumothorax.

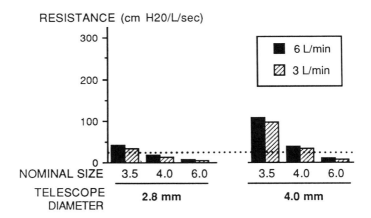

Fig. 7-4. Resistance to airflow through pediatric ventilating bronchoscopes. Replacing the 4.0-mm telescope with a smaller-diameter 2.8-mm telescope in child bronchoscopes significantly decreases airflow resistance in the nominal-size 3.5 bronchoscope. The dotted line represents the upper limit of normal respiratory resistance for an infant.

In cases where it is essential to examine an airway distal to a very narrow segment, as in a premature infant with subglottic stenosis, the 2.8-mm telescope can be used without the encasing sheath. Obviously, this technique will produce obstruction of the airway, and must be of extremely brief duration. It is essential that the infant not cough, as the sharp edges of the telescope may cause airway trauma. We have also on occasion used the 2.8-mm telescope as an optical stylet passed through a 3.0-mm endotracheal tube to facilitate tracheal intubation in infants with anatomic impediments that restrict airway access.

One additional piece of hardware that is provided with bronchoscope sets is a defogging sheath, a thin-walled metal sleeve that surrounds the length of the telescope. A flow of air through this sheath serves to prevent fogging of the distal lens of the telescope. Obviously, for the smaller sheaths, this represents a major encroachment on the lumen available for gas exchange. Also, the airflow serves to dilute the concentration of anesthetic gases delivered through the broncho-scope. We do not use this defogging sheath at all, relying instead on an antifog solution applied after dipping the telescope into warm saline just before use.

Open Bronchoscopy Using a Jet Ventilation Bronchoscope

The bronchoscope pictured in Figure 7-1 is referred to as a *ventilating* bron-choscope, in contrast to an *open* bronchoscope, which is essentially a hollow metal tube. The difference is that instrumentation can be performed through a ventilating bronchoscope at the same time positive pressure ventilation is being provided, whereas this is not possible with an open bronchoscope. When the telescope is removed from a ventilating bronchoscope, and the proximal end is not sealed with a glass window or a fingertip, this instrument is functionally converted into an open bronchoscope (Figs. 7-5 and 7-6).

Use of open bronchoscopes in paralyzed patients will lead to hypercarbia if too much time is spent by the endoscopist in instrumentation relative to the time spent providing positive pressure ventilation through the bronchoscope. Toward the goal of allowing simultaneous instrumentation and ventilation through an open bronchoscope, Sanders attached a 16-gauge needle to the prox-imal end of an open bronchoscope and delivered intermittent bursts of oxygen under a pressure of 50 psi through the open bronchoscope.[4] The inflation pres-sure measured at the distal end of the bronchoscope was not high, as there was a transfer of kinetic energy from a relative small mass of oxygen under high pressure to a much larger mass of gas in the lumen of the bronchoscope. As this column of gas was accelerated forward, a Venturi effect was created at the prox-imal end of the bronchoscope and a volume of room air many times larger than the volume of high-pressure oxygen was entrained through the bronchoscope. Thus, adequate tidal volumes at normal inflation pressures were delivered to the patient. The needle is now referred to as a jet injector, and many different sizes and positions have been evaluated.[5-9]

Use of these techniques in pediatric patients has been associated with pneu-mothoraces resulting from excessive airway pressures. The problem lies in the

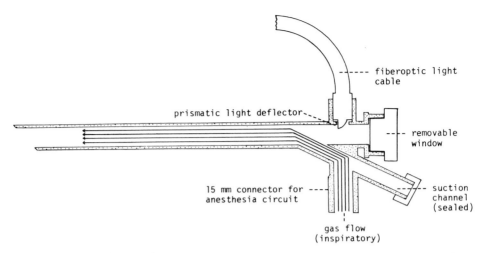

Fig. 7-5. Schematic of the Storz ventilating bronchoscope. With the proximal openings sealed, fresh gas delivered into the lumen will exit at the distal end. During exhalation, gases follow this same route in reverse. When the proximal window is removed and replaced with a telescope, a semiclosed system is still maintained.

physics of the jet injector. As the lumen of the bronchoscope gets smaller and smaller, it more and more approximates an extension of the jet injector, as there is less and less gas in the lumen of the bronchoscope for transfer of kinetic energy from the high-pressure gas. This same principle occurs when instruments are passed through the bronchoscope. Narrowing of the lumen leads to higher inflation pressures. Jet techniques require an unimpeded channel for the egress of gas from the lung through the open lumen of the bronchoscope. If the lumen is significantly narrowed, two things happen that can rapidly be catastrophic. The inflation pressure increases and the lung is unable to empty. If this is not

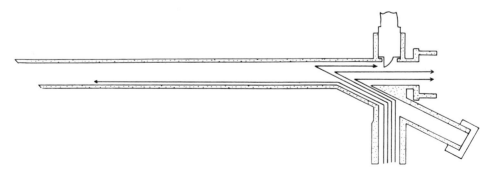

Fig. 7-6. Schematic of the Storz ventilating bronchoscope. Opening the proximal window allows most delivered gas to escape into the atmosphere. Providing positive-pressure ventilation in this case will blow anesthetic gases into the face of the endoscopist rather than the lungs of the patient.

recognized immediately, dangerous overexpansion of the lung will occur, leading to hemodynamic instability and pneumothorax.

Jet ventilation techniques represent a fairly complex solution to a fairly simple problem, which is not enough time spent providing ventilation during bronchoscopy in paralyzed patients. In our experience, the only time the endoscopists have a need for working for prolonged periods with the bronchoscope open is during difficult foreign body extractions. However, we do not advise the use of jet techniques in such cases, as potentially high inflation pressures can propel endobronchial foreign bodies even deeper into the airway. Use of jet techniques with small bronchoscopes requires a high degree of vigilance and an extensive knowledge of the flow and pressure characteristics of the particular system utilized. It is a technique used by a limited number of experts, and should not be attempted except under the guidance of such an individual.

Flexible Bronchoscopes

The ideal flexible bronchoscope for use in children would provide: clarity of vision; a movable tip under the control of the operator; a channel for instrumentation and suctioning; and a small-enough outer diameter to allow adequate airflow between the instrument and the encircling airway. However, as smaller and smaller diameters are sought, certain of these functions must be sacrificed. For example, the Olympus LF-1 has a shaft diameter of 4.0 mm and includes a 1.2-mm suction channel and a tip that can be flexed 120 degrees up and 120 degrees down; the Olympus LF-P is a 2.2-mm instrument with identical flexion and extension of the distal tip but with no suction channel. A 1.8-mm flexible bronchoscope is available that has neither a movable tip nor a suction channel.

The main use of flexible bronchoscopes by anesthesiologists has been as an aid in tracheal intubation, functioning as an optical stylet. Forcing a flexible bronchoscope through an endotracheal tube with a tight fit can damage the outer casing of the instrument. Thus, an instrument that will pass through an appropriate-size endotracheal tube is necessary. The 2.7-mm flexible bronchoscope will pass through a 3.0-mm tube, while the 1.8-mm flexible bronchoscope can be passed through a 2.5-mm tube. Since this latter instrument has no flexion capability, it may be necessary to use Magill forceps to facilitate advancement of the endotracheal tube into the trachea under endoscopic vision, with the tip of the bronchoscope not extending beyond the distal end of the endotracheal tube. If lubricants are used to facilitate passage through an endotracheal tube, water-based products or silicone are recommended. Petroleum products may injure the flexible plastic covering of the bronchoscope.

The small-diameter instruments are very easily damaged, particularly when used as a stylet to guide passage of an endotracheal tube. The shaft of the bronchoscope must be not be twisted or bent sharply, and the tip must not be moved against resistance. Such mistreatment will break optical fibers and damage the mechanical gear mechanisms. Use by inexperienced operators will almost surely prove very costly.

A potential complication of the flexible bronchoscope relates to the possibility of transmission of infection. It is more difficult to sterilize a flexible bronchoscope than a rigid one. Cracks in the flexible sheath or the suction channel can allow colonization of the interior of the shaft with pathogens that may not be destroyed by recommended sterilization procedures. This is more likely to be a serious problem in an immunocompromised host.

Preoperative Assessment of the Patient

Most pediatric patients presenting for airway endoscopy have some degree of respiratory compromise involving the airway or the lungs or both. One purpose of the preoperative assessment is to locate and quantify any areas of pathology so that an anesthetic plan can be formulated that seeks to minimize the adverse consequences related to these abnormalities.

Many infants and children will have had previous bronchoscopies, and much can be learned from their past medical records, particularly the anesthetic record and the operative report. Could the larynx be visualized? Did airway obstruction worsen in any particular position or during induction of anesthesia? Was there any difficulty with ventilation or oxygenation during bronchoscopy? Why? What anesthetic techniques were used? How effective were they? Of importance would be the size of bronchoscope and endotracheal tube used and whether these were appropriate. A child who developed postoperative stridor requiring reintubation would probably benefit from the use of a smaller instrument, unless significant growth had taken place since the previous procedure. Even in this case, a smaller tube or sheath should be introduced until it is established that the airway is also larger. Despite body growth, the airway could actually be smaller due to scar contraction.

A prior medical history may be suggestive of concomitant lung disease that is not clinically apparent. This is most frequently encountered in infants and children with a history of prematurity and respiratory distress syndrome of infancy, also known as hyaline membrane disease. These neonatal intensive care unit graduates are frequently seen for serial evaluation and management of subglottic stenosis related to tracheal intubation. Years after discharge, many of these children will continue to have abnormal pulmonary function.[10] Management of these patients for bronchoscopy is considered in detail in a subsequent section in this chapter. Children with a history of wheezing at any time in the past should be considered to have abnormal airway reactivity, and medications to treat bronchospasm should be available.

Airway obstruction can present with a wide variety of signs and symptoms, including stridor, wheezing, cough, hoarseness, changes in posture and handling of secretions, cyanotic attacks, tachypnea, and hemoptysis. Descriptions of the child's respiratory symptoms during sleep, feeding, crying, or with postural changes may be suggestive of the etiology and location of an airway obstruction. Inspiratory stridor is usually associated with extrathoracic lesions, while expiratory wheezes and biphasic stridor are more indicative of an intrathoracic obstruction.[11] An H-type tracheoesophageal fistula may produce cough and wheezing associated with feeding or the prone position, as food or secretions pass from

Table 7-4. Etiology of Recurrent or Persistent Cough in Children

Foreign body in the airways or esophagus
Asthma
Psychogenic disturbance
Cystic fibrosis
Upper airway drainage
Aspiration due to pharyngeal incoordination, tracheoesophageal fistula, or a
  tracheolaryngoesophageal cleft
Bronchiectasis
Bronchitis
Endobronchial or endotracheal tumor
Extrinsic compression by a vascular structure, cyst, tumor, or lymph node
Infection of a viral, bacterial, fungal, or mycobacterial etiology

(From Vaughn et al.,[48] with permission.)

the esophagus into the trachea. Mild tracheomalacia may result in stridor only when the patient is crying. A child who develops airway obstruction when sleeping may be expected to do the same when pharyngeal muscle tone is decreased by the induction of anesthesia.

The presence of a recurrent and persistent cough may be indicative of a wide range of congenital or acquired lesions (Table 7-4). It can also often represent a concomitant respiratory tract infection unrelated to the underlying airway lesion. In many cases, it may be the presence of an otherwise innocuous "cold" that precipitates the symptoms of airway obstruction, as in a child with unrecognized subglottic stenosis.

In examining the child preoperatively, attention is appropriately focused on the airway and respiratory tract. Upper airway lesions can often be well localized by listening over the throat with a stethoscope with the headpiece removed, placing the hollow tube directly on the skin.

Diminished or absent breath sounds over a significant portion of one hemithorax may be found in conditions producing an obstructed bronchus or with lobar alveolar disease. Such situations will slow the induction of general anesthesia with potent inhalational agents. These findings may also be indicative of potential ventilation/perfusion inequalities, which may complicate anesthetic management.

The child who has a difficult airway due to anatomic factors, such as macroglossia or micrognathia, presents special problems for bronchoscopy due to inability to visualize the larynx. Children with deformities of the cervical spine may not have the necessary range of neck extension to permit passage of the rigid bronchoscope. In such cases, use of a flexible fiberoptic bronchoscope should be considered.

Although the respiratory system is of major concern in terms of preoperative evaluation, other organ system dysfunction must not be overlooked. For example, infants and children with cardiac lesions other than corrected patent ductus arteriosus or corrected atrial septal defect require subacute bacterial endocarditis prophylaxis with penicillin. In a child with a cardiac lesion and significant periodontal disease, additional coverage with an aminoglycoside is warranted.

Laboratory data may be helpful or necessary in certain cases. A hemoglobin level gives an estimate of the oxygen carrying capacity of the blood. Even though bronchoscopy is rarely associated with blood loss, significant preoperative anemia may result in impaired tissue oxygenation. Especially in sick children with severe pulmonary disease, anemia should be corrected prior to an elective endoscopic procedure.

Radiographic studies, including xeroradiography, fluoroscopy, and tomography, are often helpful in the evaluation of possible airway lesions and any concomitant pulmonary impairment. Radiolucent foreign bodies can be localized. Use of forced expiratory chest films has been used to demonstrate unilateral obstructive emphysema in cases of airway foreign bodies that are not radiopaque. A preoperative chest radiograph is often helpful postoperatively for comparative purposes in assessing the efficacy of the bronchoscopic procedure, or in evaluating postoperative radiographic abnormalities such as an infiltrate. We routinely obtain both preoperative and postoperative chest radiographs in pediatric patients undergoing bronchoscopy.

Pharmacologic Agents

The main purpose of pharmacologic agents for patients undergoing airway endoscopy is the blockade of a host of undesirable physiologic responses associated with airway manipulation, including coughing, gagging, breathholding, laryngospasm, bronchospasm, hypertension, bradycardia, tachycardia, and increased airway secretions. To this end, there are five classes of drugs that are essential components of the pharmacologic armamentarium of the anesthesiologist who provides care for children undergoing airway endoscopy: anticholinergics, local anesthetics, narcotics, inhalational agents, and sedatives/hypnotics. In addition, drugs to alter the pH and volume of gastric fluid may be useful.

Anticholinergics

Anticholinergic medications prior to bronchoscopy provide the dual benefit of decreased airway secretions and attenuation of vagally mediated bradycardia associated with mechanical stimulation of the airway. A dry airway improves topicalization with local anesthetic, as the concentration is not diluted by abundant secretions. Contrary to the opinion of many endoscopists, anticholinergics do not affect the viscosity of secretions, only the volume.[12] It is the use of dry gases in the airway that tends to dehydrate bronchial secretions and make them more difficult to suction.

The incidence of laryngospasm and coughing during induction of anesthesia is lessened by reducing the amount of secretions that might trigger these protective airway reflexes. Drying agents also reduce the amount of suctioning time required of the endoscopist. The significance of this is that suctioning removes oxygen from the lung and can promote atelectasis. In additions, anticholinergics are helpful in blocking reflex bronchoconstriction. For these reasons, we consider anticholinergics an essential component of all bronchoscopic procedures.

Atropine is well absorbed from the gastrointestinal tract, and has been reported to be effective by this route within 10 minutes of administration.[13] Glycopyrrolate, because of its quaternary ammonium structure, is poorly absorbed following oral dosing. For this reason, an oral dose of glycopyrrolate that is five times larger than the parenteral dose is recommended. However, the same polar structure that impairs gastric absorption of glycopyrrolate also prevents it from crossing the blood-brain barrier. Thus, unlike atropine and scopolamine, it has no central nervous system effects.

It must be stressed that bradycardia during bronchoscopy means hypoxia until proven otherwise, and assurance of oxygenation and ventilation must be the first response to bradycardia, not the administration of an anticholinergic drug.

Local Anesthetics

Local anesthetics can be used both topically and intravenously to obtund airway reflexes. Because of its proven efficacy and wide margin of safety, lidocaine is the most commonly used local anesthetic for airway anesthesia. Absorption through the pharyngeal and laryngeal mucosa is slow, with peak levels occurring 15 to 25 minutes after topical administration.[14] Local anesthetic delivered into the trachea, however, may be rapidly absorbed if it reaches the alveoli in the liquid phase. This can occur in any patient with an impaired cough reflex, as with general anesthesia, narcotic sedation, neuromuscular blockade, or brain injury. In this case, blood levels more closely resemble those following intravenous administration, and there is a greater risk for toxicity shortly after dosing.

It is best to apply the local anesthetic only to the areas where it is needed, rather than to the entire oro- and hypopharyngeal region. This is often best accomplished after induction of anesthesia using a fingertip dipped in viscous lidocaine and then applied to the larynx and epiglottis. Alternatively, under direct laryngoscopy, lidocaine can be sprayed directly onto these structures using a small syringe with a 25-gauge needle attached. This syringe can also be used to deliver lidocaine into the trachea through the glottic opening.

When application is limited to the portion of the airway above the vocal cords, dosages of 3 to 5 mg/kg of lidocaine can be safely used. The amount delivered through the vocal cords into the trachea should be limited to 2 mg/kg. Newborns, particularly those born prematurely, have decreased levels of the proteins that bind lidocaine, and 25 to 50 percent reductions in total drug dose is probably prudent in such infants.

Our preference for topical use is 4 percent lidocaine. As this concentration has 40 mg of drug in each milliliter, in a 3-kg infant we would limit our laryngeal dose to 15 mg (slightly less than 0.3 ml) and our tracheal dose to 6 mg (0.15 ml). The utility of a 1-ml tuberculin syringe in such cases is obvious. In a baby with normal liver function, an additional laryngeal dose of 3 mg/kg or a tracheal dose of 1 mg/kg may be administered 30 minutes after the initial dose, if needed.

There is a formulation of 10 percent lidocaine available in a metered aerosol sprayer. This delivers 10 mg of lidocaine per activation of the sprayer. In newborns and infants, one must be very careful when using it, since two or three sprays to the airway may result in toxic blood levels of lidocaine.

Narcotics

Narcotic medications are useful for airway endoscopy because they provide a high degree of suppression of airway reflexes with a minimum degree of cardiac depression. However, in cases in which spontaneous ventilation is desired, the use of narcotic medication is limited by the associated depression of respiratory drive.

Narcotics or other sedative medications should not be administered as premedication to children with airway obstruction unless they are under the continuous supervision of an expert in airway management. In some children with significant obstructive pathology, narcotic sedation may actually improve gas exchange. Crying increases airflow rates and turbulent flow. This produces increased airway resistance; the increased respiratory effort required to overcome this causes exaggerated pressure changes in the airways and can worsen the degree of obstruction. Narcotic sedation of such a child may improve alveolar ventilation by facilitating slower, deeper breaths. Conversely, sedation may only make the child more tolerant of either hypoxia or hypercarbia, and while calming the patient, may worsen gas exchange. We stress again that the potential usefulness of narcotics in cases of airway obstruction requires their administration under the continuous supervision of an expert in airway management. A major factor favoring the use of narcotics in such situations is the ease of reversibility. Morphine can be given intravenously in dosages of 0.05 to 0.1 mg/kg. Fentanyl may be administered in 1-μg/kg increments.

Inhalational Agents

Inhalational agents are also effective in obtunding airway reflexes, but quite high brain levels are required for this. The airway reflexes are very primitive and very essential for survival, and not readily blocked. One study found that at an end-tidal halothane concentration of 1.46 percent, tracheal intubation still caused movement in 50 percent of children.[15] This represents a doubling of the anesthetic requirement necessary to prevent a similar degree of movement in response to a surgical incision. Even higher concentrations are necessary if one wants to prevent 95 percent of patients from moving, or if it is necessary to block the body's adrenergic response to tracheal stimulation.

End-tidal concentrations of halothane that approach 2 percent are associated with moderate myocardial and respiratory depression. While this may be well tolerated in a healthy, well-hydrated child, it may result in inadequate cardiac output in children with less reserve. Thus, most anesthesiologists find that a combination of inhalational agent, topical local anesthetic, and intravenous narcotic provide adequate blockade of airway reflexes without undue depression of respiration or cardiac function.

Sedatives and Hypnotics

Centrally acting sedatives and hypnotics such as midazolam, methohexital (Brevital), and sodium thiopental can be used for sedation as well as induction of anesthesia. However, the same concerns apply to these medications as to narcotics in cases of significant airway obstruction, and their use in an unmonitored environment is not advisable.

In many cases a parent is as effective in calming a child as pharmacologic agents, and with less risk. This knowledge has led many anesthesiologists to adopt the practice of having the parent hold the child in the induction area or operating room while anesthesia is induced, particularly in cases involving tracheal foreign bodies or acute epiglottitis.

Agents to Reduce Gastric Acidity and Volume

Fortunately, aspiration of gastric contents appears to be an uncommon complication of bronchoscopy, despite the fact that the airway is often unprotected during a procedure frequently associated with uncertain levels of anesthesia. Although there is no consensus on the need for routine use of medications to neutralize gastric acidity prior to bronchoscopy, there are many situations in which this is indicated, especially in light of the very favorable risk:benefit ratio of the agents commonly used.

Ranitidine, a highly selective H_2-receptor antagonist, has been shown to increase gastric pH in children following oral doses of 2.5 mg/kg.[16] pH values above 4 can be expected within 2 hours after oral administration. However, by 4 hours after oral dosing, the gastric pH is likely to have returned to a value below 2.5, thus presenting increased risk for lung injury should aspiration of gastric contents occur. Ranitidine has been found to have no effect on gastric volumes in children. The drug is now also available in an intravenous preparation.

Sodium citrate (0.3 M) works more rapidly to increase gastric pH than does ranitidine, but is distasteful and most children will decline to drink it. An alternative is Alka-Seltzer Gold (contains no aspirin), tablets of which can be fractionated and dissolved in a small volume of water and flavored with grape or orange syrup.

Another potentially useful drug is metoclopramide. This agent speeds gastric emptying, inhibits the vomiting center in the brain stem, and increases the lower esophageal pressure.[17] The pediatric dose range is 0.1 to 0.2 mg/kg orally or intravenously. Onset of action is within minutes following intravenous administration, and within 30 to 60 minutes following oral dosing. The actions of metoclopramide appear to be mediated by acetylcholine, and are abolished by anticholinergics. Since these latter agents are an important component of airway endoscopic procedures, it is advisable to administer the metoclopramide well in advance of any anticholinergic if the purpose is to accelerate gastric emptying.

Anesthesia

Monitoring

For pediatric patients undergoing bronchoscopy, a pulse oximeter, an electrocardiograph monitor, an automatic blood pressure monitor, and a precordial stethoscope are essential monitoring equipment. In addition, a Doppler ultrasound device, a capnograph, and gas monitors are recommended as being very useful in certain situations.

The critical issue during bronchoscopy is oxygenation, and the pulse oximeter is currently the best monitor for continuous assessment of oxygen saturation. While arterial blood gas analysis gives precise information, the information obtained is always intermittent and delayed. The transcutaneous oxygen electrode is not as accurate as the pulse oximeter and has a slower response time.

The Doppler ultrasound device, with the sensor placed over a distal artery, provides a beat-to-beat assessment of blood flow, and a change in this signal reflects a change in either cardiac output or vascular resistance. If positive pressure is applied through the small ventilating bronchoscopes when the telescope is in place, it is possible to unknowingly hyperinflate the thorax and impair cardiac return. This will be detected earliest by changes in the audio signal from the Doppler.

End-tidal carbon dioxide waveforms provide a great deal of useful information regarding gas exchange. During induction, a capnogram will provide an immediate indication of airway obstruction, should it occur. Capnography is helpful in documentation of tracheal intubation. Capnography may be misleading in certain situations during bronchoscopy, especially if one merely looks at numbers rather than evaluates the shape of the CO_2 waveform in relation to the known alterations in airflow. For example, if significant air trapping occurs when a telescope is introduced through an infant bronchoscope, one is likely to see a lowering of the peak expired CO_2 concentration, and possibly a loss of the end-tidal plateau of the waveform. While one might think that ventilation was improved due to a lowered expired CO_2 value, this value is not a true end-tidal measurement, but one that is diluted by an increased proportion of dead space gas. Thus, the infant may be quite hypercarbic while the capnograph indicates a low expired CO_2 concentration.

Gas monitors may be helpful in providing information on inspired and expired gas concentrations. When using low flow rates in conjunction with the small pediatric bronchoscopes, some anesthesia machines deliver much lower concentrations of anesthetic vapor than indicated by the dial on the vaporizer. This can result in an inadequate plane of anesthesia. In other cases gas monitors can be misleading. When there is a mismatch of ventilation and perfusion, as there may be in cases of foreign body aspiration, end-tidal gas concentrations may overestimate brain tensions.

Advance Preparation

Prior to anesthetizing a child for airway endoscopy, the endoscopist must be in the operating area with all endoscopic equipment checked and ready for possible emergent use. A backup light source should be available. Instruments for an emergency cricothyrotomy should be in the room. The room should be warmed if the patient is an infant, and additional heating devices may be necessary to avoid cold stressing a neonate. The anesthesiologist should have an assistant skilled in airway management and vascular access techniques. Syringes with premeasured doses of essential drugs should be prepared, and potentially necessary drugs should be immediately available.

Our preference is the use of a pediatric circle apparatus with small, lightweight hoses. This semiclosed system allows delivery of known concentrations of potent anesthetic agents with effective scavenging.

General Considerations

The anesthetic goals for pediatric endoscopy include the following:

1. Adequate oxygenation and ventilation, with as much oxygen reserve as possible
2. A still patient whose airway reflexes are sufficiently depressed so that there is no coughing, laryngospasm, bronchospasm, or breathholding during the procedure
3. The avoidance of dysrhythmias and extremes of blood pressure
4. Maximal protection of the airway from gastric contents or undue mechanical trauma
5. The rapid return of consciousness and airway reflexes following the procedure
6. Absence of recall of parental separation or painful procedures

There is no single anesthetic technique that can satisfy all these requirements in all patients. The nature of the airway obstruction, the presence of concomitant lung disease, and the child's level of understanding are all variables that may require modification of technique. It is in such cases that the skill and experience of the anesthesiologist are crucial to an optimal outcome.

Foreign Bodies

Foreign body aspiration is a leading cause of accidental death in children under the age of one year, and evaluation and treatment of suspected foreign body aspiration is one of the most frequent indications for rigid bronchoscopy in this age range. For this reason, and due to a number of controversial issues associated with the management of these patients, we consider this topic in some detail, while also using it as a framework to present more general aspects of anesthesia for endoscopy.

A foreign body in the airway is a surgical emergency. There was a time when some clinicians recommended "conservative management"—bronchodilator therapy, postural drainage, and chest physiotherapy—for several days in the hope that the child would cough up the foreign body and avoid a bronchoscopic procedure.[18,19] While this approach was successful in some children, in others it resulted in cardiopulmonary arrest.[18,20] There are a number of possible explanations for total airway obstruction in such cases. Bilateral bronchial ob-

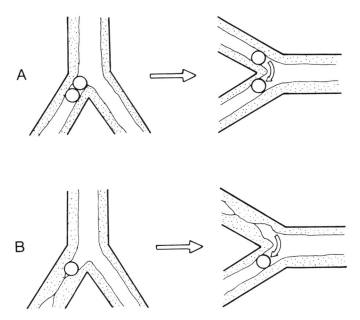

Fig. 7-7. Mechanisms of bilateral bronchial obstruction following foreign body aspiration. **(A)** Two objects are in the right main bronchus, and when the patient assumes the left lateral decubitus position, one of them enters the opposite bronchus. **(B)** There is swelling distal to a foreign body. When the object is dislodged and enters the opposite bronchus, total obstruction results.

struction can occur when there are multiple foreign bodies in the airway (not a rare event) and one or more is dislodged by coughing (Fig. 7-7A). Alternatively, single objects, such as a bean or a peanut, may split into two fragments and block both bronchi.[21] Another explanation is that inflammation and suppuration distal to a mainstem bronchial foreign body may render one lung nonfunctional; when the foreign body is dislodged by postural drainage and percussion, it may enter the opposite mainstem bronchus and produce bilateral obstruction (Fig. 7-7B). A final possibility is that an inhaled foreign body may obstruct the subglottic region when coughed from a bronchus, possibly due to an increase in size as a result of water absorption. It is now clear that prompt bronchoscopic removal constitutes the conservative approach, rather than techniques that are less invasive but potentially catastrophic.

The timing of bronchoscopy is such that there is often uncertainty regarding gastric contents. Since the most commonly aspirated items are foodstuffs, it is likely that there is also food in the stomach immediately following an aspiration event. Most cases, however, are not acute, and the child is brought for medical attention days or weeks after an unrecognized aspiration. Some of these patients will have eaten recently and the question will arise as to the advisability of delaying bronchoscopy to allow for gastric emptying. In this situation, in which the toddler is probably highly stressed by a strange environment and interactions with strangers, one cannot assume normal gastric emptying times. And, as discussed above, there is a certain degree of risk associated with delay in cases of foreign body aspiration. Thus, the anesthesiologist must be prepared to manage children based upon the assumption that the stomach may contain food particles as well as acidic gastric juices. The risk:benefit ratio of metoclopramide and ranitidine is such that their use in this setting is recommended.

Once a diagnosis of an endobronchial foreign body is made, either clinically or radiographically, the child should ideally be kept on his side with the involved airway in the dependent position. This will decrease the likelihood of a dislodged foreign body falling into the uninvolved bronchus. Should bilateral obstruction occur, the child's best chance for survival lies in being able to cough and clear the airway. Since it is likely to have been a cough that dislodged an endobronchial foreign body in the first place, the foreign body may well obstruct the opposite bronchus at end exhalation and thus block re-expansion of the lung. This will greatly impair the effectiveness of the cough reflex, and the child will rapidly become cyanotic. It also makes artificial cough maneuvers such as the Heimlich maneuver futile and probably counterproductive. In such a catastrophic situation, the most readily available therapeutic intervention that may be of benefit lies in intubation of the trachea and pushing the endotracheal tube beyond the carina. If it enters a previously obstructed but still atelectatic side, this may allow for re-expansion of enough lung to facilitate resuscitation. If the tube goes into the freshly obstructed bronchus, it may be able to either pass around the foreign body, or possibly push it deeper into a segmental bronchus and expose an upper lobe bronchus. The limited amount of ventilation afforded may be life-saving while preparing for an emergent bronchoscopy and possible thoracotomy.

In light of the experience with delaying bronchoscopy for alternative therapy, our initial approach to the child with a history consistent with an acute aspiration may need to be reevaluated. Specifically, in the case of a toddler who is brought to the emergency room after a "choking spell" associated with eating peanuts, should radiographic studies, particularly forced expiratory films, be undertaken? Such studies may be normal, particularly in the first 24 hours following aspiration, and, in our judgment, this child would warrant bronchoscopy based solely upon the history. Also, should this child be continually accompanied by personnel skilled in airway care? Although these episodes of in-hospital bilateral bronchial obstruction are apparently rare, it is still in the best interest of the child to take measures to minimize this risk.

Induction and Maintenance of Anesthesia

The pulse oximeter sensor and electrocardiograph electrode patches should be applied before induction in patients with obstructive airway lesions, preferably while the parents are still holding the child. The stimulation associated with the placement of monitoring equipment during the early phase of an inhalational induction can trigger undesirable airway reflex activity.

In cases of acute foreign body aspiration, in which significant mucosal swelling has not yet occurred, it is possible to move the foreign body deeper into the airway if positive-pressure ventilation is used. For this reason, we prefer the use of anesthetic techniques that allow for continuous spontaneous ventilation. If one does not have the benefit of capnography, worsening of airway obstruction is usually more readily assessed in a spontaneously breathing patient. Thus, in cases of acute foreign body aspiration, we recommend an inhalational induction, even in a child with an indwelling venous catheter. This is often facilitated by the judicious use of prior sedation with midazolam, sodium thiopental, or methohexital as previously discussed. The child is allowed to breathe a mixture of 70 percent nitrous oxide, 30 percent oxygen, and halothane, which is incrementally increased every 20 seconds by 0.25 to 0.5 percent until 4 percent inspired halothane is reached. For a child with obstructive emphysema, which frequently accompanies acute foreign body aspiration, induction will be delayed and the rate of increase in halothane concentration should be slowed to lessen the risk of airway irritation, coughing, and possible laryngospasm. We have experienced no difficulty in administering nitrous oxide to children with obstructive emphysema and unilateral lung hyperinflation, although this has been warned against.[22] A lung that is hyperinflated is still a ventilated lung, but one in which emptying is delayed. If ventilation ceases, the lung becomes atelectatic. Therefore, the hyperinflated lung distal to a foreign body does not constitute a closed gas space analogous to an obstructed bowel or a tension pneumothorax. Also, nitrous oxide is only used for a short time to hasten the induction of anesthesia and is then discontinued as soon as consciousness is lost.

When it appears that an adequate depth of anesthesia has been reached with the patient spontaneously breathing halothane and oxygen, and intravenous access has been established, the anesthesiologist should begin topicalization of the airway with lidocaine at the dosages and concentrations previously described. Spraying local anesthetic on the larynx and into the trachea under direct laryngoscopy allows the anesthesiologist to assess the depth of general anesthesia prior to insertion of the bronchoscope. This is an important step, since coughing with the bronchoscope in place has been associated with pneumothoraces.[23]

At this stage, considerable patience is required. It may take 20 minutes or more for the child to reach a sufficient depth of anesthesia to allow bronchoscopy. Clinically, this is suggested by the appearance of shallow respirations. End-tidal halothane concentrations of approximately 1.5 percent, coupled with topical lidocaine to the larynx and trachea, should be adequate in most cases. Recall from the section on capnography that mismatching of ventilation and perfusion can lead to erroneous assessments of tissue tensions of anesthetic. It is important that cardiac output be supported with adequate intravenous fluid administration and anticholinergic medication, the latter to maintain the heart rate.

A shoulder roll facilitates proper alignment of the airway axis, particularly in infants and small children, whose head size relative to trunk size is larger than in older children. The upper gums and teeth should be protected from direct pressure by the bronchoscope.

If there is concern regarding gastric contents, cricoid pressure should be maintained until an appropriate size endotracheal tube is passed to protect the airway.

The stomach cavity should be suctioned using a large-bore orogastric tube. The pH of the gastric aspirate should be obtained, and if less than 4.0, sodium bicarbonate 5 to 10 ml should be given through the orogastric tube and the pH rechecked. While a pH of 2.5 is definitely associated with lung injury in cases of gastric fluid aspiration, there are no human studies to document that values slightly above this level are not injurious, and a pH of 4 provides an extra measure of safety. After bicarbonate administration, the stomach cavity should again be suctioned.

At this point the airway is turned over to the endoscopist. Using a laryngoscope, the larynx is exposed for inspection, and then the bronchoscope sheath is inserted through the glottic opening, either with or without the telescope in place, depending on the preference of the endoscopist. If the patient coughs or breathholds, the anesthetic depth is inadequate. This is most rapidly treated with intravenous fentanyl 1 µg/kg or sodium thiopental 1 mg/kg at this stage, particularly if maximum recommended dosages of topical lidocaine have already been applied. In this situation, these doses should not produce significant apnea, and positive-pressure ventilation can usually be avoided if so desired. Once the patient resumes normal respirations, more time should be allowed for inhalational agents to reach appropriate tissue tensions. Inadequate anesthesia is one of the major causes of difficulty in endoscopic procedures.

Once the bronchoscope is in the trachea, ventilation must be accomplished through the lumen of the bronchoscope. Problems with ventilation through the smaller bronchoscopes with a telescope in place have already been discussed. Because much bronchoscopic exploration and manipulation is done under telescopic vision, the anesthesiologist should anticipate impaired ventilation when these instruments are used, and the endoscopist should periodically remove the telescope and allow several minutes of spontaneous ventilation with the proximal end of the bronchoscope sealed. If the bronchoscope is deep in a bronchus, it should periodically be withdrawn to a more central position. These steps are important to prevent severe hypercarbia and to maintain an adequate depth of anesthesia. Use of various instruments or catheters through the side channel will further obstruct the lumen and increase resistance to airflow.

The anesthesiologist must be constantly evaluating the adequacy of gas exchange using all available modalities. Is the bag moving with respirations? Is the chest moving? Is the child's color good? Are breath sounds audible? It is during such periods that pulse oximetry is particularly useful in confirming one's clinical impressions regarding gas exchange. As discussed in the section on monitoring, capnography may providing misleading information if there is not proper interpretation of the waveform.

Foreign Body Removal

Once the foreign body is located, the endoscopist should examine the other main airways to make sure that they are patent. Suppuration in the airway should be removed using suction. Topical vasoconstrictors are helpful if edema is severe enough to impede removal of the object. Phenylephrine (0.5 percent) can be delivered through a tiny catheter, or nebulized racemic epinephrine can be delivered through the side arm of the bronchoscope.

The nature of the foreign body will determine what type of instrument the endoscopist will use to grasp and remove it. In many cases, the foreign body forceps must be used through the open bronchoscope. This requires that the rear window be open during the actual retrieval process, and allows expired gases to be exhausted into the operating room. Inspiration with the sheath open will produce significant room air entrainment if gas flow rates are very low, diluting both oxygen and the anesthetic agent. If high gas flow rates are used, entrainment is minimized, but at the expense of operating room pollution, since a large portion of the flow will be directed toward the open proximal end.

Grasping a peanut has long presented a challenge to endoscopists. This is due to its rounded shape, smooth surface, and tendency to fragment. One technique that has been reasonably successful employs a Fogarty balloon catheter. The lubricated catheter is advanced beyond the peanut, the balloon is inflated, and the peanut is pulled to the tip of the bronchoscope and held there by the balloon. The peanut is usually too large to enter the lumen of the bronchoscope, and the peanut, balloon catheter and bronchoscope must be removed as a unit. With smaller objects that can be grasped with one of the specially designed forceps, the foreign body can be extracted through the lumen of the bronchoscope, which is left in place in the airway. Dry vegetable matter, such as a bean, may swell due to water absorption and become too large to pass through the upper airway. In such cases the object is often fragmented and removed in pieces.

Once the endoscopist has the foreign body in a secure grasp, gentle positive pressure may be applied to deepen anesthesia. This step is also important to facilitate re-expansion of atelectatic lung, particular after bronchial suctioning. A supplemental dose of intravenous lidocaine is helpful at this point, with the dose dependent on the timing relative to prior topical application of lidocaine.

Regardless of the technique used, it is essential that the anesthesiologist ensure an adequate depth of anesthesia prior to attempted delivery of the foreign body through the upper airway. If the bronchoscope has been deep in one bronchus for an extended period, the patient is likely to be both hypercarbic and inadequately anesthetized. The same may occur if the proximal end of the bronchoscope has been open for an extended period. Some recommend paralysis with succinylcholine at this time to guarantee abducted vocal cords and a relaxed larynx.[22] The narrow subglottic region and the cords can easily dislodge a foreign body from the often tenuous grasp of the endoscopist. However, paralysis is still no assurance of an unobstructed passage through the upper airway, as illustrated by the report of a case in which the foreign body was lost five times while attempting withdrawal through the vocal cords using a paralysis technique.[24] We do not routinely use paralysis prior to removal of the foreign body, preferring to avoid the necessity for positive-pressure ventilation should the object be dislodged as it passes through the narrow upper airway. However, we stress that adequate anesthesia is essential, and if this cannot be provided, then muscle paralysis is advisable.

The great concern with bringing a foreign body through the glottic region of a child is the possibility that the object may become dislodged and fall into the previously patent mainstem bronchus at a time when the other bronchus is still obstructed, producing complete obstruction. One way to lower this risk is to tilt the child so that the obstructed lung is lower than the lung supporting gas exchange. In the event that a foreign body should be lost during removal, it is essential that it be located immediately. While the endoscopist is inspecting the pharynx, the trachea and the bronchi, the anesthesiologist should evaluate the key issue—is the lost object causing critical airway obstruction? This is done more easily in a spontaneously breathing patient. If the airway is critically obstructed, and the foreign body is lodged high in the trachea, it is usually best to push the object back down into the same bronchus from which it was extracted, unless it can be readily grasped and removed. Should the lost foreign body fall into the only patent bronchus and result in total airway obstruction, the most important task for the anesthesiologist is to provide the endoscopist with a motionless, anesthetized patient so that the foreign body can be expeditiously retrieved. If the patient was adequately anesthetized prior to attempted extraction, this will not be a problem. If not, and since ventilation is now obstructed, obtaining anesthesia will require use of rapidly acting intravenous agents. If the object cannot be grasped, possibly because of a different presenting part, it may be possible to retrieve it by using the Fogarty balloon catheter technique already described. If this is not possible, either the foreign body must be pushed deeper into the airway to expose a lobar bronchus, or a small bronchoscope may be passed around the foreign body. In most cases, it will be possible to simply grasp the previously held foreign body and pull it out of the bronchus, provided the endoscopist is given adequate working conditions.

Once a foreign body is removed, the endoscopist will reinsert the bronchoscope and make sure there are no additional fragments not previously visualized. Any pus or accumulated secretions should be suctioned out.

It should be pointed out that a number of investigators do not share our concern over the possible hazards of positive-pressure ventilation, and routinely use controlled ventilation with muscular paralysis.[24,25] A high success rate is reported for all techniques, and it is difficult to demonstrate the superiority of any one technique. The main point is that the patient and the airway must be under control at all times. A moving, coughing patient presents the danger of airway injury and obstruction.

Emergence and Postoperative Care

The child whose stomach is considered to be empty can be allowed to breath oxygen through a face mask until he is awake. Otherwise, an appropriate-size endotracheal tube should be passed. Gastric suctioning is optional, but may be beneficial if positive-pressure mask ventilation was used during the case.

The endoscopist and the bronchoscopes should remain in the operating room during emergence. This may be prolonged, as airway endoscopy usually ends with the child at a deep level of anesthesia. Also, the same obstructive pathology that delays induction of anesthesia can delay emergence. Once full airway reflexes have returned and the child is awake, the endotracheal tube can be removed. The operating room is the best place to manage airway difficulty, not the corridors, and it is essential that the child be breathing spontaneously with airway reflexes intact before transport to the recovery area.

Humidified oxygen is administered routinely. Postoperative stridor is not an uncommon problem following bronchoscopy for any cause, and will usually be apparent within 30 minutes of extubation of the trachea. The likelihood of postoperative airway edema is usually related to the degree of airway manipulation. If the stridor is significant, racemic epinephrine delivered via a nebulizer is indicated. Corticosteroids, while not acutely of benefit, may be useful as an adjunct to the short-term benefits afforded by the epinephrine. Due to the fact that it takes 20 to 30 minutes before steroids are effective, we prefer to administer dexamethasone 0.5 to 1.0 mg/kg prior to the procedure if traumatic manipulation of the airway is expected, as in dilatation of a narrowed subglottic segment. A certain percentage of children will require reintubation owing to upper airway edema. This should be done with a smaller endotracheal tube than previously used in order to avoid additional trauma. The child must be observed in a critical care area until there is a large leak around the endotracheal tube, indicative of reduced airway swelling.

In most cases, a chest radiograph should be obtained while the child is still in the recovery area. A number of children will need to be admitted to the hospital for treatment of pneumonia related to chronic obstruction by a foreign body or for other pulmonary pathology. A child with normal airway anatomy who has had bronchoscopy following an acute foreign body aspiration can usually be discharged from the hospital after 6 hours of observation if there are no symptoms of airway obstruction and the postoperative chest radiograph is clear.

Infants With a History of Respiratory Distress Syndrome

Infants and children with a history of prematurity and respiratory distress syndrome are particularly likely to require bronchoscopy for evaluation and treatment of laryngotracheal injuries resulting from prolonged intubation or tracheostomy. It is the infants with the most severe lung disease who require long-term respiratory support, and who are most likely to develop airway complications, usually subglottic stenosis. In addition to tracheal narrowing, these patients will have varying degrees of abnormal pulmonary function, which will persist for years.[10]

Bronchopulmonary dysplasia (BPD) is the name given to the chronic lung disease that develops in some infants after extended mechanical ventilation with high pressures and high concentrations of oxygen. It is characterized by bronchial smooth muscle hypertrophy, interstitial pulmonary edema, and lung that is hyperaerated in some areas and atelectatic in others. Damage to small airways results in airflow obstruction, and lung fibrosis and scarring renders the lungs noncompliant. Dead space is increased, and minute ventilation must be increased to maintain normocarbia. All these factors increase the work of breathing, and result in increased caloric requirements. However, the pulmonary status requires fluid restriction, and the nutritional status is often compromised. Growth is inhibited, and recovery is often agonizingly slow. Supplemental oxygen is often required for months or years. Varying degrees of right heart failure may be present.

In such patients, bronchoscopy and general anesthesia can be a harrowing experience for all concerned, particularly during the first year of life. It is often necessary, however, since these infants with marginal pulmonary function may not tolerate the added insult of upper airway narrowing due to subglottic scarring. The bronchoscopic approach to this problem is directed at enlarging the narrowed lumen through mechanical distension using serial dilators.

The anesthetic management of these infants is complicated by the frequent presence of gross abnormalities of ventilation and perfusion and extreme airway hyperreactivity. These children may develop severe bronchospasm in response to any stimulation of the airway, including anesthetic induction, tracheal intubation, or tracheal extubation. Thus, pharmacologic measures to maximize bronchodilation and to minimize airway reactivity are essential. In many cases, this may merely be additional doses of medications that the child is already receiving on a chronic basis.

Bronchodilators are an important component of therapy for children with BPD. Traditionally, bronchodilators have not been used routinely in children under the age of 18 months who develop wheezing, as these agents have not been found to be effective in reducing symptoms of bronchoconstriction. This most likely relates to the lack of airway smooth muscle in this age group. However, BPD is characterized by peribronchiolar smooth muscle hypertrophy, and infants with this condition have been shown to respond to isoproteranol inhalation with lowered airway resistance and increased specific airway conductance.[26] Inhaled β_2-agonists such as albuterol and terbutaline can be administered preoperatively and intraoperatively via an oxygen nebulizer. Metered-dose aerosol inhalers can also be utilized intraoperatively with special adapters to allow delivery into the breathing circuit. β_2-Agonists can also be administered intravenously, with the dose limited by excessive tachycardia (heart rate above 180 beats/min) or dysrhythmias. Even if the infant is not on chronic bronchodilator therapy, perioperative administration of bronchodilators is warranted in the presence of a history of BPD.

Anticholinergics are given intravenously to decrease airway secretions, to block vagal responses, and for their bronchodilatory benefits. Doses twice recommended levels may be useful in these patients.

Most infants with BPD will be on chronic diuretic therapy. Their lung disease is characterized by excessive fluid movement from the pulmonary capillaries into the interstitium and alveoli, and this is treated by fluid and sodium restriction and diuretics. In addition to its diuretic properties, furosemide (Lasix) has been shown to acutely decrease airway resistance and increase specific airway conductance and dynamic pulmonary compliance in infants with BPD.[27] This effect occurs within minutes, and appears to be unrelated to the diuretic action. Furosemide is thus useful as an adjunct to bronchodilator therapy, and also serves to promote a decrease in interstitial lung water. Because of chronic exposure, rather large doses of furosemide may be required. Our usual dose is 1 mg/kg IV.

Lidocaine is applied topically to the airway as previously described for bronchoscopy, and in addition, a dose of 1 mg/kg IV is given 2 minutes prior to intubation of the trachea. Fentanyl 1 to 3 μg/kg is given as an additional agent to blunt airway reflexes and suppress coughing. The use of steroids remains controversial, but the potential benefits appear to outweigh the risks. Dexamethasone 0.25 to 1 mg/kg is given preoperatively. This agent has very little mineralocorticoid activity, so should create no problems with sodium and fluid retention.

It can be seen from the above recommendations that an IV catheter is necessary prior to the induction of anesthesia. Vascular access in these chronically ill infants is often extremely difficult. Lack of access reduces one's options in managing complications arising during induction. Also, the time required to place an IV after induction may result in an unnecessarily prolonged anesthetic in an unstable patient. If a peripheral line cannot be established percutaneously, a cutdown under local anesthesia or a centrally placed line via the internal jugular, subclavian, or femoral vein is necessary. These infants tend to be extremely sensitive to small shifts in fluid balance, and intraoperative fluids must be administered precisely. This requires an in-line measuring canister.

Despite potential dysrhythmogenic interactions with patient medications such as theophylline and catechols, we prefer halothane for induction because it is less of an airway irritant than the other potent agents. Using intravenous barbiturates in sedative doses, plus additional narcotic if necessary, a mask is gently applied and the infant is allowed to breathe increasing concentrations of halothane in a mixture of 50 percent nitrous oxide in oxygen. As soon as consciousness is lost, the nitrous oxide may be discontinued. Induction will usually be delayed owing to the lung disease, and the rate of increase in the delivered halothane concentration should be adjusted to reflect this. One cannot expect episodes of bronchoconstriction occurring during induction to be responsive to the bronchodilatory effects of potent anesthetic agents, since severe bronchoconstriction will prevent sufficient gas from reaching the alveoli to produce the desired effect on the airways. In spite of the above medications and precautions, bronchospasm and hypoxia may still occur. Management includes more of the above agents in doses and combinations that mainly reflect the skill and experience of the anesthesiologist rather than any prescribed formula. A similar round of pharmacologic assault may be necessary prior to extubation. Our preference is to leave the endotracheal tube in until the patient is fully awake. This may require the treatment of bronchospasm triggered by the tube. However, this is preferable to an early extubation and then development of laryngospasm and bronchospasm with no direct access to the distal airways. Mucous plugging is always a source of potential bronchial obstruction and subsequent hypoxemia.

Flexible Bronchoscopy

In contrast to rigid bronchoscopy, most flexible bronchoscopies in infants and children can be performed without general anesthesia.[28] These procedures are done transnasally (unless there is nasal obstruction) and topical local anesthetic is essential. The use of sedatives and narcotics for airway procedures depends on the age and medical condition of the patient and requires the presence of personnel skilled in overall pediatric perioperative management and the availability of facilities for postoperative observation. A mandatory feature of flexible endoscopy in children is the presence of a trained observer to monitor the patient while the endoscopist's attention is focused inside the airway. The use of pulse oximetry to document adequate oxygen saturation is also essential in infants and sedated children.

Flexible bronchoscopes with a 4-mm shaft diameter can be readily passed through the nasal passages of pediatric patients, including premature infants. This diameter is the same as that of a 3.0-mm endotracheal tube. However, the shaft of the flexible bronchoscope occupies a large portion of the tracheal airway, and neonates will be unable to overcome the greatly increased airway resistance. As with rigid bronchoscopes, it is the smallest patients who are at greatest risk for compromised ventilation.

The risk for hypoxia during endoscopy can be decreased by the administration of supplemental oxygen delivered via a face mask with a special port for the flexible bronchoscope, or delivered intermittently through the suction channel at a flow rate of 1 L/min. This will not prevent hypercarbia in small patients, and the bronchoscope should be withdrawn after 30 to 45 seconds and the infant allowed several minutes of ventilation with supplemental oxygen before continuing.

There are cultural differences in the use of the flexible bronchoscope for specific applications. For example, flexible endoscopists in English speaking countries tend to recommend that foreign body extraction not be attempted with a flexible bronchoscope,[28,29] whereas in Japan, flexible bronchoscopy appears to be the method of choice for airway foreign body extraction.[30] Flexible bronchoscopes have the advantage of being able to reach foreign bodies in airways too distal for a rigid bronchoscope, although this is rarely of concern in pediatric patients as most objects lodge in the proximal airways. Rigid bronchoscopy provides better access to the airway and more diverse instruments to aid in foreign body removal. Even in cases where the flexible bronchoscope is used to retrieve objects from distal airways, a rigid instrument is still usually used (outside Japan) for removal once the foreign body is brought back into a central airway using the flexible bronchoscope. The use of the flexible bronchoscope in airway foreign body removal in mentally retarded and physically handicapped patients has been reported.[31] This special population of individuals is more likely to have anatomic impediments to rigid bronchoscopy, such as cervical spine deformities, as well as cardiopulmonary abnormalities that increase the risk of general anesthesia.

In experienced hands, there are few if any absolute contraindications to flexible bronchoscopy. However, advancing a flexible bronchoscope through a narrowed airway segment will produce total airway obstruction. While the interruption of ventilation may be of little consequence if the procedure is brief, there remains the concern that passage of the flexible bronchoscope through a narrowed airway segment may produce enough trauma and subsequent edema to cause severe obstruction following the procedure. In such cases, one must be prepared to closely observe the patient postoperatively and personnel and facilities for prompt tracheal intubation and ventilatory support must be immediately available. Bleeding disorders represent a relative contraindication to flexible bronchoscopy, particularly if appropriate platelet or factor therapy fails to correct the abnormality. Infants in respiratory distress also must be carefully considered in terms of the balance between risks and benefits, since flexible bronchoscopy will in almost all cases be associated with a worsening of gas exchange during the procedure.

The incidence of reported complications of flexible bronchoscopy is very low. Epistaxis occurs occasionally, but is rarely significant in the absence of a coagulopathy. Pneumothorax is an uncommon complication, but is increased when the procedure involves trauma to the airway mucosa, as in dilatation of a stenotic area or a transbronchial biopsy. Bradycardia is unusual, and is usually seen in infants, related to either hypoxia or vagal stimulation.

In adults, the suction channel has been used to provide jet ventilation.[32] Exhalation must still occur along the outside of the bronchoscope. Because of the size of the airway in small children, such techniques are more likely to result in dangerously high airway pressures. In the event of a suspected pneumothorax intraoperatively, the bright fiberoptic light source has been used to transilluminate the chest to make an immediate diagnosis without waiting for radiographic confirmation.[33]

As during rigid bronchoscopy, suctioning removes oxygen from the patient's airway and decreases lung volume, promoting atelectasis. Unless one is monitoring the patient using pulse oximetry, the extent of hemoglobin desaturation produced by excessive suctioning may not be appreciated.

BRONCHOGRAPHY

Bronchography involves the instillation of radiopaque material into the conducting airways to allow radiographic imaging (Fig. 7-8). There are very few indications for this procedure in children; persistent right middle lobe syndrome tends to be the most common reason for performing bronchography at our institution. Suspected bronchiectasis is now evaluated by computed tomography scan rather than bronchography.

Patients presenting for bronchography may have extensive underlying lung disease, or they may be asymptomatic, having only radiographic evidence of lung pathology. Symptoms of cough and fever raise the possibility of an active infection, which is a relative contraindication to general anesthesia and bronchography on account of the possibility of airway edema and airway hyperreactivity.

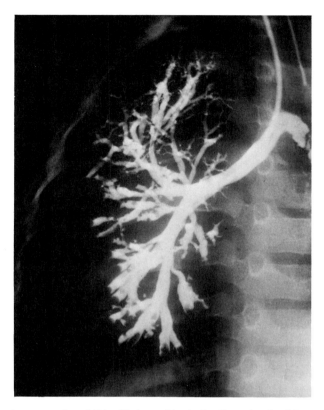

Fig. 7-8. Bronchogram of a child with bronchiectasis. Note the flexible catheter through which the contrast medium has been instilled.

Bronchography is usually performed in a radiology suite where fluoroscopy is also available. It is important that the remote location not be allowed to compromise patient safety, and all standard equipment for operating room bronchoscopy should be available.

Bronchography Under General Anesthesia

Preoperative preparation and induction of anesthesia is carried out as previously described for endoscopy. The placement of a precordial stethoscope should be such that the radiographic field is avoided. A pediatric esophageal stethoscope placed transnasally usually does not interfere with the procedure. Bronchoscopy is performed prior to bronchography to allow directed suctioning of the airway to remove secretions that might obstruct the dispersion of the contrast material.[34] After the airway has been adequately suctioned, it is important to allow several minutes of ventilation to restore lung volume and alveolar oxygen levels, which are both impaired by suctioning. It is also helpful for the endoscopist to apply 4 percent lidocaine topically to the area of the airway

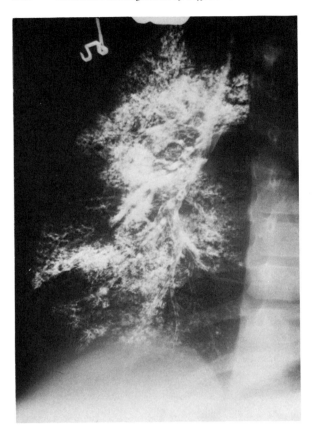

Fig. 7-9. Alveolarization of contrast material resulting from a patient coughing during bronchography.

to be studied. The suction catheter can then be used to mechanically stimulate the airway to test for adequacy of anesthesia. The purpose of the local anesthetic is to depress the cough reflex. If the patient coughs while the contrast material is being instilled in the airway, the result is diffuse alveolarization of the contrast agent and an inadequate study (Fig. 7-9).

The rigid bronchoscope is then withdrawn and replaced with an appropriate-size endotracheal tube, which is less likely to cause trauma to the airway as the patient is moved from side to side to distribute the contrast material. Strapping the child to a radiolucent papoose board facilitates the positional changes required. A right angle connector with a port covered by a perforated rubber diaphragm is used to connect the endotracheal tube to a pediatric circle apparatus. Using fluoroscopy, a radiopaque catheter is advanced through the endotracheal tube and positioned in the desired bronchus. The contrast material, a viscous iodized oil, is injected through the catheter. The patient is then turned and tilted as necessary to allow the oil to drain into the desired bronchi under fluoroscopic guidance.

Best results are obtained by allowing the patient to breathe spontaneously. The suction effect of inspiration provides more uniform distribution of the oil than positive pressure, which is more likely to produce a patchy distribution.[35] It is essential that the depth of anesthesia be such that the child does not cough during the procedure. Weak inspiratory efforts resulting from an excessive depth of general anesthesia also fail to provide good dispersal of contrast material. The combination of adequate topical anesthesia to the airway plus inhalational anesthesia allows both good inspiratory effort as well as depression of airway reflexes. Moderate doses of narcotic provide additional suppression of airway reflexes, and while opiates slow the respiratory rate, respiratory mechanics are not significantly altered. Once the contrast material is adequately deposited along the bronchial walls, permanent radiographs are taken.

During bronchography there is significant mechanical obstruction of small airways by the viscous contrast material, and high concentrations of oxygen are used to lessen the risk of hypoxia. Monitoring with pulse oximetry during this period is essential. Because of the pulmonary impairment produced by the contrast agent in the airway, it is advisable that both sides of the airway not be studied simultaneously in patients with significant bilateral lung disease.

Neuromuscular blockade with succinylcholine is used by some to prevent reflex coughing and provide apnea for improved radiographs.[36,37] While effective for these purposes, the loss of spontaneous inspiration to disperse the contrast uniformly tends to offset these benefits.

The oily contrast material is minimally absorbed, and clearance from the airway is primarily mechanical. This can be facilitated by directed suctioning of the bronchi at the end of the procedure, again using pulse oximetry to detect unsuspected hypoxia. Once the patient demonstrates the return of an adequate cough reflex, the endotracheal tube can be removed.

Humidified oxygen should be provided in the recovery room. Positioning changes will help clear the remaining contrast material, but it is the child's cough that is most effective. Postoperative chest radiographs will often demonstrate retention of contrast medium in areas of diseased lung, particularly distal to a stenotic bronchus.

Bronchography Under Local Anesthesia

Wilson and associates have described a technique for obtaining bronchograms on awake children using topical anesthesia.[38] A nebulizer is used to deliver lidocaine 6 to 10 mg/kg to the airway. As previously discussed, only a fraction of this dose is deposited on airway mucosa and subsequently absorbed. A transnasal catheter is passed blindly into the trachea, and under fluoroscopic vision this catheter is used for suctioning and contrast instillation.

Lundgren and colleagues have utilized a flexible bronchoscope in adults for bronchography under local anesthesia.[39] There appear to be several problems with extending this technique to children as described for adults. The size of the required flexible pediatric bronchoscope occupies a large portion of the airway of a small child, and ventilation may be inadequate during a prolonged procedure. Also, the suction channel on the pediatric instrument is quite small, and it is difficult to administer the viscous contrast oil through this narrow lumen.

Lundgren points out that the contrast material obscures the view through the flexible bronchoscope, and that fluoroscopic guidance is necessary for repositioning the bronchoscope, although radiation causes detrimental changes in the optical fibers of the flexible bronchoscope. In spite of these limitations, Wood reports the successful use of the flexible pediatric bronchoscope for bronchography in patients as small as 2.5 kg.[28]

The flexible bronchoscope does offer the advantage of inspection and directed suctioning of areas too distal to be reached using a rigid bronchoscope. In such cases one can pass a long catheterization wire through the suction channel, and then remove the flexible bronchoscope from the airway. Having localized the tip of the wire in the area of pathology under direct bronchoscopic vision, a radiopaque catheter can then be advanced over the wire under fluoroscopy and, after removal of the wire, contrast material injected. This directed instillation of contrast allows for use of less agent, thus reducing adverse pulmonary effects. Following the bronchogram, the flexible bronchoscope can be used to suction contrast medium from the airway. The child should be observed postoperatively in the same manner as after general anesthesia for bronchography.

LARYNGOSCOPY
Diagnostic Laryngoscopy

Flexible fiberoptic instruments are increasingly being used for diagnostic upper airway examinations in infants and children. These procedures are usually very brief and rarely require general anesthesia. Using only topically applied 4 percent lidocaine and, in many cases, mild preoperative sedation, it is possible to observe the dynamics of the upper airway during spontaneous ventilation without the tissue distortion produced by a laryngoscope blade.

Alternatively, for "quick-look" procedures in which spontaneous ventilation is not required for diagnostic purposes, laryngoscopy can be performed following the administration of adequate preoxygenation, thiopental 4 to 6 mg/kg, and succinylcholine 1 to 2 mg/kg IV. The laryngoscopy is performed while the patient is apneic and paralyzed. After 30 to 60 seconds, the procedure is interrupted and the child is ventilated with a bag and mask. Such techniques should not be used in cases of suspected upper airway foreign bodies or other conditions in which the ability to maintain an airway in the anesthetized state is uncertain.

Operative Laryngoscopy

Operative procedures involving the larynx generate an inherent conflict between the need of the surgeon to have unimpeded access to the operative site and the need of the anesthesiologist to maintain a secure airway. There is no ideal solution to this problem, and most cases involve some degree of compromise by both parties. When the airway is shared, mutual respect is essential, and patient safety must always be the paramount consideration. The following section presents a number of different approaches that are utilized for anesthesia for laryngeal surgery.

Awake Procedures

On occasion, optimal surgical results are obtained when the patient is in an awake state, as for injections into the vocal cords. Operative procedures in the glottic region usually require the use of a laryngoscope blade to depress the tongue for adequate visualization. Topical anesthesia alone is inadequate for blocking the gag reflex in response to pressure on the root of the tongue, since the receptors for this reflex are quite deep to the surface mucosa. However, this reflex is mediated through the glossopharyngeal nerve (cranial nerve IX) and can be blocked in the palatoglossal arch (anterior tonsillar pillar) as it crosses from the lateral pharyngeal wall to the tongue.[14,40] Because this procedure requires needle injections in the oral cavity, we confine its use to older, cooperative children. Our technique for blockade of the glossopharyngeal nerve is as follows.

The patient's tongue is gently retracted medially, exposing the palatoglossal arch (Fig. 7-10). It may be helpful to also retract the buccal mucosa laterally. Using a 23-gauge $\frac{5}{8}$-inch needle attached to a 3-ml syringe, the arch is pierced approximately 1 cm from the lateral margin of the root of the tongue, at the

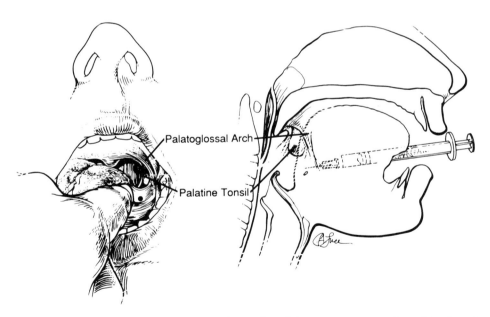

Fig. 7-10. Glossopharyngeal nerve block. Retraction of the tongue exposes the palatoglossal arch as it inserts into the root of the tongue. The black dot indicates the site of injection. A short $\frac{5}{8}$-inch needle is essential for safety. Injections must be performed on both sides. Aspiration tests should be performed prior to injection. There should be no resistance to injection, and minimal discomfort. If either occurs, the needle may be in tongue muscle rather than in the palatoglossal arch.

point where it joins the floor of the mouth. The needle is inserted to half its length and an aspiration test for blood or air is performed. Lidocaine (1 percent) is slowly injected and the procedure is repeated on the opposite side. A total dose of 0.5 mg/kg is adequate for the block, and the usual dose is approximately 2 ml per side. The injection is submucosal, and there should be minimal resistance to injection. The muscular tissue of the tongue must be avoided. Within a few minutes the posterior third of the tongue should be anesthetized adequately to allow direct laryngoscopy with minimal discomfort or gagging, taking care to avoid contact with the epiglottis. This structure, as well as the central portion of the posterior third of the tongue (the vallecula) is also innervated via the superior laryngeal nerve (cranial nerve X) and thus may elicit gagging if stimulated. Supplemental topical anesthesia to the larynx, epiglottis, and pyriform sinuses can be applied before or during laryngoscopy. The duration of glossopharyngeal nerve blockade when using lidocaine is approximately 15 minutes; epinephrine 5 μg/ml may be added to prolong the duration of the block to 20 to 25 minutes.

It is essential that a short needle be used and that the injection be made just lateral to the tongue. This will prevent injection into the internal carotid artery, which descends in the neck lateral to the pharyngeal wall. In the approach described here, the needle never leaves the oral cavity, and always remains on the medial aspect of the pharyngeal wall.

General Anesthesia

Endotracheal Tubes

Whether or not to use an endotracheal tube is an important decision that must be made when providing general anesthesia for operative laryngoscopy.

An endotracheal tube is the best assurance of a secure airway. It allows use of a semiclosed anesthetic circuit so that operating room pollution with anesthetic gases is avoided. A cuffed tube may also protect the lower airways from tumor particles and tissue debris.

On the negative side, the presence of a tube obstructs surgical access to the posterior commissure. Of potentially greater concern is the fact that all nonmetal tubes currently in use are combustible, and may be ignited during laser surgery by a direct strike with the laser beam. An enriched oxygen mixture being delivered through the tube may then be turned into a blow torch in the patient's airway. Even when the outer portion of a nonmetal endotracheal tube is protected by wrapping with laser-resistant material, the tube can be ignited indirectly from flaming tissue near the tip of the tube. In addition to thermal burns, the products of combustion of some endotracheal tubes may also cause lung injury.

Metal endotracheal tubes

There are several varieties of metal endotracheal tubes currently available. The Laser-Flex (Mallinckrodt, St. Louis, MO) endotracheal tube is metal, flexible, thin walled, and airtight. It is formed by crimping and stretching a single length of stainless steel tubing. There is a double cuff that, prior to use, is filled with saline to serve as a heat sink to prevent ignition in case the laser beam strikes the cuff. Should the upper cuff be penetrated, the lower cuff remains intact to protect the lower airway. Adding a drop of methylene blue to the saline allows ready detection of cuff penetration. The smallest-size tube currently available with a dual cuff has a 4.5-mm internal diameter and an outer diameter of 7 mm. This outer diameter is about the same as a 5.0-mm standard polyvinyl chloride tube, which means that it can be used in the average 3-year-old child.

For smaller patients, there are Laser-Flex tubes without cuffs that have internal diameters of 3.0 mm, 3.5 mm, and 4.0 mm, with corresponding external diameters of 5.2 mm, 5.7 mm, and 6.1 mm. The smallest tube, the 3.0 mm, has an external diameter that is slightly smaller than a 4.0-mm polyvinyl chloride tube, which means that it can be used in most children over the age of 1 with an age-appropriate airway size, and sometimes in even younger patients.

The Porch tube is formed in a similar manner to the Laser-Flex tube, but it has an internal diameter of only 3 mm, and an external diameter of 7 mm. The manufacturer recommends that the tube be used only with a jet injector, in which case ample space between the tube and the surrounding airway must be present to allow for egress of gases. Because of the large external diameter, the Porch tube is not suitable for use in small children.

The Norton tube is spiral wound strip of stainless steel with overlapping edges, and is not airtight. Sizes range from 2.14 mm internal diameter to 6.4 mm, with corresponding external diameters of 4.2 mm and 8.5 mm. The only advantage compared to the Laser-Flex tube is the availability of a neonatal-size tube.

Protected endotracheal tubes

Metallic tape and wet muslin have been used to protect nonmetal endotracheal tubes from the high-energy laser beam, but without total success. Only the outside of the tube is protected, and burning material that reaches the inner lumen can still ignite the tube. Wrapping a tube with reflective aluminum tape can present hazards of its own. Rigid tape can impair tube flexibility, and spiral-wrapped metallic tape can present sharp edges to the tracheal mucosa when the tube is bent. Tape can become detached from the tube and become an airway foreign body with the potential for obstruction. Laser beams reflected off the shiny aluminum maintain their intensity, and can damage normal tissue. Also, there is a wide range of difference in the performance characteristics of different aluminum tapes, particularly since the tape that is commercially available is not made for this purpose, and manufacturers do not want such use to be made of their product owing to liability concerns. Thus, a brand of tape that is laser resistant may be modified by the manufacturer with no notification to medical users. Each roll of tape must be laser-tested before it is used to wrap a tube.

Wet muslin absorbs the laser energy and thus protects the outer surface of the endotracheal tube. It is also soft and will not injure the trachea.

A new product, Laser Guard (Americal Corporation, Mystic, CT), combines the benefits of metallic tape and muslin. A laser-resistant sheet of foil with adhesive on one side and sponge on the other is used to wrap the endotracheal tube. The tube remains flexible and there are no sharp edges. The sponge is to be kept moist during the laser procedure. Of course, there is still the possibility of fire if glowing material reaches the unprotected inner surface of the tube.

Unprotected endotracheal tubes

It is possible to safely perform laser surgery using flammable polyvinyl chloride (PVC) endotracheal tubes if certain rules are followed. The oxygen concentration should be kept below 30 percent. Nitrous oxide, while not flammable, supports combustion as readily as oxygen, and must not be used to dilute the oxygen flow. Helium 60 percent retards PVC endotracheal tube ignition following a laser strike better than air as long as the laser intensity remains below 10 watts.[41] Thus, the laser should be used at the minimum possible power settings, and never above 10 watts, when there is flammable material in the airway. The laser should be activated intermittently, with the duration of any power burst limited to 10 seconds. The barium sulfate stripe on the endotracheal tube is quite flammable, and tubes without stripes are preferable. The endotracheal tube must be constantly observed for evidence of laser damage.

Pharyngeal Insufflation

Pharyngeal insufflation uses a high flow of anesthetic gases delivered by a small nonflammable tube aimed at the patient's larynx, and positioned as close as possible while remaining above the vocal cords. Spontaneous ventilation by the patient is required.

The absence of a tube gives the surgeon unimpeded access to the entire larynx. The risk of an endotracheal tube fire is also removed. However, the absence of a tube leaves the anesthetized patient with an unprotected airway, and decreases the level of control that the anesthesiologist has over the airway. The risk of airway obstruction is increased. If the tip of the insufflation tube becomes displaced, it can direct its flow into the esophagus, distending the stomach. One method for reducing the risk of inadvertent malpositioning of the insufflation tube involves delivering the gases through the suction channel of an Andrews anterior commissure retractor.[42] The channel is designed to permit suction removal of smoke arising from vaporizing tissue in the airway, but this capability is not needed since the fresh gas flow disperses the smoke. The retractor sits at the level of the cords in continuous view of the surgeon, reducing the likelihood of unrecognized displacement.

Another disadvantage of insufflation techniques is the pollution of operating rooms with anesthetic gases. Activated charcoal masks adsorb halogenated agents but not nitrous oxide. Nitrous oxide levels have been found to be 75 ppm during pharyngeal insufflation for laser surgery, with the recommended maximum permissible level being 25 ppm.[43] By placing high suction near the patient's mouth, effective scavenging can reduce room nitrous oxide levels to 7 to 10 ppm. This same technique can also decrease pollution with potent agents. Procedures using insufflation should be done in an operating room with a high rate of room air turnover.

Tracheal Jet Ventilation

In tracheal jet ventilation, a catheter is passed through the vocal cords and intermittent bursts of high pressure gas are used to ventilate the patient. This technique allows controlled ventilation so that intravenous anesthetic agents can be used, thus eliminating the problem of operating room pollution. The surgical field is readily accessible.

With a jet below the cords, obstruction to expiratory flow for even a brief period can produce a tension pneumothorax owing to the high pressures generated. The jet in the trachea can also create a Venturi effect and entrain air and surgical debris from the upper airway. If the tip of the jet is directed at the tracheal wall, mucosa injury can result. The Benjamin jet tube uses petals at the tip to keep it centered in the tracheal lumen.[44] Also, since the driving gas is oxygen, if the jet tube material is flammable it is still possible to have an airway fire.

Tracheostomy

With a mature tracheostomy, surgical access is excellent and the airway is secure. Effective scavenging of anesthetic cases is facilitated. Postoperative upper airway obstruction is no longer a problem. However, there are problems inherent with any tracheostomy, including vascular injury with hemorrhage and possible tracheal scarring resulting in stenosis. Also, in patients with papillomas in the airway, there is concern that tracheostomy may lead to seeding of the distal airway with tumors.

Anesthetic Management for Laryngeal Microsurgery Using the CO_2 Laser

One of the most frequent uses of the CO_2 laser in the pediatric airway is in the surgical management of juvenile laryngeal papillomatosis. These presumably viral tumors are seen most often in preadolescent children. They typically arise from the vocal cords, and the first presenting complaint is usually hoarseness. As the tumors multiply and spread, they may produce significant airway obstruction manifested by stridor. Surgical destruction of the tumors is only palliative, since there is a high rate of recurrence. Multiple procedures over a period of years are frequently required to maintain a patent airway. Fortunately, the tumors tend to regress spontaneously with the onset of puberty.

The preoperative assessment and monitoring of patients undergoing laryngeal procedures is essentially the same as for bronchoscopy, and has been covered elsewhere in this chapter. If it is anticipated that the procedure may cause even modest edema in a narrowed airway, it is reasonable to administer dexamethasone 0.5 to 1 mg/kg prior to the procedure. The main anesthetic problem that these children present is the presence of a narrowed airway, and the fact that the surgeon needs operative access to this compromised airway. In many cases, a combination of approaches to airway management are utilized. For example, a metal endotracheal tube may be used to allow laser resection of papillomata in the supraglottic area and along the anterior aspect of the vocal cords, and then the trachea can be extubated and pharyngeal insufflation used to allow access to the posterior commissure and subglottic areas.

Because of the risk of eye injury by the laser beam, patients should have their eyes covered with wet sponges or metal eye patches, and all operating room personnel should wear appropriate eye protection.

Prior to induction of anesthesia in patients with significant airway compromise, a rigid bronchoscope set with a range of pediatric-size instruments should be checked and immediately available. The thin-walled bronchoscope sheath provides a larger lumen than an endotracheal tube of the same outer diameter, and may be necessary in cases of a severely narrowed airway. In such cases, the rigid bronchoscope can then be used as the airway for the induction of anesthesia. In addition, instruments for an emergent cricothyrotomy must also be on hand, and the surgeon should be scrubbed and in the operating room during induction. A plan for the management of complete obstruction of the airway during induction should be discussed in advance, so all members of the operating team know their role should such an incident arise.

During induction of anesthesia, upper airway obstruction by papillomata frequently worsens. For this reason, we prefer to have an IV established prior to induction, even though a mask induction is planned. This also allows the use of sedative doses of thiopental 1 mg/kg if necessary to calm an extremely frightened child. Adequate preoxygenation prior to induction helps to increase the margin of safety in this situation. Spontaneous ventilation should be maintained during the induction of anesthesia until it is certain that an airway can be maintained in an anesthetized state. If severe obstruction develops during induction, it is not wise to immediately paralyze the patient with the idea of promptly intubating the trachea. Muscle relaxants may convert a partial obstruction into complete obstruction. Also, it may be difficult to identify the tracheal opening due to the abundance of papillomata. In such cases, it may be helpful to gently compress the chest and watch for air bubbles emanating from the airway.

A child who develops severe obstruction during a mask induction may be helped by providing positive end-expiratory pressure manually, while still allowing the child to breathe spontaneously. Extrathoracic obstructions tend to be improved by distension of the hypopharynx. If this allows adequate ventilation, the anesthesiologist can proceed with an inhalation induction. If not, the safest course may be to allow the patient to awaken and attempt another technique.

One such alternative would be topicalization of the upper airway followed by flexible laryngoscopy in the awake patient. This procedure can be done with a child in the sitting position if necessary, as this position tends to cause less obstruction than the supine position. If the airway is large enough to admit an endotracheal tube that will pass over the flexible bronchoscope, the larynx can be further topicalized and the child intubated awake. If the airway is readily visualized with distinct landmarks and an adequate glottic opening, the anesthesiologist has the option of resuming a more conventional inhalational induction, with the option of using a muscle relaxant if necessary. If direct or flexible laryngoscopy reveals an extremely narrow airway obscured by numerous papillomata, it may be necessary to pass a small rigid bronchoscope in a topicalized, sedated but awake and spontaneously breathing child.

Topicalization of the upper airway may be impaired by dense papillomata that prevent the local anesthetic from making contact with the airway mucosa. Intravenous procaine has been used as a supplement to general anesthesia in such cases, and has been shown to effectively decrease laryngeal irritability and suppress the cough reflex.[45] It is rapidly hydrolyzed by pseudocholinesterase. This requires that procaine be administered as a constant infusion (1 mg/kg/min of a 2 percent solution). The short half-life allows rapid recovery of airway reflexes at the end of the procedure.

Postoperative management is similar to that previously discussed for patients undergoing bronchoscopy.

Management of an Endotracheal Tube Fire

Should an endotracheal tube fire or explosion occur, the gas flow should be interrupted and the patient's trachea extubated at once to remove the fuel source and to prevent further thermal injury from the hot tube material. This is facilitated by having tabs at the end of the tape used to secure the tube. The patient should be reintubated with a new tube and laryngoscopy and bronchoscopy performed immediately to assess airway injury and to remove any charred material.[46] Systemic steroids should be begun, and the patient transferred to an intensive care area for close monitoring of pulmonary status.

Anesthetic Management for Laryngeal Foreign Body Removal

Laryngeal foreign bodies differ from bronchial foreign bodies in several respects. They are much less common, occurring in 2 to 4 percent of foreign body aspirations reported in several large series.[24,25,47] Laryngeal foreign bodies are almost always symptomatic, with a brassy cough being the classic finding in cases of partial laryngeal obstruction. The cough associated with bronchial foreign bodies is not brassy, and may be absent altogether. Laryngeal foreign bodies are much more likely to result in total obstruction of the airway. Foreign bodies lodge in the larynx either because they are sharp, such as egg shell fragments, or because they are too large to pass the narrow subglottic region. Fragments of hot dogs tend to be the most frequent cause of total laryngeal obstruction and death in children.

The main anesthetic problem presented by a laryngeal foreign body relates to the potential for worsening airway obstruction. The obstruction caused by the acute aspiration of a foreign body that lodges in the larynx can be expected to progressively worsen owing to secondary edema. Thus, the nature and location of upper airway foreign bodies is more critical than in cases of lower airway foreign bodies. Older children may be able to give a history of aspiration and point to a specific area of pain. Unfortunately, laryngeal foreign bodies usually occur in children too young to talk. Anteroposterior and lateral neck radiographs can be useful in cases in which the clinical condition of the patient permits such studies. However, many foreign bodies are not radiopaque. A child with a suspected tracheal foreign body should be treated in the same manner as a child with suspected epiglottitis, and should be accompanied at all times by an expert in pediatric airway management.

Localizing a foreign body to the larynx or adjacent areas of the hypopharynx has important implications for the induction of anesthesia. Foreign bodies obstructing the entrance to the trachea are medical emergencies, and may require anesthesia in a child with a full stomach. The use of externally applied cricoid pressure may produce further damage to the airway or surrounding structures. Figure 7-11 is a radiograph taken of a child with a tack in his hypopharynx. His presenting symptom was difficulty in swallowing. Pressure applied directly over this tack could have produced further tissue injury and possibly perforation of vascular structures. In this case, in which the foreign body was not actually obstructing the airway, the anesthesiologist used a rapid-sequence intravenous induction after adequate preoxygenation, but avoided cricoid pressure. When the object is in the larynx, a mask inhalation induction with spontaneous ventilation would appear to be the safest technique. This has the benefit of avoiding gastric distension and allowing for continual assessment of airway patency. In all cases, strong suction with a large-bore tube capable of admitting particulate gastric contents must be immediately available.

In some cases, in which the child is not in severe distress and the nature and the location of the foreign body are unknown, evaluation of the upper airway using a flexible fiberoptic instrument and topical anesthesia prior to the induction of anesthesia may be helpful.

Children with foreign bodies causing severe upper airway obstruction producing cyanosis or changes in level of consciousness should be given no anesthetic at all, and direct laryngoscopy should be performed on an awake but restrained child. Topicalization of the upper airway may be helpful. In all cases of upper airway obstruction, instruments and personnel for an emergency cricothyrotomy must be in the operating room during the induction of anesthesia. In cases of an impacted laryngeal foreign body in which a difficult extraction is anticipated, and in which there is a high risk of bleeding in the airway, it may be advisable to perform a cricothyrotomy under local anesthesia in order to establish an airway prior to manipulation of the foreign body.

If the child is able to move sufficient volumes of air past the laryngeal obstruction, general anesthesia can be induced by inhalation with spontaneous ventilation. As with laryngeal papillomata, obstruction may worsen during the induction of anesthesia as muscle tone is lost. Positive end-expiratory pressure maintained by manual compression of the breathing bag may diminish the degree of obstruction in such cases. Topicalization of the larynx is an important part of the procedure, because the protective airway reflexes can, when stimulated, produce laryngospasm and further airway obstruction. This can also impede removal of the object. Although such responses can be effectively blocked by adequate doses of neuromuscular blocking agents, we avoid paralyzing such patients prior to the establishment of a secure airway. Topically applied lidocaine 5 mg/kg or intravenous lidocaine 1.5 mg/kg should adequately suppress these airway reflexes while still allowing spontaneous ventilation. It is purely a judgment decision as to whether a full stomach should be suctioned prior to attempted extraction of a laryngeal foreign body. The danger is that such manip-

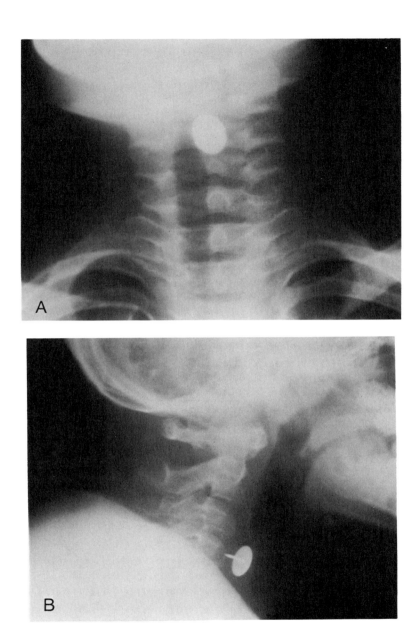

Fig. 7-11. (A) Anteroposterior and **(B)** lateral neck radiographs showing a tack in the hypopharynx of a child. Cricoid pressure could result in further tissue injury.

ulation adjacent to the airway may worsen the degree of obstruction or impaction.

In almost all cases of laryngeal foreign bodies, it is inadvisable to attempt to pass an endotracheal tube. To do so risks further airway injury. This means that the extraction procedure will be performed with the airway unprotected, and with the possibility of obstruction being always high. For this reason, we recommend using oxygen and halothane, and avoid nitrous oxide in order to provide the patient with the greatest margin of safety. If an adequate airway has been maintained throughout the induction of anesthesia, it is advisable to allow at least 10 additional minutes to reach a high degree of tissue saturation with anesthetic agent. This will avoid rapid lightening of anesthesia when the airway is turned over to the surgeon. While it is possible to insufflate an anesthetic mixture into the hypopharynx via a catheter, there is a risk that the flow may be misdirected and inflate the stomach, increasing the risk of vomiting. Such techniques also present problems with operating room pollution. We prefer to obtain an adequate depth of anesthesia, including topicalization of the airway, and then allow the surgeon unimpeded access to the airway of a spontaneously breathing patient. If the surgeon is unable to remove the foreign body within 3 minutes, the child's airway should be returned to the anesthesiologist to reestablish the previous depth of anesthesia. Should complete obstruction occur during these maneuvers, only a brief period of attempted removal should be attempted before the performance of an emergency cricothyrotomy.

After the foreign body is removed, the trachea should be intubated with an appropriate-size tube and the stomach emptied using a large-lumen catheter. It is also advisable to check the pH of the gastric contents, and if it is below 4.0 sodium bicarbonate can be administered down the same catheter to neutralize the gastric contents. Any excess volume can be removed by suction. If there is marked edema of the upper airway, the child should remain intubated and be admitted to an intensive care unit. Such swelling should resolve within 24 hours. If there is no marked swelling, the child can be extubated when awake. However, additional swelling resulting from the procedure itself may occur postoperatively, and such patients should remain in the recovery area for at least 1 hour after extubation.

REFERENCES

1. Woods AM, Gal TJ: Decreasing airflow resistance during infant and pediatric bronchoscopy. Anesth Analg 66:457, 1987
2. Lockhart CH, Elliot JL: Potential hazards of pediatric bronchoscopy. J Pediatr Surg 19:239, l984
3. Rah KH, Salzberg AM, Boyan CP, Greenfield LJ: Respiratory acidosis with the small Storz-Hopkins bronchoscopes: Occurrence and management. Ann Thorac Surg 27:197, 1979
4. Sanders RD: Two ventilating attachments for bronchoscopes. Delaware Med J 39:170, 1967

5. Miyasaka K, Sloan IA, Froese AB: An evaluation of the jet injector (Sanders) technique for bronchoscopy in paediatric patients. Can Anaesth Soc J 27:117, 1980
6. Spoerel WE, Grant PA: Ventilation during bronchoscopy. Can Anaesth Soc J 18:178, 1971
7. Carden E, Chir B, Burns WW, et al: A comparison of Venturi and side-arm ventilation in anaesthesia for bronchoscopy. Can Anaesth Soc J 20:569, 1973
8. Eriksson IA, Sjostrand UH: High frequency positive pressure ventilation during bronchoscopy and laryngoscopy. Int Anesth Clin 21:63, 1983
9. Komesaroff D, McKie B: The "bronchoflator": A new technique for bronchoscopy under general anesthesia. Br J Anaesth 44:1057, 1972
10. Smyth JA, Tabachnik E, Duncan WJ, et al: Pulmonary function and bronchial hyperreactivity in long-term survivors of bronchopulmonary dysplasia. Pediatrics 68:336, 1981
11. Maze A, Bloch E: Stridor in pediatric patients. Anesthesiology 50:132, 1979
12. Eschenbacher WL, Bethel RA, Boushey HA, Sheppard D: Morphine sulfate inhibits bronchoconstriction in subjects with mild asthma whose responses are inhibited by atropine. Am Rev Respir Dis 130:363, 1984
13. Brzustowicz RM, Nelson DA, Betts EK, et al: Efficacy of oral premedication for pediatric outpatient surgery. Anesthesiology 60:475, 1984
14. Woods Am, Longnecker DE: Endoscopy. In Marshall BE, Longnecker DE, Fairley HB (eds): Anesthesia for Thoracic Procedures. Blackwell Scientific Publications, Boston, 1988
15. Yakaitis RW, Blitt CD, Angiulo JP: End-tidal halothane concentration for endotracheal intubation. Anesthesiology 47:386, 1977
16. Pilato MA, Bissonnette B, Finley GA, et al: Effect of time on the serum concentration of ranitidine and gastric fluid pH and volume in young children. Anesthesiology 71:A1040, 1989
17. Manchikanti L, Colliver JA, Marrero TC, Roush JR: Ranitidine and metoclopramide for prophylaxis of aspiration pneumonitis in elective surgery. Anesth Analg 63:903, 1984
18. Burrington JD, Cotton EK: Removal of foreign bodies from the tracheobronchial tree. J Pediatr Surg 7:119, 1972
19. Law D, Kosloske AM: Management of tracheobronchial foreign bodies in children: A reevaluation of postural drainage and bronchoscopy. Pediatrics 58:362, 1976
20. Kosloske AM: Tracheobronchial foreign bodies in children: Back to the bronchoscope and a balloon. Pediatrics 66:321, 1980
21. Ward CF, Benumof JL: Anesthesia for airway foreign body extraction in children. Anesth Rev Dec:13, 1977
22. France NK: Anesthesia for pediatric ENT. In Gregory GA (ed): Pediatric Anesthesia. Churchill Livingstone, New York, 1983
23. Gallagher MJ, Muller BJ: Tension pneumothorax during pediatric bronchoscopy. Anesthesiology 55:685, 1981
24. Kosloske AM: Bronchoscopic extraction of aspirated foreign bodies in children. Am J Dis Child 136:924, 1982
25. Cohen SR, Herbert WI, Lewis GB, Geller KA: Foreign bodies in the airway: Five-year retrospective study with special reference to management. Ann Otol Rhinol Laryngol 89:437, 1980
26. Lenny W, Milner AD: At what age do bronchodilator drugs work? Arch Dis Child 53:532, 1978
27. Kao LC, Warburton D, Sargent CW, et al: Furosemide acutely decreases airways resistance in chronic bronchopulmonary dysplasia. J Pediatr 103:624, 1983

28. Wood RE: Spelunking in the pediatric airways: Explorations with the flexible fiberoptic bronchoscope. Pediatr Clin North Am 31:785, 1984
29. Nussbaum E: Flexible fiberoptic bronchoscopy and laryngoscopy in children under 2 years of age. Crit Care Med 10:770, 1982
30. Oho K, Amemiya R: Practical Fiberoptic Bronchoscopy. Igaku-Shoin, New York, 1984
31. Cunanan OS: The flexible fiberoptic bronchoscope in foreign body removal. Chest 73:725, 1978
32. Satyanarayana T, Capan L, Ramanathan S, et al: Bronchofiberscopic jet ventilation. Anesth Analg 59:350, 1980
33. Gallagher MJ, Muller BJ: Tension pneumothorax during pediatric bronchoscopy. Anesthesiology 55:685, 1981
34. Levy M, Glick B, Springer C, et al: Bronchoscopy and bronchography in children. Am J Dis Child 137:14, 1983
35. Bell H: Bronchography in children. Arch Dis Child 42:55, 1967
36. Webster AC: Anesthesia for operations on the upper airway. Int Anesth Clin 10:61, 1972
37. Cameron EW, Holloway AM: Bronchography in children aged 3 years and under. S Afr Med J 54:271, 1978
38. Wilson JF, Peters GN, Fleshman K: A technique for bronchography in children. Am Rev Resp Dis 105:564, 1972
39. Lundgren R, Hietala S, Adelroth E: Diagnosis of bronchial lesions by fiberoptic bronchoscopy combined with bronchography. Acta Radiol Diag 23:231, 1982
40. Woods AM, Lander CJ: Abolition of gagging and the hemodynamic response to awake laryngoscopy. Anesthesiology 67:A220, 1987
41. Pashayan AG, Gravenstein JS: Helium retards endotracheal tube fires from carbon dioxide lasers. Anesthesiology 62:274,1985
42. Johans TG, Reichert TJ: An insufflation device for anesthesia during subglottic carbon dioxide laser microsurgery in children. Anesth Analg 63:368, 1984
43. Rita L, Seleny F, Holinger LD: Anesthetic management of gas scavenging for laser surgery of infant subglottic stenosis. Anesthesiology 58:191, 1983
44. Benjamin B, Gronow D: A new tube for microlaryngeal surgery. Anaesth Intensive Care 7:258, 1979
45. Lawson NW, Rogers D, Seifen A, et al: Intravenous procaine as a supplement to general anesthesia for carbon dioxide laser resection of laryngeal papillomas in children. Anesth Analg 58:492, 1979
46. Keane WM, Atkins JP: CO_2 laser surgery of the upper airway. Surg Clin North Am 64:955, 1984
47. Rothman BF, Boeckman CR: Foreign bodies in the larynx and tracheobronchial tree in children. Ann Otol Rhinol Laryngol 89:434, 1980
48. Vaughn VC, McKay RJ, Behrman RE: Nelson Textbook of Pediatrics. WB Saunders, Philadelphia, 1979

8

ACUTE AIRWAY OBSTRUCTION, WITH SPECIAL EMPHASIS ON EPIGLOTTITIS AND CROUP

Frederic A. Berry

Acute airway obstruction represents one of the true emergencies facing pediatric patients and the medical teams responsible for their care. The vast majority of these children are completely well until the time of their illness. With the illness, they face a life-threatening problem that must be handled with dispatch through a team approach. Almost all of these children will recover with proper therapy, and in a very short time will return to their previous state of health. There are very few other life-threatening medical problems in which this is true.

The anesthesiologist is occasionally called upon to leave the security of the operating room to provide diagnostic and therapeutic assistance in the emergency management of the pediatric patient with acute airway obstruction. This chapter focuses on the problems of acute epiglottitis and croup. Foreign body obstruction, subglottic stenosis, and other sources of obstruction are discussed in Chapter 7.

THE USUAL PRESENTATION OF ACUTE AIRWAY OBSTRUCTION

The spectrum of presentation of acute airway obstruction ranges from mild inspiratory stridor in a child who is still able to take food and fluids to cardiopulmonary arrest. Many times the situation is not well defined or under control, and the anesthesiologist is called because the child needs cardiopulmonary resuscitation. Several diagnostic possibilities should be considered during the resuscitation, but the bottom line is resuscitation first, diagnosis to follow. Often the rescue squad or emergency room physician has been able to obtain a brief history. If the history of illness is negative up until the time of acute upper airway obstruction, the most likely diagnosis is aspiration of a foreign body. Another possibility is an anaphylactic reaction to an insect envenomation or a drug. The history may reveal that the child was only sick a few hours and then suddenly deteriorated. This clinical course favors acute epiglottitis. A history of a longer, more gradually developing (2 or 3 day) illness favors laryngotracheobronchitis (infectious croup).

Graduates of the neonatal intensive care unit who have been intubated often have varying degrees of laryngeal injury and subglottic stenosis. In one series, 47 percent of these patients had laryngeal damage.[1] These infants may be asymptomatic upon discharge from the nursery. They are particularly susceptible to frequent respiratory infections, which may precipitate an episode of acute airway obstruction. The respiratory infection will produce secretions and edema, and in conjunction with the pre-existing laryngeal pathology the airway may become compromised and the subglottic stenosis become symptomatic.

The condition of the child determines the sequence of diagnosis and therapy. The child in extremis needs immediate resuscitation and supportive care. Often, but not always, the diagnosis becomes evident at this time. Immediate airway management is the first priority. Attempts should be made to ventilate the child with a bag and mask. If the child can easily be ventilated, time can be taken to start an IV and bring the situation under control. If the child cannot be ventilated, the anesthesiologist must be prepared to perform a laryngoscopy and intubate the patient. At this time, the various diagnostic possibilities may become evident. If the anesthesiologist is unable to manage the airway, the airway must be secured surgically. It is the consensus today that a cricothyrotomy is the technique of choice to establish an emergency airway if endotracheal intubation is impossible. (Chapter 6 carries a discussion and description of the surgical establishment of an airway.) It becomes evident from the above scenario that there must be a systematic approach to this problem. For this reason it would seem appropriate at this point to discuss briefly the preliminary planning that has to be done.

THE MANAGEMENT PLAN FOR THE PATIENT WITH ACUTE AIRWAY OBSTRUCTION

Although this is a book about pediatric patients, there has to be an overall management plan for any patient who arrives in the emergency room with acute airway obstruction. In adults, the causes of this are more likely to be either trauma or loss of consciousness, whereas in children the most frequent causes are infection, trauma, a foreign body, and a loss of consciousness. Table 8-1 gives an extensive differential diagnosis of airway obstruction. A plan has to be developed by the representatives of the anesthesiology, pediatrics, and otolaryngology departments for the management of the patient with acute airway obstruction. If there is no otolaryngology department, a general surgeon, pediatric surgeon, or plastic surgeon must be involved with this plan. The plan starts with the identification of the child who has an acute upper airway ob-

Table 8-1. Causes of Airway Obstruction in Infants and Children

Foreign body
Laryngotracheobronchitis
Epiglottitis
Vocal cord paralysis
Choanal atresia
Subglottic edema
    Postintubation
    Allergic
Subglottic stenosis
    Congenital
    Postintubation
Tracheal stenosis
    Vascular ring, posttracheostomy, postintubation
Neoplasms
    Cyst, granuloma, lymphangioma
Hypoplasia of mandible
    Pierre Robin syndrome
Inhalation burns
Hypertrophied tonsils/adenoids

struction, and proceeds with a system to call members of all of the involved departments immediately. As suggested in the introductory paragraph, the first priority is that of supportive care, starting with the airway. The spectrum of airway management may vary from the child with early minimal symptoms in mild distress who needs careful observation and a diagnosis to the child who has already suffered a cardiopulmonary arrest and needs resuscitation or who is on the brink of such a disaster. If the airway can be managed, the second priority is a diagnosis. Once the child arrives in the emergency room with acute airway obstruction, a person with airway expertise must stay with the child until the diagnosis is made, therapy initiated, and the child admitted to the appropriate nursing unit for intensive observation (Fig. 8-1).

DIAGNOSIS OF ACUTE AIRWAY OBSTRUCTION

An immediate examination of a child with acute respiratory distress often reveals the existence of stridor. Stridor is defined as high-pitched, harsh respiratory sounds that may occur upon inspiration, upon expiration, or both. Stridor signifies obstruction; it is not a diagnosis. The basis for the obstruction may be an acute inflammation, either from a foreign body or from an infectious process. A congenital anomaly or an acquired problem, such as subglottic stenosis or a laryngeal web, may become evident when the child develops a respiratory infection. In general, inspiratory stridor is caused by airway obstruction stemming from an extrathoracic abnormality; it occurs in acute epiglottitis and with foreign bodies lodged at the level of the larynx. Airway obstruction in the subglottic or intrathoracic area leads to inspiratory and expiratory stridor, and may be as-

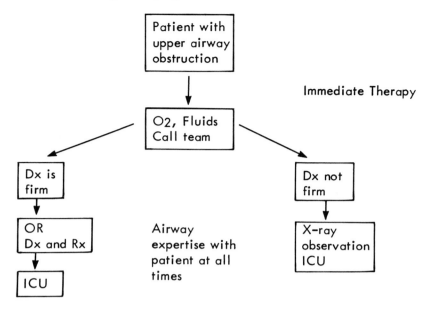

Fig. 8-1. Team management plan for children with upper airway obstruction.

sociated with wheezing; occasionally, it is diagnostically confused with acute asthma or reactive airway disease, in which the child has bronchospasm, which may be confused with stridor. I have seen several children with acute epiglottis who were initially thought to have asthma and were treated with epinephrine.

There are certain diagnostic steps, such as obtaining a radiograph, that should be considered in the child with an acute airway obstruction. However, if acute epiglottitis is considered to be the reason for the obstruction, the child should be taken to the operating room and intubated. There is no need for any type of radiograph if the working diagnosis is acute epiglottitis, since the patient will have a definitive diagnostic and therapeutic procedure. On the other hand, if the diagnosis is in question and there is no danger of immediate respiratory failure, certain diagnostic procedures should be considered. The procedure for diagnosis of an acute airway obstruction involves physical diagnosis, radiography, and at times, endoscopy. Children presenting with an acute airway obstruction usually have either epiglottitis or croup, with the next most frequent cause being a foreign body. The problem of the premature nursery graduate with subglottic stenosis who becomes symptomatic during respiratory infection is being seen with increasing frequency, and may be confused with the previously mentioned diagnosis.

There has been recent interest in the use of pharyngoscopy in the differentiation of infectious croup from epiglottitis.[2] The differential diagnosis is extremely important, since the majority opinion is that children with acute epiglottitis need prompt airway management with an endotracheal tube, whereas the majority of children with infectious croup need supportive care, racemic epinephrine, and at times, steroids. The report of Mauro et al.[2] suggested that the approach to this problem should be as follows: if the child is suspected of having epiglottitis, an anesthesiologist is called and the patient is taken to the operating room for laryngoscopy and intubation.[2,3] If the child is thought to have infectious croup, the pediatrician or emergency room physician does a pharyngoscopy with an anesthesiologist standing by. The steps for direct inspection of the epiglottis are done in a sequential fashion depending on the success of visualization. The first step of the technique involves having the child sitting and leaning forward, and simply opening the mouth and inspecting the epiglottis using a light. If this is unsuccessful, the next step is to use a light and wooden tongue depressor with the child still in the sitting position. Mauro et al.[2] reported that the epiglottis could be seen successfully and the diagnosis made at this point in approximately half of the children with either croup or epiglottitis. If the epiglottis still cannot be seen, a laryngoscope is used on the tongue with the child remaining in the sitting position and restrained as necessary. If this is unsuccessful, the child is placed in the supine position and restrained and a laryngoscope used. The entire length of the tongue is depressed using either the tongue blade or laryngoscope with care taken not to touch the epiglottis. Using this technique, there was no instance of acute airway obstruction associated with the procedure. One of the great fears that has pervaded the literature through the years has been that of a rapid acute airway obstruction following examination of the oral pharynx in children with acute epiglottitis. The exact cause of the acute airway obstruction has never been determined, but possibilities include either trauma to the epiglottis with resulting rapid inflammation or the activation of a vagal reflex with apnea and bradycardia. The other possibility is that the acute airway obstruction was due to the normal course of the disease, which at times may be extremely rapid and may have occurred with or without an examination of the airway. Using the system of Mauro et al.,[2] all six cases of suspected acute epiglottitis were confirmed, whereas 2 of 151 children thought to have infectious croup were discovered to have epiglottitis. This study is ongoing, and it is hoped that it will provide the medical community with a reasonable approach to the management of the differential between croup and epiglottitis. One of the important observations that was made in this study was that spontaneous coughing during this observation period signified infectious croup.

The patient with an undiagnosed acute obstruction should have a chest x-ray as well as a lateral neck film. Plans should be made for persons with airway expertise and support personnel to accompany the patient to the radiology department.

ACUTE EPIGLOTTITIS

Even though acute epiglottitis is often considered a disease of childhood, it may present at all ages, as indicated in the following case presentation.[4]

A 67-year-old retired general was completely well until approximately 2 to 3 AM, when he awakened with dysphagia and dyspnea. His symptoms increased in severity, and at 7 AM he summoned his farm manager and requested the administration of certain home remedies. He had a therapeutic maneuver of 0.5 L. The home remedies brought no relief. Shortly thereafter, his wife noticed that she had difficulty understanding him because his voice was muffled. He was given a mixture of molasses, vinegar, and butter that he could not swallow. He then had repeated the previous therapeutic maneuver and this provided minimal if any relief. Later on he was given a mixture of sage, tea and vinegar, and this almost caused him to suffocate. He found that he was unable to lie down, and had to sit up, leaning forward in order to be more comfortable. He had two more therapeutic maneuvers performed during the late afternoon. Several physicians were consulted. One considered the possibility of performing an immediate tracheostomy, but this was not performed because of the inexperience of the physicians and concern for possible criticism should it fail. He was treated with "blisters of cantharides" on his legs and throat, all to no avail. The patient's last words were, "I feel myself going. I thank you for your attention, but I pray you take no more trouble about me. Let me go off quietly. I cannot last longer." The patient died quietly, 21 hours after the beginning of his illness.

The four therapeutic maneuvers that were performed on this gentleman were bloodlettings. The amount of blood that he lost eventually totaled 2,000 ml. At that time and ever since, there has been some question about the diagnosis and appropriate therapy for the retired general, former President, and Father of Our Country, who died on December 14, 1799, at Mount Vernon, Virginia, at the age of 67. However, a perusal of the clinical course would indicate that the most probable diagnosis is that of acute epiglottitis. This rather dramatic case history of an adult should forewarn the anesthesiologist that acute epiglottitis can occur in any age group and at any station of life.

Diagnosis of Epiglottitis

Acute epiglottitis is primarily a bacterial infection of the supraglottic area. The term *epiglottitis* is somewhat of a misnomer, since the disease involves not only the epiglottis but the entire supraglottic region. It should really be called *supraglottitis*. The bacteria involved is *Haemophilus influenzae* type b. The clinical course is biphasic, starting with or without a very mild coryza, fever, a slight cough, and dysphagia. The tissues in the supraglottic region become inflamed and edematous. The second phase of the illness occurs when the supraglottic tissues become so edematous that there is airway obstruction. Any movement of the base of the tongue, such as occurs with swallowing and talking, causes the movement of these painful tissues, which is the reason for the dysphagia and the muffled voice. Because of the dysphagia, the child or adult will not swallow secretions, and instead will lean forward and drool (Fig. 8-2). As the patient leans forward, the supraglottic structures will move forward, off the posterior wall of the hypopharynx, easing the patient's discomfort and improving the airway. This obstruction is characterized by tachypnea, dyspnea, and inspiratory stridor. When the full-blown picture develops, the patient will lean forward, drooling, in respiratory distress with a high fever, and will have a quite

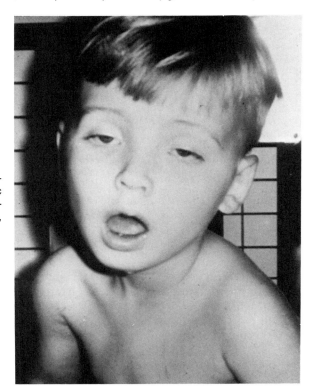

Fig. 8-2. Child with acute epiglottitis demonstrating classic picture of open mouth, drooling, forward-leaning position, and dehydrated appearance.

anxious appearance. There is usually no spontaneous coughing in the patient with acute epiglottitis, which is in contradistinction to the classic cough of infectious croup. Table 8-2 compares the main features of the two conditions.

The temperature of the patient with acute epiglottitis may vary between 38° and 40°C. The clinical course in children is complicated by the inability to take fluids, which leads to dehydration. The work of breathing and the septicemia that increases the temperature combine to increase the metabolic demand for both fluid and oxygen. The child becomes toxic, more dehydrated, and more fatigued as the airway obstruction persists (Table 8-3). The amount of drooling may well decrease as the child becomes severely dehydrated. The eyes become sunken, and if the child is young enough, so do the fontanelles. If the diagnosis of acute epiglottitis is probable because of the history and appearance of the child, a laryngoscopy must be done for diagnosis and the insertion of an artificial airway.

If the child is made to lie in the supine position for the drawing of blood, starting of an IV, or for any other reason, complete obstruction and cyanosis often occur. Such maneuvers are not only unnecessary but are also life-threatening, and should be avoided. The child should be immediately taken to the operating room accompanied by an anesthesiologist. A surgeon or physician who can perform an emergency cricothyrotomy and another anesthesiologist or

Table 8-2. Differential Diagnosis of LTB and Epiglottitis

	Epiglottitis	Croup
Etiology	Bacterial	Viral[a]
Age	1 year–adult	1–5 years
Obstruction	Supraglottic	Subglottic
Onset	Sudden (hours)	Gradual (days)
Fever	High	Low grade
Dysphagia	Marked	None
Drooling	Present	Minimal
Posture	Sitting	Recumbent
Toxemia	Mild → severe	Mild
Cough	Usually none	barking, brassy
Voice	Clear to muffled	Hoarse
Respiratory rate	Normal → rapid	Rapid
Larynx palpation	Tender	Not tender
Clinical course	Shorter	Longer

[a] Occasionally complicated by bacterial tracheitis (pseudomembranous croup).

pediatrician who can start an IV immediately after the induction of anesthesia should be standing by. If an IV can be started while the child is in the sitting position without compromising the airway, this should be done. On the other hand, if the IV cannot be started easily, or if attempts at doing so cause crying and cyanosis, the infusion should be started after the induction of anesthesia. At times the child will be in severe distress in the emergency room. If so, intubation should be done at that location.[5]

Epiglottitis in Young Infants

Epiglottitis most frequently occurs in children ages 2 to 7 years. However, it may also appear in those who are much older and infrequently in children who are much younger. Blackstock et al. recently reported a clinical study of 14 cases of acute epiglottitis in children less than 2 years of age.[6] The youngest child was a 7-month-old infant. The major differences in these young infants was that 3 of the 14 had a barking cough, which is more typical of croup, and 3 of the 14

Table 8-3. Clinical Problems in Acute Epiglottitis

Anatomic obstruction
    Edema, inflammation
    Secretions
Respiratory failure
    Hypoxia, respiratory acidosis
Fatigue (depends on length and severity of increased
    respiratory effort)
Circulatory status
    Dehydration → metabolic acidosis
Toxic and febrile
    Increased oxygen demand
    Decreased central nervous system function

had a coryzal illness for 3 to 7 days before the appearance of respiratory distress. The other interesting finding was that the presenting complaints in many were fever and irritability. All of the infants had respiratory distress and most of them were drooling. Several also had varying degrees of dysphonia.

Treatment of Acute Epiglottitis

Induction of Anesthesia

The techniques for the induction of anesthesia depend on the condition of the child, the cooperation of the child, and the experience and training of the anesthesiologist.

There are many different opinions and acceptable techniques for the induction of anesthesia, intubation, sedation, and extubation in the child with acute epiglottitis.[7-9] The most important part of any anesthetic plan is to have several contingency plans well thought out and prepared and to have assistance immediately available in the event of difficulty. Another physician, who may be needed to perform an emergency cricothyrotomy or rigid bronchoscopy, should be in the room.

In certain institutions the parents are allowed to accompany the child to the operating room and a general inhalational induction is performed. The parents are gowned and are allowed to come into the operating room to comfort the child. As soon as the child loses consciousness, the parents leave and the intubation is performed. Obviously not all anesthesiologists will be comfortable with this technique and the potential advantages of a calmer child must be weighed against the disadvantages of increasing the stress of the anesthesiologist by the presence of the parents.

If the child is cooperative, an inhalational induction with nitrous oxide and halothane can be accomplished. There is some degree of disagreement about the use of nitrous oxide. There are those who recommend using halothane and oxygen because of the increased need for oxygen in children with acute epiglottitis. However, a 70/30 or 60/40 nitrous oxide/oxygen mix to begin the induction, followed by slowly increasing incremental doses of halothane with decreasing concentrations of nitrous oxide, can be a very gentle way to induce anesthesia while at the same time increasing the F_IO_2. Then, as the patient tolerates the halothane, the nitrous oxide is completely discontinued and the induction is completed with halothane/oxygen. If the child is very cooperative, a small amount of lidocaine spray can be introduced into the oropharynx before induction. This will decrease the irritability of the airway, but may cause coughing and more obstruction. Clinical judgment is needed in the use of such a spray. Halothane is the volatile agent of choice because it is the least irritating of all of the volatile agents. If the child is not cooperative and has an IV in place, small doses of thiopental (1 to 2 mg/kg) can be administered incrementally to obtain cooperation. The remainder of the induction then can be accomplished as above.

If the child is very uncooperative, does not have an IV in place, and becomes cyanotic from struggling during attempts at an inhalational induction, the most gentle and quickest way to accomplish induction is to use ketamine 3 mg/kg IM in the deltoid muscle. Pretreatment with atropine is not necessary. Regardless of the technique used, the surgeon, pediatrician, or whomever should rapidly establish an IV as soon as the child will tolerate it. Since children with acute epiglottitis are dehydrated, a bolus of 20 to 25 ml/kg of a balanced salt solution should be administered.

Position for Induction

Anesthesia is induced with the child in the sitting position, since this is the most comfortable position in epiglottitis and it avoids risking the airway obstruction that may occur if the child is placed in the supine position. It is extremely unusual for children with acute epiglottitis to have complete airway obstruction, and once anesthesia is induced it is usually possible, with skillful upper airway manipulation, to ventilate them. If an oral airway is inserted too early, it may precipitate an episode of coughing, laryngospasm, and obstruction. On occasion, the anesthesiologist cannot manage the airway and complete obstruction occurs, often due to laryngospasm. At this point, there are three options open to the anesthesiologist: (1) My preference is to paralyze the patient with succinylcholine 2 mg/kg, thereby relaxing the muscles of the airway, and then ventilate the child and carry out the intubation. (2) Give lidocaine 1.5 mg/kg IV, ventilate the child, and then proceed with intubation. (3) If the first two options fail, immediately perform a cricothyrotomy or rigid bronchoscopy. This is an unusual circumstance, but must be part of the contingency plan. In the majority of instances the airway can be controlled and anesthesia induced.

Intubation

When induction proceeds smoothly the next step is intubation. Two options are available to the clinician: relaxation with a volatile agent followed by intubation and relaxation with succinylcholine and intubation. There is a difference of opinion about which of these two routes is best. Both techniques are acceptable, and both depend on the judgment and skill of the clinician. The decision of which to use is left to one's own judgment. The clinician who is relatively inexperienced with children might feel more comfortable using an inhalational agent to obtain the relaxation needed for laryngoscopy and intubation. A variation of this technique is to use the volatile agent for relaxation, laryngoscope the child, topicalize with lidocaine 3 mg/kg, ventilate for 1 to 2 minutes, and then intubate. Another alternative is to administer lidocaine 1.5 mg/kg IV just before intubation to deepen the anesthesia.

There are three options for intubation: (1) oral intubation, (2) oral intubation followed by nasal intubation, and (3) nasal intubation. If there is difficulty with maintaining an airway or with laryngoscopy, an oral endotracheal tube should be inserted initially and control of the airway obtained. Some clinicians recommend this as a routine approach, regardless of the ease of airway management. If there is great difficulty in laryngoscopy, either because of a very difficult airway or the lack of experience of the anesthesiologist, oral intubation without changing to nasal intubation is appropriate for the definitive management of the airway. On the other hand, if the situation is under control, the second option, to initially insert an oral endotracheal tube, ventilate the patient, decongest the nasal mucosa with phenylephrine, and then proceed with nasal intubation is appropriate. If the airway is under control, the third option, initial placement of a nasotracheal tube is acceptable. In this circumstance, after the induction of anesthesia, the nasopharynx is sprayed with phenylephrine to constrict the vascular bed of the nasopharynx, and a nasotracheal tube is then introduced. Regardless of which option is taken, the anesthesiologist must realize that laryngoscopy may be very difficult and that there may be a great deal of edematous tissue that will have to be identified. It is extremely important to follow the routine method for laryngoscopy, slowly introducing the laryngoscope blade along the right side of the tongue until it arrives in the vallecula, identifying the epiglottis, and then lifting the epiglottis with either a straight blade or a MacIntosh blade, placing the tip of the blade in the vallecula and exposing the vocal cords. The edema may well have spread into the supraglottic region as well as the false vocal cords. At times it becomes very difficult to identify the larynx. If the patient is breathing spontaneously, one can sometimes hear breath sounds coming from the appropriate orifice. Otherwise, gentle pressure on the chest can force an air bubble out through the edematous tissue. The air bubble marks the larynx, and the endotracheal tube can be introduced through this area of edema. For oral intubation it is quite helpful to have a stylet in the endotracheal tube. Regardless of the intubation technique used, an endotracheal tube with a stylet in place must always be ready for emergencies. After the endotracheal tube is securely fastened and its position verified, blood cultures can be taken and antibiotic therapy begun. If an IV is established in the emergency room, antibiotics should be started at that time. Cultures in acute epiglottitis are positive for *H. influenzae* type b in 70 to 90 percent of cases. The antibiotic chosen depends somewhat on whether or not a penicillin-resistant organism is reported in the area. The usual therapy is to begin with high-dose ampicillin (400 mg/kg/day) and chloramphenicol (100 mg/kg for the first dose) and to then reduce the dose of chloramphenicol to 50 mg/kg/day. If the culture is negative or if a resistant organism grows, the chloramphenicol is continued. Molteni[10] reviewed the incidence of extraepiglottic infections in acute epiglottitis. He reviewed 72 cases of epiglottitis between 1958 and 1975 and found a 25 percent incidence of both pneumonia and cervical lymphadenitis. The other major infection in acute epiglottitis is meningitis. Fortunately, this occurs very rarely. A chest x-ray should be taken to verify the position of the endotracheal tube and to determine whether pneumonia is present. This can be done either in the operating room or in the nursing area in which the patient is to be monitored. Securing the endotracheal tube is extremely important in these children. One technique is to spray the endotracheal tube and patient's face with an agent that enhances adhesiveness and to then use circumferential tape around the tube and entirely around the child's face and neck. Reversed tape or padding is placed on the back of the neck so that the tape does not adhere to the patient's hair. Two circumferences of tape are used, after which a safety pin is placed 2 mm

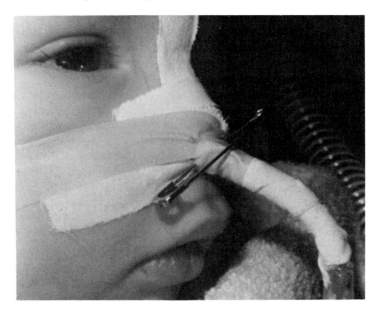

Fig. 8-3. Child with nasotracheal tube firmly secured in nose with circumferential tape and safety pin through tape and edge of tube.

from the nares through the endotracheal tube and the tape (Figs. 8-3 and 8-4). The safety pin goes through the side rather than the middle of the endotracheal tube so that a suction catheter can easily be passed into the tube. The arms should be restrained to prevent extubation. The endotracheal tube is then shortened so that approximately 2 to 3 cm extends outside the nose. This is attached to some form of T-piece so that humidity, oxygen, and, when indicated, positive end-expiratory pressure can be administered during the period of observation and therapy. Another method for providing postoperative oxygen and humidity is to place the child in a croup tent after intubation. This way the endotracheal tube is not attached to any other piece of equipment, such as a T-piece. It is believed that this may reduce the incidence of accidental extubation.

Supportive Care of an Artificial Airway

An endotracheal tube or tracheostomy tube inserted into the airway, although life-saving, can defeat nature's mechanisms for keeping the tracheobronchial system humidified and clean. Also, the tube causes a reduction in the functional residual capacity (FRC). Because the presence of the endotracheal tube makes it most difficult for the child to remove secretions, attention must be paid to adequate suctioning of the tracheobronchial system. When relatively unhumidified gas is inspired, there is desiccation of the tracheobronchial system, resulting in an increased viscosity of secretions, an inhibition of ciliary activity, and damage to the cell structures. Increasing the humidity of the gas with a small moisture-trapping humidifier will provide the appropriate humidification

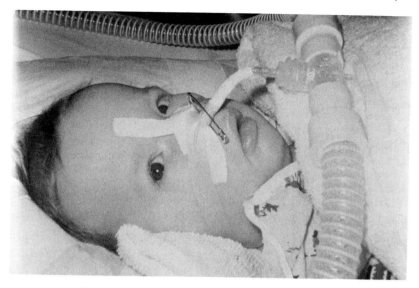

Fig. 8-4. Child with nasotracheal tube and T-piece.

to minimize these derangements. Additionally, the presence of an artificial airway will decrease the FRC and may also decrease the PaO_2. Children with acute epiglottitis should also have their FiO_2 increased to approximately 35 percent so that if the endotracheal tube should accidentally be removed the increased oxygen reserve will be sufficient until the child can be reintubated or until airway control can be accomplished.

Postobstructive Pulmonary Edema

Patients who have experienced acute airway obstruction and hypoxia and have had this obstruction acutely relieved are candidates for developing a relatively infrequent but nonetheless potentially dangerous form of pulmonary edema.[11,12] This is discussed in greater detail in Chapter 13. The treatment is administration of oxygen and positive end-expiratory pressure.

Controversies in Treatment of Acute Epiglottitis

The Treatment of Acute Epiglottitis With a Bag and Mask

The treatment of acute epiglottitis by ventilatory assistance with a bag and mask rather than by intubating the patient has been suggested.[8,13,14] Two other measures are part of the treatment regimen: intravenous administration of antibiotics and steroids (dexamethasone 0.4 mg/kg). This regimen has been recommended in two circumstances: as a definitive therapy, requiring the presence of an experienced airway management team at all times during the acute phase of the illness, and in the situation in which the medical team may be unqualified to establish an airway and supportive care is needed to transport the patient to a medical center where the condition can be managed. The latter circumstance is discussed below. The majority opinion today is that if a diagnosis of acute epiglottitis is made, the patient needs an artificial airway.

The issue of what to do for the patient with the life-threatening problem of acute epiglottitis when qualified medical care is not available for definitive airway management has received scant attention. The recent focus on the technique of cricothyrotomy has appropriately emphasized the relative simplicity and increased speed with which an airway can be secured as compared to tracheostomy. However, the performance of this procedure requires some degree of training. Perhaps the best compromise in this very difficult situation is a "full-court press," with supportive care to transport the child to a definitive medical center in the company of a physician or someone familiar with cricothyrotomy who can perform it if it becomes impossible to manage the airway otherwise. The "full-court press" includes:

1. Antibiotics (ampicillin 200 mg/kg IV and chloramphenicol 100 mg/kg IV)
2. Intravenous fluids (a 25-ml/kg bolus of a balanced salt solution followed by an infusion at the rate of 10 ml/kg/hr for an infant or young child and 6 ml/kg/hour for an older child or adult)
3. A positive-pressure mask and administration of 100 percent oxygen with assisted ventilation and/or positive end-expiratory pressure
4. Steroids (dexamethasone 1 mg/kg IV)

The role of steroids is somewhat controversial, but theoretically they may reduce the edema and inflammatory response that mark epiglottitis.

Cricothyrotomy or Tracheostomy in Epiglottitis

The question occasionally arises about the circumstances under which a cricothyrotomy or tracheostomy might be an acceptable form of definitive therapy. This situation might arise if there is no one who is capable of introducing an endotracheal tube into an obstructed airway. This would be a marginal situation at best; administration of local anesthesia for a rapid cricothyrotomy while the patient was being given oxygen with a bag and mask would be the treatment of choice.

Sedation

There is a difference of opinion as to whether or not to sedate the patient, and if so, how. I prefer to sedate with small incremental doses of morphine 0.05 mg/kg IV. The object of sedation is not to render the child comatose, but rather to titrate in incremental doses of sedation so that the child stops attempting to remove the endotracheal tube or thrashing about in bed. Morphine is a good sedative, and also provides analgesia for better tolerance of the discomfort of the nasotracheal tube. If, however, the respiratory rate of the child begins to fall below a reasonable number for the child's age and yet the child struggles and threatens the placement of the endotracheal tube between these periods of slow ventilation, one of several options can be taken. The first is to give valium or midazolam in incremental doses (0.05 mg/kg IV). The second is to completely restrain the child and ignore the periods of thrashing about. The third option is to paralyze and ventilate. This last option is often used in the infant under 2 years who cannot be easily sedated. One possible reason for a child's not being sedated with what appears to be a reasonable dose of morphine is the presence of hypoxia, which can be ascertained by use of a pulse oximeter. If an oximeter is not available, a blood gas sample should be drawn to evaluate the patient's state of oxygenation and ventilation. One advantage of using morphine for sedation is that it is easily reversible. This is quite important at the time of planned extubation, since any apparent hangover from the narcotic can easily be reversed. Also, if the child is within the time range of extubation and suddenly self-extubates, or if there is an accidental extubation, the immediate reversal of the narcotic might avoid the need for reintubation. The narcotic should be reversed with incremental doses of naloxone (Narcan). The initial dose is 0.01 mg/kg IV, and when the desired effect is achieved the same dose is administered intramuscularly for a more prolonged effect, since the effect of intravenous naloxone lasts only 30 to 60 minutes, whereas that of morphine may last 4 to 6 hours.[15]

Timing and Criteria for Extubation

The next area of difference of opinion in the treatment of acute epiglottitis concerns the criteria for extubation. At present, there are two opinions.[8,16,17] One opinion is that the child should be extubated when the clinical signs have greatly improved. The other opinion is that there is a need to visualize the supraglottic structures to determine if there has been an appropriate reduction in swelling before extubation is accomplished. The technique that I prefer is to base the timing of extubation on clinical criteria (i.e., when the child looks more alert, the signs of dehydration have disappeared, the temperature is returning to normal, and the time of day is appropriate for the staff). This technique usually takes between 12 and 24 hours. The child is extubated in the nursing unit, with emergency airway support available, and the narcotic is reversed as indicated. The temperature does not have to return entirely to normal since the febrile part of the illness may last up to 36 to 48 hours. The need to reintubate patients with epiglottitis who have been electively extubated is extremely rare, and in one study was due to the trauma of the intubation rather than the disease process.[8] Approximately 10 percent of the children in this study had postextubation stridor: 21 were observed, 9 received a dose of racemic epinephrine, and the one mentioned above required reintubation.

The other opinion holds that there is a need to visualize the supraglottic structures to determine if there has been a reduction in the swelling before extubation.[17] Three techniques have been described for accomplishing this. One is to topicalize the nose and hypopharynx and use a fiberoptic laryngoscope to examine the supraglottic structures. The second is to give the patient a sleep-inducing dose of sodium thiopental or a paralyzing dose of succinylcholine and directly visualize the supraglottic structures with a laryngoscope. The third technique is to physically restrain the child and do a laryngoscopy without any additional medications. The location in which to perform the visualization procedure is either the operating room or the nursing unit. There are certain disadvantages to visualizing the supraglottic structures. These include: (1) the enormously increased cost to the patient; (2) the need, in the second technique, for a general anesthetic for a procedure that has never been proved to be necessary for the treatment of acute epiglottitis; and (3) if restraint is used, the relatively uncomfortable nature of the procedure for any child. Those who favor this approach believe that the anatomic obstruction must be markedly reduced before extubation will be successful. Those who do not favor visualization believe that there are many reasons why intubation is needed, including partial airway obstruction, toxemia, dehydration, and fatigue. All of these factors are improved with the therapy of intubation, oxygenation, antibiotics, fluids, sedation, and rest. As a result, the causes of the airway obstruction have been treated, which makes visualization of the epiglottis is unnecessary.

CROUP
Postintubation or Traumatic Croup

The most frequent type of croup, and the one with which most anesthesiologists are familiar, is postintubation croup.[18] This is discussed in Chapter 16.

Spasmodic Croup

Spasmodic croup is a very mild form of croup that develops in an otherwise asymptomatic child after he has been put to bed at night. Its etiology is unknown. The child is afebrile and well when put to bed, but develops a brassy cough that may awaken the entire household. The condition seems to recur on several successive nights, becoming milder each night until it finally disappears, much to everyone's relief. During the daytime the child is well and shows no other evidence of illness. Spasmodic croup is thought to be more frequent in children with allergies. There are many forms of recommended treatment for it. It is quite different from laryngotracheobronchitis, in which the child is obviously ill.

Laryngotracheobronchitis

Laryngotracheobronchitis (LTB) is also known as infectious croup, subglottic laryngobronchitis, and acute obstructive laryngitis. A basic point to remember about this disease is that it involves not only the immediate subglottic area but also the remainder of the tracheobronchial tree. Children with LTB present with stridor, cough, and fever. The differential diagnosis of acute airway obstruction must always be considered in full in any child with stridor. This differential diagnosis is listed in Table 8-1.

The etiology of LTB is thought to be primarily viral.[19] The viruses that have been documented to cause LTB include influenza A and parainfluenza 1 and 2 viruses, adenoviruses, and myxoviruses. An interesting aspect of LTB is that the severity of the infection varies enormously depending on the viruses prevalent that year. This variation may be one reason why therapeutic techniques for the treatment of LTB have had such variable results.

LTB is caused by a viral inflammatory process that leads to airway obstruction. The obstruction is caused by two sequelae of the inflammatory process: submucosal edema and secretions of varying tenacity. The edema and secretions may involve the entire laryngotracheobronchial tree. As the patient becomes increasingly dehydrated, the secretions become more tenacious and difficult to expel by coughing. In some children the disease is quite mild and can be treated on an outpatient basis. However, in some outbreaks, approximately 10 percent of the children who develop LTB will have to be hospitalized, and approximately 0.1 to 1 percent may need an artificial airway.

The major differential diagnosis in LTB is that of epiglottitis. Table 8-2 lists the major symptoms and signs of the two processes. Both may start with what would appear to be a mild coryza or sore throat. Some cases of epiglottitis do not appear to have a prodromal coryza and have an explosive onset, whereas with LTB the symptoms usually develop more slowly over a period of days. Also, because of its viral etiology, LTB lasts considerably longer (i.e., up to 7 to 10 days). As noted earlier, the patient with acute epiglottitis will be agitated, sitting up, leaning forward, and drooling, whereas the usual patient with LTB may be lying down and not in as much distress. The child with LTB often has a classic barking, brassy, seal-like cough. The early clinical course of the two illnesses may be indistinguishable. There are two approaches to this problem. One, which has already been mentioned, is to examine the child's airway in the emergency room with an anesthesiologist standing by.[2,3] The other opinion is that if there is this much question about the diagnosis, the child should be taken to the operating room, anesthetized and laryngoscoped, and the correct diagnosis made. However, the matter is one of clinical judgment. It is far preferable to diagnose the occasional case of LTB by this method than to miss the occasional case of acute epiglottis, thinking it is LTB.

If LTB is thought to be the diagnosis, time can be taken to obtain a lateral radiograph of the neck.[20] There are classic radiographic signs for differentiating between acute epiglottitis and LTB, however, even in the best of hands the radiographic diagnosis of LTB or epiglottitis is not 100 percent successful. Mention should be made of the thumb sign in acute epiglottitis: as the epiglottis becomes swollen, it resembles the thumb. The neck radiograph of the child with LTB demonstrates subglottic narrowing, often called ''pencilling,'' and may demonstrate one of the secondary signs of airway obstruction: distention of the pyriform sinus with inspiration. Figure 8-5 is a representative radiograph of acute epiglottitis and Figure 8-6 is a representative radiograph of LTB. When looking at the lateral radiograph in a case of acute airway obstruction, the epiglottis can be found by first identifying the hyoid bone (marked by an arrow in Figures 8-5 and 8-6). The epiglottis is found at the base of the hyoid bone. In acute

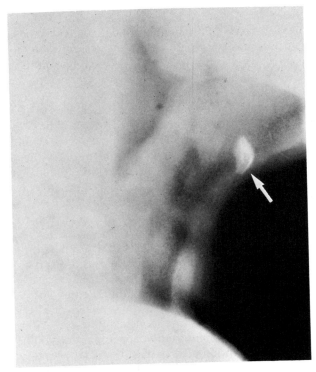

Fig. 8-5. Acute epiglottitis. Arrow points to hyoid bone.

epiglottitis, the epiglottis will be quite swollen and edematous, whereas the airway below it will be normal. In LTB, on the other hand, the epiglottis is normal but the area below it is narrowed. Both figures demonstrate distention of the pyriform sinus with inspiration. Unfortunately, not every radiograph is technically perfect and not every radiologist can correctly interpret pediatric radiographs. In a study reported by Mills,[20] approximately 13 percent of the radiographs were technically unsatisfactory; a nonpediatric radiologist read the films correctly 50 percent of the time, whereas a pediatric radiologist read the films correctly 92 percent of the time. Reading a radiograph correctly 50 percent of the time is not much better than flipping a coin. If the diagnosis of acute epiglottitis cannot be ruled out or in, the child should be taken to the operating room for a diagnosis.

Clinical Evaluation of the Child With Laryngotracheobronchitis

Downes[21] has described an excellent scoring system that allows an objective evaluation of the child with LTB. The system is shown in Table 8-4. The information can be used to assist in the clinical management of the child and may be transferred from one physician to another with a high degree of objectivity,

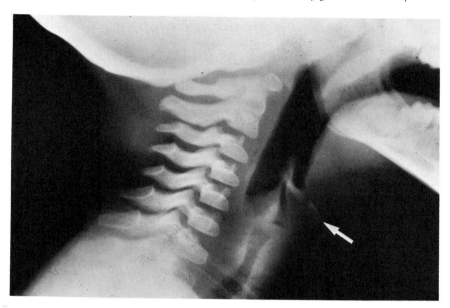

Fig. 8-6. Laryngotracheobronchitis. Arrow points to hyoid bone.

permitting changes in the child's clinical course to be more easily recognized and acted on. Another value of the scoring system is in the study of patients with LTB and the various treatment modalities. In the guidelines suggested by Downes, a score greater than 4 calls for full conservative therapy. A child with a score greater than 7 who remains hypoxic and hypercarbic despite full conservative therapy needs an artificial airway.

The vast majority of children with LTB will be treated in the outpatient department, and the anesthesiologist will never see them.[22] The only children who the anesthesiologist will see are those who are severely ill with LTB, or in whom there is a diagnostic question. This means that all of these children will have a croup score of greater than 4 and will need full conservative therapy. Such

Table 8-4. Clinical Croup Score

	0	1	2
Inspiratory breath sounds	Normal	Harsh with rhonci	Delayed
Stridor	None	Inspiratory	Inspiratory and expiratory
Cough	None	Hoarse cry	Bark
Retractions and flaring	None	Flaring and supersternal retractions	As under 1, plus subcostal/intercostal retractions
Cyanosis	None	In air	In 40% oxygen

Score >4, moderately severe obstruction: Full conservative therapy.
Score >7, with PaO_2 <70 on FIO_2 of 40 percent and PCO_2 >70: Artificial airway.
(Modified from Downes,[21] with permission.)

therapy consists of oxygen, steroids, and racemic epinephrine. Racemic epinephrine is a mixture of the levo- and dextro-isomers of epinephrine. The active form of the drug is the levo-isomer. It comes in a 2.25 percent solution (Micronefrin, Vaponefrin). It is diluted with water or saline in an 8:1 ratio. The drug is nebulized and the child inspires it through an intermittent positive-pressure breathing mask, through a hand-held nebulizer, or through a pneumatically powered nebulizer. Racemic epinephrine provides temporary relief in LTB. The action of this vasopressor is to constrict the boggy subglottic area, thereby increasing the diameter of the airway. It is quite effective as a temporary measure, with relief that lasts from 30 to 60 minutes. However, the redistribution of the mixture from the inflamed area allows the mucosa to return to its previous condition, and at times rebound swelling has been reported. This may occur up to 2 hours after the initial administration of racemic epinephrine. Therefore, any child receiving this drug must be observed for at least this period of time before being discharged. The drug may be administered every 1 to 2 hours for long periods.

Steroids and Laryngotracheobronchitis

For a long time, the use of steroids in the treatment of LTB was controversial.[23-25] The reason for this controversy was mainly twofold. First, the diagnosis of "croup" was given to any cause of upper airway obstruction, including acute epiglottitis. This confusion of diagnosis made it very difficult to know which condition was being treated. The second reason for the difficulty in evaluating the efficacy of steroids in LTB was the extreme variability in the dosages used. In the studies that declared steroids ineffective, the dose of dexamethasone was 0.1 mg/kg, whereas in the studies in which steroids were deemed effective, the dose employed was anywhere from 0.3 to 1 mg/kg of dexamethasone. Despite the fact that in every reported study in which high-dose steroids have been used their efficacy has been substantiated, there are still those who do not believe such studies and think that the use of these drugs is controversial. However, such clinicians at least do recognize that, because of the relatively low risk raised by the short-term administration of steroids, they should be given.[25] It is hoped that the report by Kairys et al. will end the controversy.[26] They did meta-analysis of the 10 published reports of randomized trials involving some 1,286 patients. Their results support the use of steroids in the treatment of LTB. The initial dose of dexamethasone is 0.5 to 1 mg/kg IV. It takes from 15 to 45 minutes for the steroids to begin to become effective. The effect will last approximately 4 to 8 hours, and the dose may have to be repeated after that time if the symptoms recur. It should be remembered that infectious croup may last for 7 to 10 days, and that steroid therapy for it may be required for several days.

At times, despite full therapy, the patient needs an artificial airway. This should be accomplished according to the same guidelines and principles as for acute epiglottitis. The size of the endotracheal tube needed is one size smaller than would be expected for the patient's age. Even then, the tube may not easily slide into the subglottic airway, and there will probably be no air leak around the tube, or at least not initially. Because the etiologic agent in LTB is a virus, it will take longer for the problem to be resolved, and attempts at extubation should therefore be guided by the development of an air leak and an improvement in the clinical condition of the patient (i.e., state of hydration, alertness, etc.). Usually, extubation is not attempted before 2 to 3 days. There is a difference of opinion about whether the patient should be extubated in the intensive care unit without a laryngotracheal examination or in the operating room under full anesthesia for diagnostic laryngoscopy. The child who has been intubated for LTB will often have varying degrees of residual edema in the immediate postextubation period, at times severe enough to require reintubation. If reintubation is necessary, the child should remain intubated for 1 or 2 days before attempts at extubation are begun again. Racemic epinephrine may be quite helpful in getting over this very difficult period. This scenario of reintubation may occur several times. On rare occasions these patients may need a tracheostomy.

BACTERIAL TRACHEITIS OR MEMBRANOUS LARYNGOTRACHEOBRONCHITIS

Another cause of childhood acute airway obstruction is a complication of the viral form of LTB. It has been referred to by various names, such as membranous LTB or bacterial tracheitis.[27,28] In this situation, a bacterial infection is superimposed on the viral infection, which leads to the formation of a membrane. The organism most frequently associated with this bacterial infection is *Staphylococcus aureus*. A membrane is formed within the tracheobronchial tree. The child may cough up stringy, brownish mucus plugs. On occasion this material may be so voluminous and tenacious that it causes complete laryngeal obstruction. In one case report the membrane was initially diagnosed by radiography as a foreign body (Fig. 8-7). In this case bronchoscopy was needed to remove the membranous cast, after which the patient made an uneventful recovery. In another case report, the mucus formed the pattern of a partial cast of the infraglottic laryngeal and tracheal area. A temporary improvement may be seen after this material is coughed up, although the patient still requires aggressive therapy. This therapy consists of the full conservative therapy already described plus aggressive antibiotic therapy, and, when indicated, laryngoscopy or bronchoscopy for removal of the obstructing membrane and then intubation. Many of the strains of *S. aureus* that cause the infection are resistant to penicillin. Therefore, one of the antistaphylococcal drugs, such as cloxicillin, and a second antibiotic to cover the other possible pathogens, such as ampicillin, are necessary. Bacterial tracheitis is a relatively uncommon disease, but has been reported to be increasing in frequency.[28]

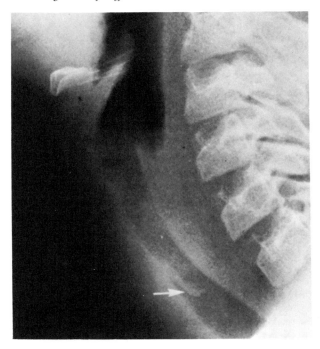

Fig. 8-7. Laryngotracheobronchitis complicated by bacterial tracheitis. Arrow points at intratracheal mass. (From Denneny and Handler,[29] with permission.)

REFERENCES

1. Jones R, Bodnar A, Roan Y, et al: Subglottic stenosis in newborn intensive care unit graduates. Am J Dis Child 135:367, 1981
2. Mauro, RD, Poole SR, Lockhart CH: Differentiation of epiglottitis from laryngotracheitis in the child with stridor. Am J Dis Child 142:679, 1988
3. The Pediatric Forum. Am J Dis Child 142:1261, 1988
4. Scheidemandel HHE: Did George Washington die of quinsy? Arch Otolaryngol 102:519, 1976
5. Adler E, Gibbons PA, Striker TW, Denson DD: Ketamine: An alternative for the anesthetic management of acute epiglottitis. Anesth Analg 65:S3, 1986
6. Blackstock D, Adderley RJ, Steward DJ: Epiglottitis in young children. Anesthesiology 67:97, 1987
7. Crockett DM, McGill TJ, Healy GB, Friedman EM: Airway management of acute supraglottitis at the children's hospital, Boston: 1980-1985. Ann Otol Rhinol Laryngol 97:114, 1988
8. Butt W, Shann F, Walker C, et al: Acute epiglottitis: A different approach to management. Crit Care Med 16:43, 1988
9. Diaz JH: Croup and epiglottis in children: The anesthesiologist as diagnostician. Anesth Analg 64:621, 1985
10. Molteni RA: Epiglottitis: Incidence of extraepiglottic infection. Report of 72 cases and review of the literature. Pediatrics 58:526, 1976

11. Travis KW, Todres ID, Shannon DC: Pulmonary edema associated with croup and epiglottitis. Pediatrics 59:695, 1977
12. Soliman MG, Richer P: Epiglottitis and pulmonary oedema in children. Can Anaesth Soc J 25:270, 1978
13. Szold PD, Glicklich M: Children with epiglottitis can be bagged. Clin Pediatr 15:792, 1976
14. Glicklich M, Cohen RD, Jona JZ: Steroids and bag and mask ventilation in the treatment of acute epiglottitis. J Pediatr Surg 14:247, 1979
15. Longnecker DE, Grazis PA, Eggers FWN Jr: Naloxone for antagonism of morphine-induced respiratory depression. Anesth Analg 52:447, 1973
16. Berry FA: Letter to the editor. Anesth Analg 63:469, 1984
17. Rothstein P, Lister G: Epiglottitis: Duration of intubation and fever. Anesth Analg 62:785, 1983
18. Koka BV, Jeon IS, Andre JM, et al: Postintubation croup in children. Anesth Analg 54:622, 1975
19. Denny FW, Murphy TF, Clyde WA, et al: Croup: An 11-year study in a pediatric practice. Pediatrics 71:871, 1983
20. Mills JL, Spackman TJ, Borns P, et al: The usefulness of lateral neck roentgenograms in laryngotracheobronchitis. Am J Dis Child 133:1140, 1979
21. Downs JJ: ASA Refresher Course. No. 111. American Society of Anesthesiologists, Chicago, 1975
22. Taussig LM, Castro O, Beaudry PH, et al: Treatment of laryngotracheobronchitis (croup). Am J Dis Child 129:790, 1975
23. Leipsig B, Oski FA, Cummings CW, et al: A prospective randomized study to determine the efficacy of steroids in treatment of croup. J Pediatr 94:194, 1979
24. Cherry JD: The treatment of croup: Continued controversy due to failure of recognition of historic, ecologic, and clinical perspectives. J Pediatr 94:352, 1979
25. Tunnessen WW, Feinstein AR: The steroid-croup controversy: An analytic review of methodologic problems. J Pediatr 96:751, 1980
26. Kairys SW, Olmstead EM, O'Connor GT: Steroid treatment of laryngotracheitis: A meta-analysis of the evidence from randomized trials. Pediatrics 83:5 683-693, 1989
27. McKenzie M, Norman MG, Anderson JD, et al: Upper respiratory tract infection in a 3-year-old girl. J Pediatr 105:129, 1984
28. Nelson WE: Bacterial croup: A historical perspective. J Pediatr 105:52, 1984
29. Denneny JC III, Handler SD: Membranous laryngotracheobronchitis. Pediatrics 70:705, 1982

9

THE CHILD WITH A RUNNY NOSE

Frederic A. Berry

One of the enigmas of pediatric anesthesia is the child with a runny nose. Webster defines *enigma* as "something hard to understand or explain; puzzling; obscure." The Greek derivation of *enigma* translates into "to speak in riddles." This definition and derivation very clearly characterize both the problem and those who try to discuss it.

A runny nose may be the signal event of an acute upper respiratory tract infection, the flu syndrome, other infections, or an allergy. By the term *cold* we refer to an infectious process of the upper airway (i.e., the airway above the vocal cords). It is another term for upper respiratory infection (URI), or nasopharyngitis. At times the terms *cold* and *runny nose* are used interchangeably, which has led to further confusion about the differential diagnosis.

There are currently major disagreements about what to do with a child with a runny nose. The first priority is arriving at an appropriate diagnosis, since many of the signs and symptoms of a mild URI are the same as those of allergic rhinitis, and it may be impossible to tell the difference clinically. For that reason, some studies do not clearly differentiate the two, and it is difficult to draw exact conclusions from them. In one study, infants and children older than 1 year of age with a URI who underwent a short halothane anesthetic without endotracheal intubation for insertion of middle-ear ventilation tubes demonstrated no increased incidence of respiratory complications.[1] As a matter of fact, a decrease in the symptoms of the illness was reported, and the authors believed there was a beneficial effect on the natural history of the respiratory infection. Other studies in children who had surgical procedures that required intubation have reported problems with anesthetic management. One such study in infants under 1 year and in some older children did report an increased incidence of "critical" incidents during anesthesia in these patients.[2] It has also been reported that infants and children with a URI who undergo anesthesia have a higher incidence of desaturation in the postoperative period.[3] The answers are not clear, and it may be that different recommendations are in order for different surgical procedures.[4,5] Children who have either frequent or chronic upper respiratory secretions regardless of their etiology often also have problems with serious otitis media and require ventilation tubes. The first study cited would suggest that this group of patients can safely undergo surgery without an increased incidence of complications. This may not hold true for different and longer surgical procedures.

The object of this chapter is to clarify some of these issues and to establish criteria for evaluating these children as well as guidelines for their management. A runny nose may be the result of a change in the weather or an emotional upset such as crying; a response to an allergen, nonspecific irritant, or infectious agent; or a further enigma. If sufficient time is allowed to pass, the cause of the runny nose may become evident or it may disappear. A diagnosis could then be made on the basis of reasonable information, and a decision made about the anesthetic implications, if any. Unfortunately, there are several problems with this scenario. We are in the era of cost containment, diagnosis-related-groups (DRGs), and ambulatory surgery. We know that there are many advantages to ambulatory surgery, such as lower costs, a shorter separation of the child from the family, a reduced exposure to hospital infections, and less upheaval of the entire family complex. We must also recognize that there are disadvantages to ambulatory surgery. These include insufficient time to allow the disease process or a potential disease process to declare itself, inadequate time to develop an extensive rapport with the patient and the family, and a dependence on the family to recognize and seek medical assistance for any postoperative complications that may occur. In dealing with ambulatory surgical patients, we do not have the luxury of time to make a diagnosis. We have to make a decision in a matter of minutes or hours. There are two reasons for this. The first is that the surgical schedule is demanding; the second is that if the child does have an infectious problem and it is communicable, we do not want to expose any more people than necessary. This includes the entire staff of the medical facility.

DIFFERENTIAL DIAGNOSIS OF A RUNNY NOSE

The two most frequent medical problems of children—allergies and viral infections—involve the respiratory tract. It has been estimated that approximately 15 to 20 percent of the American population is afflicted with some form of respiratory allergy, and that from 5 to 9 percent of the pediatric population has asthma.[6] The spectrum of this problem varies from allergic rhinitis to severe allergic asthma. The other problem afflicting all children is viral respiratory tract infection. There is evidence to suggest that the young child will have from two to four such infections per year. The end result is that very many children will have respiratory tract signs and symptoms on a relatively frequent basis. The causes can be relatively benign, as shown in Table 9-1, or potentially quite serious, as indicated in Table 9-2.

The automatic cancellation of surgery for a child with a runny nose would create a hardship for the patient, the parents, and the entire medical system,

Table 9-1. Noninfectious
Causes of Runny Nose

Allergic rhinitis
    Seasonal
    Perennial
Vasomotor rhinitis
    Emotional (crying)
    Temperature

and would be quite inappropriate. Instead, the child needs careful evaluation and management.

Allergic Disease

Allergic disease, or noninfectious or benign runny nose, is probably the most frequent medical problem in the general population. A child's earliest episodes of acute allergic rhinitis, sinusitis, or asthma may come as a surprise to the parents. However, after considering the family history and the repeated clinical course of the disease, the diagnosis of allergy both in the family and in the individual patient is usually made. Because of this, the parents are usually adept at recognizing when the child is having allergic problems or when the problem is something else (i.e., an infection). The allergic child's early years are characterized by a pattern of recurrent runny nose, frequent otitis media, frequent need for ventilation tubes, tonsillectomy and adenoidectomy, and so forth. The unfamiliar anesthesiologist, when seeing such a patient, will often become alarmed and cancel surgery. This often meets with the surprised response from the parents, "But doctor, he's this way all the time." The other factor that can complicate the diagnosis of allergic rhinitis is that after a prolonged period of chronic rhinitis, local infection with normal flora may develop and the child may have a purulent nasal discharge. This has been confused by some with respiratory tract infection, with the resulting knee-jerk response of cancellation of any type of surgery. It is for this reason that the parents must be carefully questioned, since they will be the best source of information about the child's condition.

Children with a noninfectious runny nose are candidates for elective surgery,

Table 9-2. Infectious Causes of Runny Nose

Viral infections
    Nasopharyngitis (common cold)
    Flu syndromes (upper and lower respiratory tract)
    Laryngotracheobronchitis (infectious croup)
Viral exanthems
    Measles
    Chicken pox
Acute bacterial infections
    Acute epiglottitis
    Meningitis
    Streptococcal tonsillitis

since they will often have the problem on unpredictable and frequent occasions. There are children whose allergic disease comes from identifiable causes such as seasonal pollens, and thus there is some degree of predictability about when these children will be symptomatic. Elective surgery should be scheduled in the allergic "off" season. The major concerns with elective surgery and allergic rhinitis are secretions, and that allergic rhinitis may be the prodrome of asthma.

There is no question that anesthetic complications are infrequent in the patient with a runny nose of noninfectious origin. The main cause of respiratory complications in this group of patients is sensitization of the airway by secretions, which leads to laryngospasm, coughing, apnea, and hypoxia. The other possibility is that a runny nose may be a prodrome of asthma, which certainly will have anesthetic implications. There has been an ever-increasing recognition of the fact that reactive airway disease (bronchospasm) may be associated with either viral infections or chronic sinus disease, and that this may be confused with allergic asthma.[7] Also, it is well recognized that a viral respiratory infection may precipitate an asthma attack in patients with allergic asthma.

Viral Respiratory Tract Infections

Some viruses affect mainly the upper respiratory tract; others affect mainly the lower respiratory tract, and therefore might be associated with the complication of pneumonia. The rhinovirus, adenovirus, influenza, and respiratory syncytial viruses are usually associated with URI. These infections are localized primarily to the upper respiratory tract and result in upper airway secretions and an increased reactivity of the upper airway. The influenza viruses may also spread into the lower respiratory tract and potentially result in a reactive lower respiratory tract, decreased compliance, and bronchospasm. The influenza viruses are associated with the major constitutional signs and symptoms of malaise, elevated temperature, cough, and secretions. URI usually does not cause an illness that is as severe as the flu syndromes. It usually lasts only 2 or 3 days.

In the study referred to at the beginning of this chapter, an attempt was made to objectively evaluate the patient according to the signs and symptoms.[1] The symptoms include the following:

1. Mild sore or scratchy throat
2. Mild malaise
3. Sneezing
4. Rhinorrhea
5. Congestion or stuffiness of the head
6. Nonproductive cough
7. Mild fever

In order to make a diagnosis of URI, the presence of any two of the above signs or symptoms was required. However, combinations of symptoms 1 and 2, 3 and 4, and 5 and 6 required an additional symptom to make the diagnosis. It is understandable from looking at this list of signs and symptoms why it is often difficult to differentiate URI and allergic rhinitis and to give appropriate guidelines for their evaluation and anesthetic management. If the child has a URI, it will usually last 2 or 3 days and the child will return to normal within 3 or 4 days and be left with essentially no airway residual. However, a child with a lower respiratory tract infection is sicker; the acute illness may last for 3 to 5 days and, although apparently recovering within a week or two, the child will still have the problem of reactive airway disease. These children may develop intra- and postoperative complications. Early in the course of both upper and lower respiratory tract infection, it may be difficult to differentiate one from the other.

ANESTHETIC ASSESSMENT OF THE CHILD WITH A RUNNY NOSE

It is hoped that by this time the reader will appreciate both the difficulty and the clinical importance of diagnosing a child with a runny nose. I discuss the importance of making a diagnosis as well as the possible complications with the parents so that they have an active part in the decision-making process. In addition, I have a discussion with the surgeon. The anesthesiologists and surgeons in my institution (Children's Medical Center of the University of Virginia) have developed a rapport over the years, which has allowed objective discussions and mutually agreed-upon clinical management.

The triad of anesthetic assessment consists of the history, physical examination, and the appropriate laboratory data.

History

The most important part of the assessment is the history, because most children with a full-blown illness characterized by a severe cough, an elevated temperature, malaise, nausea, vomiting, and other symptoms are not going to come to the hospital for elective surgery. The children in question are those who are early in their symptomatology and for whom the diagnosis is unclear. The parents are usually quite knowledgeable about the medical condition and past medical problems of their child. It is not sufficient, however, to simply ask whether the child has ever been sick. The parents must be specifically questioned on such items as whether the child has had a cold with a fever and a cough within the last month; whether he has ever had any wheezing associated with a cold; or whether he has ever been treated with epinephrine because of a cough. It is also important to inquire about other members of the family. If the child is of nursery or primary school age it is helpful to know whether there is anyone else in the class who is ill, or if there are any epidemics of viruses that are making the rounds of the school. Some of the questions for the parents are: Is Mary's appetite normal? Is Diane playing as usual? Is this the usual runny nose for Johnny? If Johnny didn't have a runny nose, would you think that he was perfectly well? If the parents convince me that this is the normal state of health for their child then elective surgery can be performed. However, if the parents say that they think their child has something different or is "coming down with something" then it's time to huddle with the parents and the surgeon and make a decision. It is important to inform the parents about the potential problems with a respiratory infection so that they are aware of the possible complications. Understanding that these complications pose a risk has a tendency to improve the parents' memories.

Physical Examination

The physical examination of a patient who is in the early stages of an infectious process may or may not be helpful. The examination of the respiratory tract must be especially thorough, with a specific search for viral ulcers in the oropharynx, for tonsillitis, and for other evidence of disease. Although positive findings may indicate an infectious process, negative findings do not rule it out. A purulent or semipurulent nasal discharge may be associated with acute nasopharyngitis or it may be caused by chronic allergic rhinitis in which a local infection leads to a chronic purulent nasal discharge and cough. The parents can be very helpful in making the differential diagnosis. The examination of the chest can be quite revealing if positive, but does not rule out a problem if negative. The specific findings being sought are decreased breath sounds, rales, and wheezing. Particularly in small children, viral respiratory tract infections may be associated with reactive airway disease.

Evaluation of the Child's Temperature

There is a relatively wide range of normal temperatures, extending from 36° to 38°C. Each child has his own normal diurnal variation in temperature. The parents often know if a temperature of 38°C is within the usual temperature range for their child, and their historical knowledge of the child's normal temperature patterns may be of help diagnostically. Nevertheless, the vast majority of parents have no such knowledge. A temperature of 38°C represents a temperature of 100.4°F and is the temperature that I consider highly suggestive of a respiratory tract infection when associated with a runny nose and cough. Although it is an arbitrary selection, it is easy to remember, and it is the number that has been picked by many as signifying the probability of some form of infectious process. There is no question that a small number of children have a normal temperature of 38° or 38.2°C. However, when a child presents with a runny nose, cough, and a temperature of 38.0°C, the chances are good that it will have an infectious process. On the other hand, if a child has a temperature of 38°C without any other signs or symptoms, it may well be normal for that child, or represent a slight degree of dehydration. The key point to remember is that a temperature of 38°C in the absence of any other positive finding may be considered normal and elective surgery may be performed, whereas the same temperature with the associated findings of a runny nose, cough, malaise, and so forth are highly suggestive of an infection, and in the opinion of many a reason for cancelling elective surgery, unless it is for insertion of ventilation tubes without intubation.

Laboratory Information

Anesthesiologists and surgeons frequently disagree about what should constitute the routine laboratory work for surgery. The Joint Commission on Accreditation of Hospitals answers the question quite clearly in stating in their manual that the "laboratory evaluation should be that which is appropriate for the situation." No laboratory work may be needed preparatory to elective surgery on a healthy child. On the other hand, either the patient's condition or the type of surgery may strongly suggest the blood work needed. What about the child with a runny nose, cough, and fever? Early in the course of a viral infection the white blood cell count (WBC) may be below normal. By contrast, with bacterial infections the WBC is usually above normal (i.e., greater than 12,000). Unfortunately, the WBC is all too often normal, and thus of no particular value. Therefore, I usually do not order a complete blood cell count in this situation.

Should a child being prepared for surgery have a "routine" chest x-ray. Three studies[8-10] have been done in an attempt to answer this question; two concluded that a "routine" chest x-ray was not indicated, whereas the third suggested that it was. The reasons for this difference of opinion become obvious with a careful reading of the papers. The definition of "routine" is critical. In the two most quoted reports,[8,9] which suggest that a routine chest x-ray is not needed, the children were screened with a history and physical examination. If either of these assessments was positive, the chest x-ray was considered to be "indicated." If the history and physical examinations were negative, the chest x-ray was called a "routine" chest x-ray for screening purposes. In this situation, the chest x-rays proved to be negative as far as significant physical findings were concerned. A difference of opinion was registered by Sane et al. in the one study that recommended routine preoperative chest x-rays on all children.[10] However, one must carefully examine these investigators criteria for what they consider a "routine" chest x-ray. They did a prospective study of 1,500 consecutive chest x-rays without concern for the history or physical examination. In this group of children approximately 5 percent had a significant physical abnormality. However, if these patients had had a history and physical examination, they might well have fallen into the category of patients for whom a chest x-ray is indicated.

What are the criteria for a chest x-ray? The bottom line is that any recent history of a significant fever and cough is an indication for a chest x-ray. If the x-ray is positive, it is certainly quite helpful in the decision-making process. However, if it is negative, the clinician still must make a judgment call.

CLINICAL MANAGEMENT OF THE CHILD WITH A RUNNY NOSE

The clinical management of the child who presents with a runny nose is guided by the information obtained in the history, physical examination, and laboratory evaluation. If the parent says that in addition to the runny nose there is something different about the child's condition and the temperature is 38°C, this is strongly suggestive of an infectious process. The presence of a severe, persistent cough tends to support the possibility that the disease process has already extended into the lower respiratory tract. A runny nose, cough, malaise, sneezing, and other symptoms are by themselves not definitive for an infectious process, since they may also be found in an allergic child. It is very important to differentiate between the two. Even with a complete evaluation of the patient, unavoidable errors in diagnosis will be made. There will be children whose surgery is cancelled because it is thought that they have an early infectious process who later prove to have nothing. There will also be patients who are thought to have an allergic process or mild URI who will turn out to have a more serious infectious process. This is where one's own judgment comes into play in the practice of anesthesia, and is unavoidable. It is important that the parents be made aware of these possibilities, and this step (known as *informed consent*) documented on the chart. The practice of medicine is characterized by the need to make judgment calls. (Unfortunately, the legal profession recognizes this concept in theory but not in practice.) These calls differ from one clinician to the next, depending on information, experience, and skill. When considering the natural course of a respiratory tract infection, pneumonia is certainly one of the expected complications. However, if a child is diagnosed as having a respiratory tract infection, and if elective surgery is then done and the child develops pneumonia, there is a great possibility that a plaintiff's expert witness would testify that the pneumonia was secondary to the administration of the anesthetic, and not the natural course of a lower respiratory tract infection. This is why, in today's medicolegal climate, it is so important to discuss with parents the possible sequelae of the disease and of anesthesia in a child with a respiratory infection, and document it on the chart. The anesthesiologist has an obligation to the parents to discuss these possibilities. If a complication then occurs, the parents have been informed and will have a better understanding of the process.

ANESTHETIC MANAGEMENT IN SHORT PROCEDURES IN THE CHILD WITH A URINARY TRACT INFECTION

Tait et al. have thoroughly evaluated a group of children with URI symptomatology who they diagnosed as having URI.[1] These children presented for the insertion of ventilation tubes in the ears. The surgery was short (i.e., 15 to 20 minutes). The anesthetic consisted of halothane/nitrous oxide and there was no intubation of the trachea. In those circumstances, they reported no increase in symptomatology compared to a control group. As a matter of fact, they found an improvement in symptoms. They stressed that their findings should not be carried over to longer procedures or to those that involve intubation. A study in ferrets likewise demonstrated that general anesthesia administered to ferrets infected with influenza virus carries minimal morbidity.[11] The question facing the clinician is what to do about anesthesia that may last longer than 15 to 20 minutes and that may involve endotracheal intubation. What if these children have not an infectious process, but rather an allergic process? What if they have secretions or a sensitive airway? A discussion of the anesthetic management of these patients follows.

The Child With a Sensitive Airway or Secretions

An increase in airway secretions and the presence of a sensitive airway may increase the hazards of administering an anesthetic. Increased airway secretions can lead to an increased frequency of coughing, laryngospasm, and airway obstruction. One infrequent but serious complication of this scenario is silent regurgitation and aspiration. Another complication is postobstructive pulmonary edema. The patient with lower respiratory tract disease has the potential for developing atelectasis, pneumonia, or both. There has been a difference of opinion as to whether or not a patient who has a sensitive airway with secretions should be intubated for elective surgery. On one hand, those who prefer to intubate the patient believe that better control of the airway will reduce the problems of coughing and laryngospasm. It would be most difficult to perform a meaningful prospective study that would support either point of view. If a decision is made to proceed with surgery, the next decision is whether or not to intubate the patient. If the anesthetic is to be short (i.e., under 30 minutes), I prefer not to intubate these infants and children unless indicated by other factors. However, if the procedure is going to be longer than 30 minutes, I follow the conservative approach, which is to intubate. If the decision not to intubate is made and during the early course of the anesthetic the child has significant airway management problems leading to desaturation, my choice is then to stop and intubate the child. There are pharmacologic techniques available to help modify the problems of the sensitive airway (i.e., secretions, cough, and bronchospasm). Cough and bronchospasm are reflexively mediated by the vagus nerve, which can be blocked by the anticholinergics atropine and glycopyrrolate.[12] These drugs can be given orally before surgery. It is best to have them available before the beginning of surgery. The dose for atropine is 0.02 mg/kg PO and the dose for glycopyrrolate is 0.05 mg/kg PO. The reason for the large oral dose as compared to the intramuscular or intravenous dose is that there is an incomplete absorption of these drugs from the stomach. It takes at least 30 minutes for either drug to become effective by the oral route. In addition to decreasing bronchoconstriction and airway resistance, the anticholinergics will also help to reduce the quantity of airway secretions. There is no increase in the viscosity of the secretions.[13]

Induction of Anesthesia

The induction of anesthesia in children with a sensitive airway is guided by the experience of the anesthesiologist. There are those who prefer a gentle nitrous oxide/halothane induction, whereas others might prefer an intravenous or rectal barbiturate induction. I do allow parents to be present for the induction of these children, but warn them that if the situation becomes stormy they will be requested to leave. Rectal methohexital (Brevitol) can be used for induction, but as soon as anesthesia has been induced the child should be placed on the side or prone. This is done so that any secretions will drain out of the airway and not down into the hypopharynx and larynx, where they might trigger coughing, breathholding, or other difficulties. As soon as the methohexital is effective, the child is moved expeditiously into the operating room and inhalational agents are begun. As long as the airway is under control, an IV can be started and relaxants can then be given to facilitate intubation. On the other hand, if the child begins to cough, breathhold, and become desaturated, succinylcholine 4 mg/kg IM is then administered and the patient intubated.

Inhalational inductions should be conducted slowly and gently. The presence of secretions may well lead to coughing, breathholding, and laryngospasm. Premature introduction of an oral airway or too high a concentration of anesthetic gas can precipitate these problems. Regardless of the induction technique used, an IV is started as soon as possible so that various drugs can be administered to augment the anesthetic.

Even though there are several volatile anesthetics currently recommended for use in the pediatric patient, the consensus is that halothane is the least irritating of all of these agents, and is therefore the agent of choice in this situation. If there is a clinical indication for using either enflurane or isoflurane, halothane can be used for the anesthetic induction and then a switch made to the preferred agent.

Awakening the Patient at the End of Surgery

The child with the sensitive airway will have the same problems upon awakening from anesthesia that were present upon the induction of anesthesia. The protective airway reflexes will be stimulated by the presence of secretions, resulting in coughing, apnea, and laryngospasm. The child who is awake and has intact protective reflexes is better able to avoid these problems. The goal of anesthesia is to smoothly return the child to the awake state. There are several techniques for doing this. The principles include the following:

1. Avoid stimulation of the airway. This means suctioning of the airway while the patient is still anesthetized and not at the termination of the anesthesia.
2. If the patient was paralyzed with nondepolarizing muscle relaxants, reverse with edrophonium 1 mg/kg IV. Its effect will peak in 2 minutes, whereas neostigmine will take 8 to 10 minutes to peak.
3. Glycopyrrolate would have been given as part of the preoperative medication but if there is any question about the adequacy of dose, repeat the glycopyrrolate or give another dose (0.02 mg/kg) 20 to 30 minutes before the anticipated time of extubation to help block the vagus nerve and reduce secretion, coughing, and bronchospasm.
4. Administer lidocaine 1.5 mg/kg IV at the first sign of a reaction to the endotracheal tube. The signs of this are apnea, swallowing, and coughing. The dose can be repeated once in 5 minutes.
5. Turn the nitrous oxide off before reversing the muscle relaxant.

6. Be prepared to reintubate if the patient goes into laryngospasm and becomes bradycardiac and cyanotic. The intravenous dose of succinylcholine should be calculated and should be ready before extubation is attempted. Postoperative analgesia is provided either by narcotics and/or regional techniques as indicated.

Other Potential Problems of Anesthesia in the Child With a Respiratory Tract Infection

Drying of Secretions

The use of relatively high-flow anesthetic gases that contain no moisture has the potential to dry the airway secretions of any patient. This may be a particular problem for the child with a potential for pneumonia and atelectasis, since the drying of secretions in such cases will increase their viscosity and enhance their ability to obstruct the smaller airways. For these children anesthetic gases should be humidified or an artificial nose or low-flow techniques should be used so as to minimize this possibility.

Temperature Problems

The humidification of anesthetic gases conserves some of the heat that is lost from the body and, therefore, increases the potential for developing an elevated temperature. The child with an infectious process already produces excess heat and has the potential for developing an elevated temperature. This is not a particular problem if the increase in temperature is mild. However, if the temperature rise is excessive, it will certainly increase oxygen consumption, as well as cause confusion about whether the child has malignant hyperthermia. This possibility should be kept in mind, and if there is any question, end-tidal CO_2 should be monitored and an arterial blood gas sample drawn. Metabolic acidosis, which is present in malignant hyperthermia, is not present in an uncomplicated case of an infectious process.

Complications of Infections

Meningitis is a potential complication of respiratory tract infection. Because the central nervous system of a heavily sedated postoperative patient is difficult to evaluate, this complication must be kept in mind and the patient examined closely.

Pneumonia is another potential complication. It presents postoperatively as a fever or cough.

ANESTHETIC MANAGEMENT IN CLEFT PALATE AND TONSILLECTOMY SURGERY

Of special concern when dealing with the problems of a runny nose, fever, otitis media, or other similar problems is the infant or child presenting for cleft palate surgery and/or tonsillectomy. Some of these children seem to have such symptoms almost continuously because of the nature of the defect, with the result that surgery is scheduled, cancelled, rescheduled, and so on. Often the child is given antibiotics, antihistamines, and decongestants, but to no avail. Clinical judgment would dictate an initial reasonable delay in order to achieve optimal anesthetic and operating conditions. However, if the symptoms continue, compromises may need to be made (with parental consent), since the surgical procedure may reduce these problems. These children should be treated as having a sensitive airway: premedication with glycopyrrolate; early, controlled intubation; adequate hydration, and extubation with the patient awake using the pharmacologic adjuvants described, such as lidocaine.

One of the concerns in cleft palate repair patients is postoperative airway obstruction owing to secretions, edema of the surgical area, and the effects of anesthetics. One approach to handling this airway problem is to have the child as awake as possible before extubation with the protective airway reflexes intact. One technique to accomplish this is to use local infiltration of the surgical area with 0.5 percent marcaine with epinephrine both at the beginning and the end of surgery to reduce the anesthetic requirement during surgery as well as to provide postoperative analgesia. Since the child will have postoperative analgesia, intraoperative narcotics for postoperative analgesia are omitted. In addition, the anesthetic technique is one of a volatile agent plus nitrous oxide along with muscle paralysis as indicated. Moderate hypotensive anesthesia is used to reduce the blood loss. At the termination of surgery the area is suctioned, the volatile anesthetics are tapered as the procedure is finishing, and then all of the anesthetics are stopped and the muscle relaxants reversed as indicated. The child is not extubated until the protective reflexes have returned, the eyes are open, and he's moving about. Intravenous lidocaine will reduce the irritation from the endotracheal tube until the child is ready for extubation. At this point the child is turned on to the abdomen and extubated. If there is any blood and secretions in the hypopharynx the child will cough this out instead of inhaling them into the airway, which can cause obstruction, coughing, and at times, laryngospasm. Small doses of morphine (0.05 mg/kg) can be added in the recovery room if the child still appears to have discomfort or needs sedation. This technique greatly reduces the need for prolonged intubation for airway management in patients with cleft palate repair.

Timing of extubation can also be a problem in these children. I extubate these patients when the airway reflexes are intact, which indicates that the patient is awake. At times the patient is not awake enough to be extubated but can cough and react to the endotracheal tube. Lidocaine 1 to 1.5 mg/kg IV, which can be repeated within 5 minutes, will often allow the child to tolerate the endotracheal tube until he's ready for extubation. They should also be extubated on the side or in the prone position. Postoperative analgesia for tonsillectomy and adenoidectomy can be accomplished by the surgeon injecting the tonsillar bed with a local anesthetic and by the use of small doses of narcotics either at the end of surgery or, preferably, early in the recovery room when the patient is awake and extubated. If the child has a history of sleep apnea, the narcotics are omitted intraoperatively and titrated in small doses in the recovery room when the child is awake and complaining.

RESCHEDULING SURGERY FOLLOWING A RESPIRATORY INFECTION

There are several studies in the adult and pediatric literature documenting the natural course of respiratory infections.[14,15] In the study by Empey et al., 12 adults were observed during recovery from an acute respiratory infection.[14] The authors' title for the paper suggests that this was an "upper respiratory tract infection," but a careful reading of the paper would reveal that the infection also involved the lower respiratory tract. Their hypothesis was that the influenza virus damages the "rapidly adapting airway receptors" of epithelial cells so that these receptors are sensitized to inhaled irritants. This irritation of the airway causes bronchoconstriction and cough. The reflex is mediated through the vagus nerve, and may be blunted or prevented by anticholinergics such as atropine or glycopyrrolate. Empey et al. hypothesized that the sensitization of these receptors in the airway could be an important factor in reactive airway disease. The importance of this study is twofold: (1) It documents the potential for anesthetic complications in the intra- and postoperative periods, and (2) it provides some guidelines for how long one should wait between the occurrence of a lower respiratory tract infection and the performance of elective surgery. From this report it would appear that surgery should be delayed for a period of at least 4 to 6 weeks. Collier et al. have demonstrated similar changes in children with respiratory tract infections.[15]

Criteria for Rescheduling Surgery

What are the criteria for deciding how long to wait before performing surgery on patients with a suspected respiratory tract infection? The first step in rescheduling surgery that was cancelled because of a suspected respiratory infection is to determine whether the episode was nasopharyngitis or a lower respiratory tract infection. The surgeon or pediatrician will have to follow up the episode to make a determination. If the diagnosis was nasopharyngitis, a period of 1 to 2 weeks after the cessation of symptoms would seem to be adequate. If the lower respiratory tract was involved, there should be a wait of at least 4 to 6 weeks after the cessation of symptoms. A practical problem in applying these guidelines too rigidly is that some parents, especially those with several children, cannot remember which one(s) had a "cold" or how severe it was. In the final analysis, the name of the game is clinical judgment and a degree of good fortune.

COMPLICATIONS OF VIRAL RESPIRATORY TRACT INFECTIONS

The presence of a respiratory tract infection does have the potential for various complications that involve the upper as well as the lower airway. The following two cases are presented to illustrate the problems that can occur.

Case 1

A 7-year-old boy presented for excision of a thyroglossal duct cyst. He was moderately obese. He was seen in the preoperative anesthesia clinic for an initial evaluation, and was to be admitted postoperatively. The initial history revealed no recent respiratory infections. The child was extremely afraid of needles and therefore desired an inhalational induction. The initial stages of the inhalational induction went rather smoothly, but the patient then began to cough and hold his breath, and went into partial laryngospasm. The induction was rather prolonged, with repeated episodes of coughing, breathholding, and duskiness. Finally the patient settled down. An IV was started and he was intubated on the second attempt. No drying agents had been given, and the patient appeared to have a moderate amount of airway secretions at the time of intubation. Because of his obesity, he was put on a ventilator for the duration of the $2\frac{1}{2}$-hour case. It was noted during surgery that the peak airway pressure began to rise. This was interpreted as a decrease in compliance. At the termination of the surgery the patient had another episode of coughing, breathholding, and laryngospasm, resulting in cyanosis. He also had voluminous secretions. When he was extubated, a plug was found in the endotracheal tube, and it was assumed that the patient's decreased compliance was actually a partial obstruction of the endotracheal tube. He was carefully monitored in the recovery room and was noted to have a delayed awakening. The anesthesiologist also noted that the patient was coughing up some blood-tinged secretions. A physical examination at that time revealed a slight degree of what was thought to be cyanosis, and a chest examination revealed bilateral rales and wheezing. A blood gas sample revealed a pH of 7.28, a PaO_2 of 54 mmHg, and a $PaCO_2$ of 51 mmHg. A chest x-ray showed lower and middle lung zones that were opacified bi-

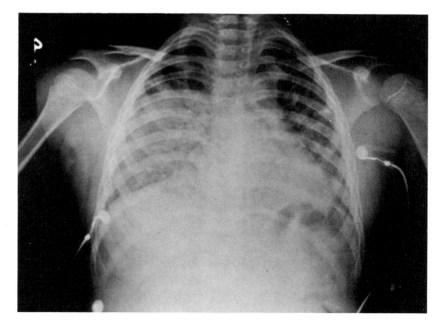

Fig. 9-1. Aspiration pneumonia secondary to a stormy induction in an asymptomatic child with an unknown history of respiratory tract infection.

laterally (Fig. 9-1). The differential diagnosis at this point was aspiration pneumonia, possible fluid overload, or postobstructive pulmonary edema. However, a check of the intravenous fluids and the patient's weight revealed that the fluid administration was on the conservative side. He was treated with a face mask and humidified oxygen. Over the next hour he became more alert and his blood gases stabilized at a PaO_2 of 80 mmHg and a $PaCO_2$ of 38 mmHg. Over the next 24 hours the patient's blood gases improved, he became more alert, and his chest x-ray cleared. He was discharged on the second postoperative day with no apparent problems.

The final diagnosis was postobstructive pulmonary edema. He may have had a degree of aspiration, which precipitated the laryngospasm and hypoxia, but there is no way to confirm this. Upon careful questioning, the mother recalled that the week before the boy had a respiratory infection associated with fever, malaise, and a cough. She had several children, and had apparently confused this child's history with that of another of her children. This is not an unheard-of problem.

Case 2

An 11-year-old boy presented with cervical lymphadenopathy with episodic fever and thrombocytopenia. He had had a previous biopsy that showed only nonspecific inflammatory disease. He was scheduled for an

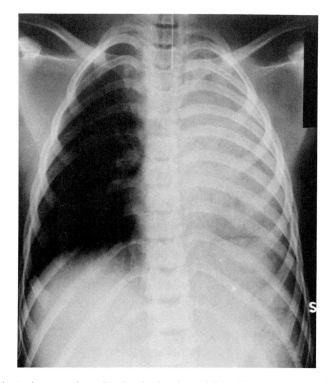

Fig. 9-2. Atelectasis occurring after intubation in a child with recurrent respiratory tract infection but who was asymptomatic at the time of surgery. A preoperative chest x-ray was negative.

extensive cervical lymph-node excision in an attempt to make a diagnosis. The procedure had been cancelled several times in the months before the proposed surgery because of respiratory infections characterized by a cough and fever lasting several days but without any long-term sequelae. The physical examination was normal except for enlarged cervical nodes, and a preoperative chest x-ray was normal. The patient had an intravenous induction and rapid-sequence intubation, which was accomplished easily. The cuff was inserted to a position just below the vocal cords. Immediately after intubation it was noted that the patient's left chest was not moving. On auscultation the breath sounds were very diminished. The patient was immediately relaryngoscoped, and the superior border of the cuff could be visualized inside the cords. A chest x-ray revealed atelectasis of the entire left lung (Fig. 9-2). A suction catheter was passed down the tube with the patient's head turned to the right in order to accomplish a left endobronchial placement. Copious whitish-yellow, muculopurulent secretions were obtained, but no specific mucus plug was found. The left lung then re-expanded and the patient's breath sounds returned. Consultation with several members of the attending anesthesiology staff revealed the usual differences of opinion. However, the majority opinion was that because of the great improvement in the patient's ventilation and the diagnostic nature of the surgery, the surgery should be performed. The operation lasted 3 hours and the patient recovered from the anesthetic without any respiratory complications. A repeat chest x-ray immediately after the surgery revealed moderate clearing of the atelectatic process (Fig. 9-3). The patient was afebrile postoperatively and was discharged 3 days later. The pathology report was again chronic inflammation.

This case caused a considerable degree of discomfort for the anesthesia and surgical team because of the rapid appearance of the atelectasis. When faced

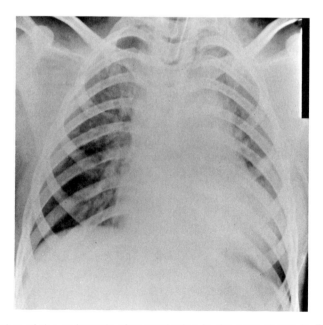

Fig. 9-3. Clearing of the atelectasis after suctioning in the case shown in Figure 9-2. The postoperative course was normal, without any respiratory complications.

with this situation, the clinician is left with a judgment call. If the atelectasis cannot be improved with tracheobronchial suction, the next step would be bronchoscopy. If the situation improves, surgery can then be performed. If the atelectasis persists and the surgery is elective, it is my opinion that it should be cancelled. If the surgery is urgent or emergent, it should be undertaken with continued hydration, suction, controlled ventilation, antibiotics, and aggressive postoperative pulmonary care.

REFERENCES

1. Tait AR, Knight PR: The effects of general anesthesia on upper respiratory tract infections in children. Anesthesiology 67:930, 1987
2. Liu LMP, Ryan JF, Coté CJ, Goudsouzian NG: Influence of upper respiratory infections on critical incidents in children during anesthesia. Reported at the 8th World Congress of Anesthesiology. Washington, DC, 1988
3. DeSoto H, Patel RI, Soliman IE, Hannallah RS: Changes in oxygen saturation following general anesthesia in children with upper respiratory infection signs and symptoms undergoing otolaryngological procedures. Anesthesiology 68:276, 1988
4. Hinkle AJ: Letter to the Editor: What wisdom is there in administering elective general anesthesia to children with active respiratory tract infection? Anesth Analg 68:414, 1989
5. Tait AR, duBoulay PM, Knight PR: Response to Letter to the Editor by AJ Hinkle. Anesth Analg 68:414, 1989
6. Dodge RR, Burrows B: The prevalence and incidence of asthma and asthma-like symptoms in a general population sample. Am Rev Resp Dis 122:567, 1980
7. Rachelefsky GS, Katz RM, Siegel SC: Chronic sinus disease with associated reactive airway disease in children. Pediatrics 73:526, 1984
8. Brill PW, Ewing ML, Dunn AA: The value (?) of routine chest radiography in children and adolescents. Pediatrics 52:125, 1973
9. Sagel SS, Evens RG, Forrest JV, et al: Efficacy of routine screening and lateral chest radiographs in a hospital based population. N Engl J Med 291:1001, 1974
10. Sane SM, Worsing RA, Wiens CW, et al: Value of preoperative chest x-ray examinations in children. Pediatrics 60:669, 1977
11. Tait AR, Du Boulay PM, Knight PR: Alterations in the course of and histopathologic response to influenza virus infections produced by enflurane, halothane, and diethyl ether anesthesia in ferrets. Anesth Analg 67:671, 1988
12. Gal TJ, Surratt PM: Atropine and glycopyrrolate effects on lung mechanics in normal man. Anesth Analg 60:85, 1981
13. Keal EE: Physiological and pharmacological control of airway secretions. p. 357. In Brain JD, Proctor DF, Reid LM (eds): Respiratory Defense Mechanisms. Part I. Marcel Dekker, New York, 1977
14. Empey W, Laitinen LA, Jacobs L, et al: Mechanisms of bronchial hyperreactivity in normal subjects after upper respiratory infections. Am Rev Resp Dis 113:131, 1976
15. Collier AM, Pimmel RL, Hasselblad V, et al: Spirometric changes in normal children with upper respiratory infections. Am Rev Resp Dis 117:47, 1978

10

ASTHMA

Douglas F. Willson

Asthma is one of the most common and potentially most frightening diseases that the anesthesiologist must deal with in children. He or she may be called on to intervene in a number of different circumstances, from anesthetizing the asymptomatic child with a history of asthma to intubating the child in status asthmaticus. While it is rare for a child with asthma to have difficulty during anesthesia, anesthetic practice extends into the preoperative period, when advice may be sought on how best to prepare the patient prior to surgery, and into the postoperative period, when issues of pain management and pulmonary function may arise. Finally, for many anesthesiologists their specialty encompasses intensive care as well. In any of these situations a thorough understanding of the pathophysiology and therapy of asthma may be immediately required to best manage what is basically a reversible disease.

Asthma comes from a Greek word meaning "difficult breathing," an appropriate description. It is the most common chronic disease in childhood, afflicting from 4 to 9 percent of children in the United States,[1] with a similar prevalence in other countries.[2] The hallmark of the disease is its episodic and reversible increased airway resistance, although most of these patients do not have normal pulmonary function even when asymptomatic.[3,4] It is the lability of the disease that is most problematic for the anesthesiologist. Emotional upset, acute exposure to allergens, manipulation of the airway, or other factors can provoke wheezing and respiratory distress acutely in a child who was previously asymptomatic.

While most children with asthma do well, the morbidity and mortality from this disease in the United States appears to be increasing, as reflected by increased rates of hospitalization and death.[5,6] The reasons for this are unclear, but similar trends have been noted in other countries as well.[7] This further emphasizes that it is important for the anesthesiologist to understand not only how to treat bronchospasm once it occurs but also the mechanisms that provoke it if the best care is to be offered to the patient. This chapter attempts to supply this information, beginning with a discussion of the pathophysiology of asthma and following with implications for therapy and anesthesia.

CLASSIFICATION OF CHILDHOOD ASTHMA

Table 10-1 is a scheme for classifying asthma in childhood based on the primary stimulus that is associated with bronchospasm. While helpful in terms of understanding the variety of stimuli that may provoke bronchospasm, such categorization breaks down when one evaluates an individual child with the disease.

Most asthma in children is thought to be "atopic" or "allergic." More than 90 percent of these children will have a positive skin test, usually to multiple allergens,[8] and most have a strong family history of atopic disease. Allergic asthma is often referred to as *extrinsic* because the stimulus that provokes bronchospasm is extrinsic to the patient. This is in contradistinction to *intrinsic* asthma—the most common type in adults—in which the inciting stimulus is considered to be within the patient (e.g., chronic bronchitis or chronic obstructive pulmonary disease). Most of these children (60 to 70 percent) have elevated IgE levels and can be shown to have IgE directed against specific antigens on radioallergosorbent testing (RAST).[9] Unfortunately, skin testing, IgE levels, and specific RAST do not always correspond to what clinically causes wheezing in a child.[10] This is not to say their asthma is not, then, "allergic" but only that viewing asthma as simply a manifestation of hypersensitivity to a given antigen may be an oversimplification.

Exercise is another common stimulus that provokes wheezing in asthmatics. In a study by Cropp[11] 85 percent of boys and 64 percent of girls with known asthma showed significant decrements in pulmonary function with vigorous exercise. The stimulus for bronchospasm appears to be airway cooling and/or changes in the osmotic environment of airway lining cells from fluid loss.[12] Changes in airway conductance have been shown to correlate directly with the magnitude of airway heat loss in several studies.[1,13,14] It appears likely that most children with significant asthma respond to exercise with some degree of bronchoconstriction. This may manifest itself as an inability to keep up with their peers or avoidance of vigorous activity. Indeed, those children whose primary complaint is wheezing with exercise but who are otherwise asymptomatic may simply be those well enough to engage in such activities.

Probably the most important factor that corresponds to exacerbations of

Table 10-1. Classification of Childhood Asthma

Atopic, "extrinsic," or allergic
Exercise-induced
Wheezing associated with respiratory illness
"Intrinsic"
Psychosomatic

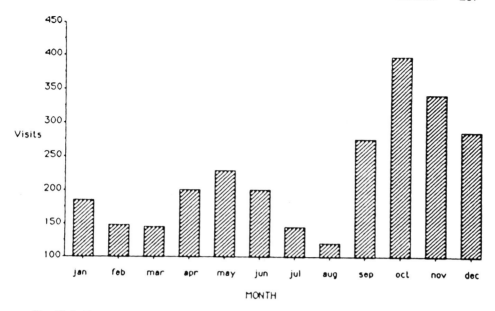

Fig. 10-1. Emergency room visits by month. (From Canny et al.,[153] with permission.)

asthma is respiratory tract infection. Viral respiratory tract infections have been shown to be associated with striking increases in bronchial reactivity even in normal individuals,[15,16] and certain viruses (e.g., respiratory syncytial virus) can provoke wheezing even in nonasthmatic children.[17] In a study by McIntosh[18] nearly half of acute episodes of wheezing in 32 known asthmatics were associated with an identifiable viral infection. As shown in Figure 10-1, hospitalizations for asthma peak at the height of the "respiratory virus season" in late fall and early winter (corresponding to return to school and increased exposure). While many children with mild asthma only wheeze "when they have a cold" and are otherwise fairly asymptomatic, severe asthmatics may be tipped over the edge into respiratory failure by the additional stimulus of a viral infection.

Emotional factors may also be inciting agents. Anyone caring for children with asthma has seen children who appear to be capable of bringing on their wheezing literally at will. Emotional stress may precipitate wheezing in some individuals, as was shown elegantly by Horton.[19] However, a study by Neuhaus[20] showed that while asthmatic children had more neurotic qualities than normal children, they were quite similar in this respect to children with other chronic diseases. In this respect it is quite understandable that a disease characterized by unpredictable episodes of difficulty breathing and feelings of suffocation would be associated with a high incidence of emotional disturbances. Clearly in some children emotional factors may be important but there is no evidence that this is the underlying cause of the disease.

Finally, "intrinsic" factors may be important (although the distinction between "extrinsic" and intrinsic" is obviously arbitrary). This is most evident in children with underlying chronic lung disease in whom there is a prominent component of reversible bronchospasm. Children with bronchopulmonary dysplasia or cystic fibrosis would be the most common examples. These children are not generally considered to have asthma per se, but frequently treatment of bronchospasm is an important aspect of their therapy. Like adults with "intrinsic" asthma, smooth-muscle hypertrophy, increased secretions, and epithelial changes are the primary underlying abnormalities. However, exacerbations may be episodic and may be responsive to bronchodilators, just as with "atopic" asthmatics.

It bears repeating that multiple factors may conspire to provoke an attack of wheezing in an asthmatic child. Categorization in terms of what appears to be the major stimulus associated with wheezing is helpful in understanding the pathophysiology but more often than not children don't fall precisely into one category. It would be more accurate and functional to classify them by degree of severity. Children with the mildest cases tend to be asymptomatic except, perhaps, when they have a viral infection or at the peak of their allergen season. More severely affected children also may have exacerbations brought on by vigorous exercise. The most severely affected are limited by their disease either by their symptoms or by the need to take medications and may require intensification of therapy with viral infection or acute exposure to their particular allergen(s).

THE PATHOLOGY OF ASTHMA

Even though asthma is a common disease, information regarding pathologic findings may be somewhat misrepresentative, as only the end result is seen at autopsy; we are lacking the intermediate stages. Despite this limitation, the construction of a pathologic sequence ranging from the early attack to the end stages of status asthmaticus has been constructed by Lopez-Vidriero and Reid[21] and others.[22-24]

Macroscopic Findings

According to Lopez-Vidriero and Reid,[21] patients who died during an acute, severe attack may exhibit macroscopically and microscopically normal lungs. Presumably they suffered overwhelming functional bronchial constriction. More typically, however, the lungs are grossly hyperinflated and do not spontaneously collapse when the thoracic cage is opened. Areas of atelectasis may alternate with areas of hyperinflation and bronchioles can be seen grossly to have thickened walls and lumens obstructed with inspissated secretions. Attempts to manually deflate the lungs are unsuccessful, reflecting distal air trapping.

Microscopic Findings

Microscopic changes have also been detailed by Lopez-Vidriero and Reid.[21] Characteristically, smooth-muscle hypertrophy, interstitial edema, and inflammation of bronchial walls are seen diffusely throughout the lung.[22] The predominant inflammatory cell is the eosinophil, but polymorphonuclear leukocytes, plasma cells, and lymphocytes are also present and are seen within mucus inspissated in bronchial and bronchiolar lumens. Charcot-Leyden crystals and Curschmann's spirals of glycoprotein may be seen within the mucus. Ultrastructurally the bronchial epithelial lining may be denuded or have a loss of cilia. The underlying basement membrane is thickened with what is seen at electron microscopy to be randomly deposited collagen fibers. Goblet cell hyperplasia is also seen.[23] More distal in the airway air trapping manifested by overdistention and rupture of some alveoli is evidenced.

Presumably these findings represent the extreme of a continuum of changes. However, marked and possibly irreversible changes can be seen in children with severe asthma even when they are asymptomatic, as shown by Cutz et al.[24] in their study of biopsy specimens of children with chronic asthma in remission.

THE PATHOGENESIS OF ASTHMA

Probably the most potent weapon a physician can have against asthma is a firm understanding of its underlying pathophysiology. More than in most diseases, our current approaches to therapy of asthma follow directly from our understanding of the pathophysiology itself—specifically, the determinants of bronchomotor tone, secretion formation and character, and inflammation. Current therapy attempts to interrupt the pathophysiologic sequence at a number of different points.

Normal Physiology

Regulation of normal bronchial diameter involves the interaction of a variety of both neural and humoral mechanisms that are incompletely understood (Table 10-2). Bronchial smooth-muscle tone is the net result of a balance between a group of systems causing bronchoconstriction (the parasympathetic system, mediator-releasing cells, and the α-adrenergic system) and a group causing bronchodilation (the β-adrenergic system and the nonsympathetic inhibitory nervous system). The relative importance of each in normal individuals can be demonstrated by the use of specific agonists and antagonists but their relationship to the pathogenesis of asthma remains to be elucidated.

According to Leff[25] direct innervation of the airways by both cholinergic and adrenergic fibers occurs in the first six generations of airways only. Parasympathetic innervation is derived from the vagus nerve with short postganglionic fibers terminating within the bronchial walls directly. Sympathetic innervation is less well defined. Fibers running from the upper thoracic region synapse mainly in the stellate ganglion. From there they travel along the airway, forming a reticulum with postganglionic parasympathetic fibers along bronchial smooth muscle.[26] A class of nonadrenergic inhibitory nerves has also been described by Richardson and Beland.[27] Stimulation results in airway relaxation that can be inhibited by tetrodotoxin but not propranolol. The importance of this is not clear.

Table 10-2. Neurohumoral Regulation of Airway Smooth Muscle Tone

System	Effect on Airway Smooth Muscle	Airways Innervated	Humoral Receptors
Parasympathetic	Constrictor	First nine generations (vagus nerve) or more; peripheral airways not innervated	All airways
Histamine			
H$_1$	Constrictor	No direct innervation	Histamine is released from respiratory mast cells; tissue concentration of histamine increased from trachea to periphery
H$_2$	May partially inhibit mast-cell release of histamine; may have a dilator effect on human airway smooth muscle	No direct innervation	
Sympathetic			
α_1 and α_2	Constrictor	No direct innervation	Major resistance significance in distal airways unknown; causes constriction after blockade
β_2	Dilator		All airway smooth muscle; causes substantial bronchodilation resulting from adrenal secretion
Nonadrenergic inhibitory	Dilator	Major resistance airways? Others?	?

(From Leff,[149] with permission.)

Table 10-3. Immunopathologic Agents Potentially Operative in Allergic Asthma

Preformed mast cell/basophil mediators
    Histamine
    Eosinophil chemotactic factors
    Neutrophil chemotactic activity
    Proteases
    Additional mediators

Arachidonic acid 5-lyposyngenase pathway
    5-HPETE, 5-HETE, leukotrienes (C_4, D_4, E_4)
    Arachidonic acid cyclooxygenase pathway
    Prostaglandins, thromboxanes, prostacyclin
    PAF acether (AGEPC)
    Bradykinin
    Cellular phase (infiltration/activation)
    Eosinophils
    Neutrophils
    Basophils
    Monocytes/macrophages
    Lymphocytes
    Platelets

(From Dolovich et al.,[43] with permission.)

While direct innervation presumably plays a major role, humoral control of adrenergic and probably cholinergic effects is also important. α- and β-sympathetic receptors, as well as cholinergic receptors, can be demonstrated on smooth muscle beyond the sixth airway generation. β-Receptors are of the β_2 subtype[25] and stimulation results in smooth muscle relaxation. The significance of α-receptors is unclear. Catecholamines with mixed agonist activity, such as norepinephrine, cause bronchodilation. Prior blockade with propranolol causes these mixed agonists to become bronchoconstrictors.[28] The specific α-antagonist prazosin, when inhaled, has little effect on resting airway tone in asthmatics and only partially blocks the bronchoconstriction with exercise.[29] The existence of distal cholinergic receptors in the lung is known but is of uncertain function because acetylcholine is not known to circulate systemically.

A host of locally released mediators are known to exert effects on bronchial smooth muscle either directly or through modulation of autonomic influence (Table 10-3). These mediators are thought to originate primarily from mast cells, although it is speculated that basophilic leukocytes and other cells may participate as well.[30] Activation of mast cells classically occurs when antigen interacts with specific IgE affixed to its surface, causing it to degranulate and release these potent mediators. The mediators (e.g., prostaglandin D_2[31]) may cause bronchoconstriction directly, and some (specifically histamine[32]) can be shown to directly activate vagally innervated irritant receptors, thus indirectly provoking bronchospasm.

Inhaled particles, including cigarette smoke, air pollution, and specific antigens, may directly stimulate irritant receptors in the airway. These receptors (Fig. 10-2) are located just underneath the epithelium of the major airways.

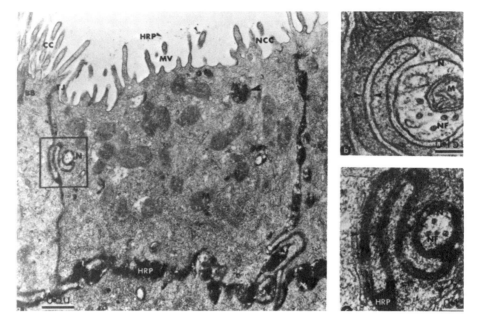

Fig. 10-2. Cigarette smoke increases mucosal permeability, allowing penetration of the tracer HRP into the mucosa as well as exposing the irritant nerve ending. **(B)** A nerve ending from a control animal showing no penetration of HRP. **(C)** An irritant receptor surrounded by HRP after smoke exposure. (From Boucher et al.,[154] with permission.)

Activation results in bronchoconstriction, mucus secretion, and cough mediated via the vagus nerve. Damage to the epithelial lining of the airway, such as with smoking and viral infection, may increase the exposure of these receptors and account for the accentuated airway reactivity seen in these conditions.[33]

In summary, regulation of bronchomotor tone involves interaction of different branches of the autonomic nervous system, local mediator effects, and irritant receptors. Presumably asthma reflects disordered regulation or imbalance among these mechanisms.

Theories of Pathogenesis

Bronchial hyperreactivity is the tie that binds all asthmatics together, and as such, any theory of pathogenesis must account for this abnormality. Whether there is a single underlying defect or several (or perhaps different abnormalities in different individuals) is not known. Possibilities include the following.

Alterations in Smooth Muscle

Asthmatics have been shown to have hypertrophy and hyperplasia of airway smooth muscle[24,34] as well as different responses to doses of inhaled broncho-constrictors.[35] This abnormality is likely secondary and fails to account for the role of immunologic, autonomic, or irritant receptor influences.

Table 10-4. Evidence of Impaired β-Adrenergic Responses in Patients With Bronchial Asthma and Atopy

I.   Increased bronchial sensitivity to methacholine and histamine
II. Decreased responsiveness to catecholamines: Metabolic: Less rise in blood glucose, lactate, and free fatty acids Cardiovascular: Higher diastolic and mean blood pressure and slower pulse rate Eosinophils: Diminished eosinopenic response Platelets: Abnormal second stage of aggregation Leukocytes: Decreased generation of cAMP cAMP: Less rise in plasma and urinary excretion
III. Abnormal responses in the skin of patients with atopic dermatitis: Enhanced sweat gland response to acetylcholine Failure of isoproterenol to inhibit DNA synthesis

(From Nelson,[150] with permission.)

Disorders of Autonomic Regulation

As early as 1915, Eppinger and Hess suggested that an imbalance characterized by "excessive cholinergic activity" might constitute the underlying physiologic derangement in asthma. Excessive cholinergic activity is supported by the consistent bronchoconstrictor response to parasympathomimetic drugs[36] as well as the exaggerated bronchodilation to parasympatholytic agents.[37,38] Conversely, multiple lines of evidence (Table 10-4) have suggested a fundamental abnormality in adrenergic responsiveness. Regardless of their veracity, to their credit these theories have made great inroads in the development of rational pharmacologic therapy in the treatment of these patients.

Epithelial Damage

Epithelial injury produced by exposure to ozone[39] or viral respiratory tract infection can produce a variable period of bronchial hyperreactivity similar to asthma. Such injury is postulated to increase the exposure of airway irritant receptors. Morphologic abnormalities have been found in the airway epithelium of asthmatics[24,40] but it is unclear whether these are primary or secondary.

Disordered Immune Function

As "allergy" is believed to be the most common mechanism in childhood asthma[8–10,41], abnormal immune function must top the list of possible mechanisms. It is speculated that early exposure to foreign protein[42] or some inherited propensity toward a "polyclonal IgE" response from altered suppressor T-lymphocyte function may result in enhanced IgE antibody formation.[43] IgE antibody affixes to mast cells in the airway and interaction with its specific antigen provokes degranulation and begins the cascade of events ending in bronchoconstriction, edema, and inflammation of the airway. Several studies have shown abnormal suppressor T-lymphocyte number and/or function in vitro in asthmatics.[44,45] This is an area of active investigation.

The Dual-Phase Response

As stated above, most asthma in children is believed to be "allergic" or antigen mediated. Interaction of a specific allergen with IgE in the airways of sensitized individuals may provoke a dual-phase response—sometimes referred to as an "immediate and late reaction." The "immediate" response, consisting primarily of bronchoconstriction, occurs within a few minutes after inhalation of allergen and subsides within 1 to 2 hours. Some individuals also develop a "late" response, which may occur 4 to 6 hours after exposure and persist for many hours[46] and which is believed to be inflammatory in nature. At the present time it is unclear if the early and late responses have different mechanisms or if the late response merely constitutes an "amplification" of the initial response based on recruitment of various cell types, including eosinophils, mononuclear cells, and platelets, which have low-affinity receptors for IgE.[47] Both responses are initiated by specific interaction of allergen and IgE affixed to mast cells but it is clear that "late responders" develop mucosal edema, increased mucus secretion, and inflammatory cell infiltration subsequent to the initial bronchoconstriction. The late response may also have the effect of "priming" subsequent response to allergen exposure, resulting in increased bronchial reactivity that may persist for days or weeks, rendering the individual symptomatic for prolonged periods.

The concept of a "dual-phase reaction" has several important practical implications. It may explain why an asthmatic episode, once elicited, can persist for days to weeks in an apparently self-sustaining fashion, even after allergen exposure is eliminated. It supports the early and aggressive use of steroids, which, while having little effect on the early-phase response, appears effective in preventing the inflammatory late-phase response. Finally, it suggests that prophylactic use of cromolyn, which inhibits mast cell degranulation, is the most logical therapy for individuals prone to the late-phase response.

Common Mechanisms and Physiology

Regardless of the underlying pathogenic mechanisms, the common result is airway obstruction from a combination of bronchospasm, edema, inflammation, and increased mucus secretion. This has several consequences on pulmonary physiology:

1. Gas trapping behind obstructed or critically narrowed airways results in steadily increasing residual volume. This places the lung at a mechanical disadvantage, increasing the elastic work of breathing while diminishing the mechanical efficiency of the respiratory muscles.
2. Gas trapping also results in mismatching of ventilation with perfusion.[13] Obstructed airways cannot participate in gas exchange. The result is arterial desaturation and increased dead space ventilation.
3. Elevated lung volumes also require the development of more negative inspiratory pressure, with a consequent increase in the transmural pressure in the pulmonary circulation and left atrium, potentially impairing venous return and cardiac output.

Changes in respiratory drive also occur in asthmatics. Clinically one frequently sees patients early in their attack who, despite adequate oxygenation, are hypocarbic. As commented by Levison et al.,[48] it is paradoxical that a patient who has to work so hard to breathe should overbreathe. The origin of this "overdrive" is thought to be vagally innervated pulmonary receptors. These are also thought to be responsible for the accompanying feeling of dyspnea.[48] The response of asthmatics to hypoxia has variably been found to be normal,[49] supernormal,[50] and depressed.[51] Clinically, an altered response to hypoxia is not apparent in children.

Summary

As we will see, much of our current therapy for asthma has been developed as a direct consequence of our understanding of the underlying pathophysiology. Research in this area has borne fruit, as a wide range of increasingly specific pharmacologic agents have been developed. Further developments will clearly spring from better understanding, particularly in the field of immunology.

CLINICAL EVALUATION OF THE CHILD WITH ASTHMA

History

The anesthesiologist will most often see the child between attacks, when he is generally well. Here a thorough history is the most important means of evaluation.

As most childhood asthma appears to be allergic in origin, it is helpful to find out what (if anything) seems to precipitate an attack. If the child is allergic to a specific airborne allergen, particular attention should be addressed to symptomatology during that season of the year. How often the attacks occur, how severe they are, and how the child does between episodes are also important. The extent of the child's physical activity is frequently helpful in determining how compromised the child is by his symptoms. Probably the most common history is that the child "only wheezes when he has a cold" and, thus, any history of a recent viral respiratory infection should be sought. If the child is on chronic medication, what he takes, how often, and what additional medications are required to break an attack should be evaluated. Patients should be counselled to continue their medications up to the time of surgery. Previous use or dependence on steroids should be ascertained, as chronic or frequent use generally indicates severe asthma. Also, intraoperative steroids may be necessary if the child is potentially adrenally suppressed. A history of prior hospitalization and, particularly, respiratory failure requiring admission to the intensive care unit or mechanical ventilation is important information. As shown by Newcomb and Akhter, children with a prior history of respiratory failure are at very high risk for repeated episodes.[52]

Clinical Signs and Symptoms

The clinical signs and symptoms seen in asthma reflect the underlying disturbed physiology. Most often, of course, the child is well and the examination is normal. The child in the throes of an acute episode, however, may demonstrate a variety of abnormalities. He may be flushed and agitated, with tachycardia and other evidence of endogenous catecholamine release. In watching the child one notes a prolonged expiratory phase of respiration with use of expiratory muscles to exhale, usually a passive process. However, he may struggle to get air "in" as much as "out" because of a feeling of dyspnea and the requirement for higher negative inspiratory pressure necessitated by air trapping. Blood pressure may show a distinct paradox, with a fall of greater than 20 mmHg in systolic pressure during inspiration being associated with severe obstruction.[53] Gross examination of the chest usually reveals hyperinflation, and wheezing may be audible without the aid of a stethoscope. A variety of adventitious sounds may be appreciated on auscultation. The most ominous sound, of course, is little or no air movement. Wheezing often becomes louder as the patient improves! Associated findings may include stigmata of allergic disease, including eczema, transnasal crease, and "allergic shiners."

It should be kept in mind that not all wheezing is asthma. Particularly in small children or those presenting with wheezing for the first time, foreign body aspiration must be considered. Other causes include tracheoesophageal fistula ("H" type), gastroesophageal reflux (particularly because of its episodic nature[54]), cystic fibrosis, bronchiectasis, and recurrent pneumonia. Wheezing associated with respiratory infection (WARI[17]) may also mimic asthma.

Laboratory Findings

Asthma is a clinical diagnosis and, as such, laboratory tests are used primarily to investigate potential complicating factors (e.g., atelectasis or pneumonia) or to follow response to therapy (e.g., pulmonary function testing). The more commonly used tests and their indications are given below.

Chest X-Ray

A chest x-ray is probably indicated in the initial evaluation of every child with asthma, if for nothing other than comparison purposes and to exclude more unusual causes of wheezing. Most often these are negative (73 percent) or show only mild hyperinflation (15 percent) or enlarged hilar vessels (12 percent).[55] Radiography for evaluation in the acute episode is a clinical decision but should be performed in the child who requires hospital admission after outpatient therapy has failed. Acute pneumothorax, mediastinal emphysema, and atelectasis occur commonly in this setting.[56] Chest x-rays prior to surgery are not routine for the child who has a history of asthma but who is currently asymptomatic.

Table 10-5. Pulmonary Functions in Children With Asthma

Flow	Status	Mean	Standard Error	Standard Deviation	Significance of Difference from Normal P
MIFR (L/sec)	Normal children	2.73	0.15	0.81	
	Acute attack	1.70	0.16	0.90	<0.01
	Symptom-free status	2.56	0.17	0.92	>0.05
MMEF (25–75%)	Normal children	2.33	0.12	0.67	
	Acute attack	0.51	0.07	0.37	<0.01
	Symptom-free status	1.43	0.12	0.68	<0.01
FEV$_1$	Normal children	1.79	0.10	0.55	
	Acute attack	0.76	0.07	0.37	<0.01
	Symptom-free status	1.58	0.11	0.59	>0.05
FEV$_1$/FVC(%)	Normal children	85.77	0.49	5.76	
	Acute attack	54.90	2.64	14.44	$0.65 > P > 0.01$
	Symptom-free status	71.83	2.16	11.85	>0.05
PEF (L/min)	Normal children	265.34	12.68	68.27	
	Acute attack	131.48	10.67	57.44	<0.01
	Symptom-free status	218.79	13.21	71.11	>0.05
MBC (L/min)	Normal children	70.53	3.53	19.32	
	Acute attack	31.85	2.63	14.39	<0.01
	Symptom-free status	60.20	3.95	21.62	>0.05

(From Weng and Levinson,[151] with permission.)

Pulmonary Function Testing

A large number of abnormalities in pulmonary function tests have been described in asthma (Table 10-5), but these tests are difficult to perform in children and, frankly, with the exception of simple spirometry, add little to the day-to-day care of these patients.

Other Laboratory Tests

Further laboratory testing should, as always, be dictated by the clinical circumstances. With the exception of theophylline levels for children taking that drug, there are few tests that should be "routine" for asthmatics. The role of allergy testing, RAST, IgE levels, or other immunologic studies is controversial and beyond the scope of this chapter.

TREATMENT OF ASTHMA

Advances in clinical pharmacology and in our understanding of the disturbed physiology in asthma have greatly improved the management of these patients. Our approach has changed substantially—even since the first edition of this book—as the importance of the inflammatory response in asthma has been emphasized. The practicing anesthesiologist may find it difficult to keep up with the newest drugs, which seem to be introduced nearly daily. There is some comfort in knowing that nearly all of these can be "fit in" to our basic understanding of the pathophysiology of the disease.

Pharmacologic Agents

Theophylline

Theophylline is the primary bronchodilator used in the United States.[57] It is a demethylated xanthene similar in structure to caffeine. Its bronchodilator effect is approximately proportional to the logarithm of the serum concentration[58] within the therapeutic range of 10 to 20 μg/ml. While dosage of theophylline must be individualized, a reasonable starting dose for children (excluding infants) is 5 mg/kg every 6 hours.[59] Dosages of slow-release oral formulations are given in Table 10-6. In status asthmaticus a loading dose of 5-6 mg/kg followed by an infusion of 1 mg/kg/hr is a safe starting point for those not currently receiving theophylline. Those already receiving the drug should have their serum level checked prior to beginning an infusion. As a rough guide, 1 mg/kg results in a 2-μg/ml elevation in serum level.[58]

The mechanism of action of theophylline was formerly thought to be inhibition of cellular phosphodiesterase. Recent work, however, has shown that theophylline is only a weak phosphodiesterase inhibitor.[59] Other mechanisms, such as direct stimulation of catecholamine release,[60] interference with intracellular calcium kinetics,[61] and antagonism of prostaglandin effects,[62] may be more important than phosphodiesterase inhibition.

Table 10-6. Absorption of Oral Theophylline Preparations

Preparation	Theophylline Content of Lot(s) Used[a]	Mean Study Dose (mg/kg)	No. Subjects Studied	Calculated Fraction Absorbed (Mean ± SEM)
Theophylline solution				
Theophyl, 225 mg/30 ml (Knoll)[b]	7.5 mg/ml	7.3	10	1.03 ± 0.09
Uncoated tablets				
Theophyl, 225 mg (Knoll)	235 mg/tab	7.6	10	0.95 ± 0.05
Theophyl Chewable 100 mg (Knoll)				
Chewed	102.9 mg/tab	7.1	14	0.98 ± 0.05
Swallowed whole	102.9 mg/tab	7.1	14	1.01 ± 0.04
Partially enteric-coated tablets				
Choledyl, 100 mg (Warner-Chilcott)	60.5 mg/tab	7.0	6	1.05 ± 0.08
Choledyl, 200 mg (Warner-Chilcott)	132 mg/tab	7.7	6	0.92 ± 0.08
Sustained-release bead-filled capsule				
Slo-Phyllin Gyrocap, 60, 125, 250 mg (Dooner)	58.7, 118.5, 240.3 mg/cap	7.8	12	1.11 ± 0.06
Theophyl S-R, 125 and 250 mg (Knoll)	126.5 and 250.4 mg/cap	7.9	14	0.99 ± 0.06
Aerolate, 130 and 250 mg (Fleming)	127 and 262.6 mg/cap	7.8	4	0.81 ± 0.08[d]
Theobid Duracap, 250 mg (Meyer)	279 mg/cap	8.5	6	0.87 ± 0.06[d]
Sustained-release tablet				
Theodur, 100 mg (Key)	100.1 mg/tab	8.7	5	1.03 ± 0.06
Theodur, 300 mg No ÷ (Key)[c]	300.3 mg/tab	9.1	5	1.05 ± 0.05
Theodur, 300 mg No. 2 (Key)	307.5 mg/tab	12.9	5	0.97 ± 0.05
Aminodur Duratab (Cooper)	244.5 mg/tab	7.2	5	0.65 ± 0.04[e]

[a] Results of USP assay of sample from the lot(s) used in the study were supplied by each manufacturer.
[b] Name of manufacturer.
[c] Two different lots of this formulation were examined; tablets from the first lot were reported by manufacturer to be pressed more firmly than those from the second, and exhibited somewhat slower in vitro dissolution. A higher dose of lot 2 was used to assure accuracy of the serum theophylline measurement, since the slower absorption of the Theodur 300 mg tablet resulted in lower serum levels from a single dose than with other products.
[d] The probability was $0.025 < P < 0.05$ that the calculated fraction absorbed would differ this greatly from 1 by chance alone.
[e] The probability was $P < 0.001$ that the calculated fraction absorbed would differ this greatly from 1 by chance alone.
(From Weinberger et al.,[152] with permission.)

As might be expected from the variety of mechanisms of action of the drug, theophylline has numerous effects beyond bronchodilatation. The most important include transient diuresis, central nervous system stimulation, cerebral vasoconstriction, increased gastric acid secretion, inhibition of uterine contractions, decreased lower esophageal sphincter tone, improved diaphragmatic function, and increased cardiac contractility.

Theophylline has a fair number of significant side effects. Work by Furukawa et al.[63] has demonstrated serious cognitive and behavioral changes in children taking theophylline and suggests that the drug should not be used as first-line therapy. More practical problems are that the drug is bitter and it is often difficult to get children to take it. Additionally, because the metabolism of the drug is so variable in children, proper dosing requires frequent drug levels in order to assure a therapeutic but safe level. Theophylline has a relatively small therapeutic index and at higher serum levels (>20 μg/ml) can cause cardiac dysrhythmias, seizures, and death.[64,65] Nausea, vomiting, and jitteriness are signs and symptoms that generally precede such toxic effects and parents must be cautioned to seek medical advice if such symptoms develop. The issue of the drug's interaction with halogenated hydrocarbon anesthetics will be discussed later in this chapter.

Theophylline can be used with at least additive effects with β-adrenergic agonists[66,67] and it is reasonable to add a β-adrenergic agonist either acutely or chronically for patients who are still wheezing despite adequate theophylline levels.

β-Adrenergic Drugs

β-Adrenergic drugs have been used in the therapy of asthma for more than 50 years. Ephedrine, an indirectly acting sympathomimetic, was the first adrenergic drug used, but was eclipsed by the more direct agonist, epinephrine. More specific β₂-agonists have now replaced epinephrine.

Regardless of whether autonomic dysfunction is an underlying mechanism in asthma (see discussion above), the autonomic nervous system contributes to bronchomotor tone and can be manipulated pharmacologically. Stimulation of β-adrenergic receptors in the lung results in bronchodilatation and enhancement of mucociliary clearance[68] and may actually increase the threshold for lung mast cell degranulation.[69] Preferential activation of β_2-receptors is now possible and allows more effective bronchodilatation with lessened tachycardia.[70–72]

β-Agonists can be given by the oral, parenteral, or aerosol route. The aerosol route is the most attractive, as it has been associated with greater bronchodilatation and fewer side effects.[73] Aerosol albuterol[74] and fenoterol[71] have been shown to be at least as effective as subcutaneous epinephrine and are generally better accepted by children. The currently available β-agonist aerosols, along with their relative selectivity, are given in Table 10-7.

Oral administration of β-agonists is also effective. Metaproterenol, fenoterol, terbutaline, and albuterol are available for oral use and have been shown more effective and longer acting than ephedrine.[72] Metaproterenol has been found comparable to aminophylline for control of symptoms in chronic asthma.[75,76]

Table 10-7. Preparations of β-Adrenergic Agonists for Aerosol Administration[a]

Agent	Relative Potency	Duration (Hours)	Mechanism of Action	Dose (Maximum)	Solution Concentration (%)
Isoproterenol	4	1–2	$\beta_1 = \beta_2$	0.02 ml/kg up to 0.5 ml qid	0.5
Metaproterenol	3	3–5	$\beta_2 = \beta_1$	0.01 ml/kg up to 0.3 ml qid	5
Isoetharine	2+	2–3	$\beta_2 \geqq \beta_1$	0.02 ml/kg up to 0.5 ml qid	1
Albuterol	4	4–6	$\beta_2 \gg \beta_1$	0.01 ml/kg up to 1 ml qid	0.5
Terbutaline	4	4–6	$\beta_2 \gg \beta_1$	0.03 ml/kg up to 1 ml qid	1
Fenoterol[b]	4	4–6+	$\beta_2 \gg \beta_1$	0.01 ml/kg up to 1 ml qid	0.5

[a] All β-agonists are diluted up to 2 or 3 ml with saline and delivered by a compression-powered neubulizer.
[b] Not yet available in the United States.
(From Galant,[70] with permission.)

Table 10-8. Preparations of β_2 Drugs for Oral Use

Agent	Relative Potency	Duration (Hours)	Mechanism of Action	Dose	Dosage Form
Metaproterenol	3	3–5	$\beta_2 > \beta_1$	0.3 to 0.5 mg/kg tid to qid	10 mg/5 ml liquid; 10 mg and 20 mg tablet
Albuterol	4	4–6	$\beta_2 \gg \beta_1$	0.10 to 0.15 mg/kg tid to qid	2 mg/5 ml liquid; 2 mg and 4 mg tablet
Fenoterol	4	4–6+	$\beta_2 \gg \beta_1$	0.01 mg/kg tid to qid	2.5 mg tablets[a]
Terbutaline	4	4–6	$\beta_2 \gg \beta_1$	0.075 mg/kg tid to qid	1.5 mg/5 ml liquid; 2.5 mg and 5 mg tablet

[a] Not available in the United States.
(From Galant,[70] with permission.)

Table 10-8 lists the currently available β_2-agonist oral preparations. Not listed are a number of β_2-agonists not yet available but which appear to promise greater selectivity, longer duration, and fewer side effects and are currently undergoing study.[77]

Table 10-9 lists currently available parenterally used β-agonists.

β-Agonist drugs should be the first-line therapy for acute asthma[70] and may be the wisest choice for individuals whose asthma attacks are infrequent, as they can be used when symptoms arise and not used otherwise.[78] They are also reasonable adjuncts to use acutely when breakthrough occurs with other modes of therapy. Side effects are generally mild in children, and include tachycardia, nervousness, tremor, and nausea. A practical problem is that the aerosol "metered-dose inhalers" require some coordination to use; thus, the oral route is probably preferable for small children.

Anticholinergic Drugs

Antagonism of cholinergic tone would seem to be a rational approach to achieve bronchodilation. Intravenous atropine does produce relatively greater bronchodilatation in asthmatics than normal individuals[37,38] but causes more tachycardia for equivalent bronchodilation than β_2-agonists.[79] Ipratropium, a quaternary derivative of atropine that is poorly absorbed from mucosal surfaces, has been found to be a useful adjunct when combined with β-agonists and delivered via aerosol. At a dose of 250 μg (1 ml) added to albuterol[80] or fenoterol,[81] the combination was found to be more effective than either β_2-agonist alone and did not increase toxicity. Other studies have failed to show any benefit.[82,83] In brief, ipratropium appears less effective than specific β_2-agonists but may be a useful adjunct to these agents, particularly in view of its minimal systemic effects.

Cromolyn Sodium (Disodium Cromoglycate)

Cromolyn sodium, or disodium cromoglycate (DCG), is a unique drug for asthma that has no intrinsic bronchodilating effect nor any direct anti-inflammatory or antihistamine effect. DCG is thought to "stabilize the membrane of the mast cell and thus prevent degranulation."[84] The mechanism is unclear. It appears to act directly on the mast cell surface, stabilizing the membrane but not interfering with antigen-antibody interaction or blocking the effects of released mediators.[58] The effects are then nonspecific regarding the type or dose of antigen and it may also block nonimmunologic stimulation of mast cells as well[85]—thus explaining its effectiveness in exercise-induced asthma.[86]

DCG is effective only as an inhaled powder and can be delivered using an inhaler device ("spinhaler") or by nebulization in saline. After inhalation the drug is not metabolized and most is excreted unchanged in bile, urine, and stool.[58] Several multicenter and long-term follow-up studies have demonstrated virtually no significant side effects[87–89] and overdose does not appear to be a problem.[58] Common minor adverse effects are related to the drug's irritating properties on the airway—namely, cough, bronchospasm, and dry throat.[58]

Table 10-9. Preparations of β-Adrenergic Agonists for Parenteral Use

Agent	Relative Potency	Duration (Hours)	Mechanism of Action	Dose	Solution Concentration (%)
Epinephrine	3	1–2	α, β_2, β_1	0.01 ml/kg max. of 0.3 ml q 15 min × 3	0.1
Terbutaline	4	4–6	$\beta_2 \gg \beta_1$	0.01 ml/kg max. of 0.25 ml q 15 min × 2	0.1
Isoproterenol	4	Varies	$\beta = \beta_2$		

(From Galant,[70] with permission.)

Prior inhalation of a β-agonist drug is commonly employed to prevent bronchospasm and improve the distribution of the drug in the lung.

In this country use of the drug in children has not gained popularity, most likely because it is expensive and, unlike the newer theophylline preparations, has to be taken four times a day (thus the child has to take the inhaler to school, among other inconveniences). Also, 2 to 4 weeks of use are usually required before clinical improvement is seen. The dosage is one capsule (20 mg) four times per day. If using an inhaler, proper technique is important,[90] although the availability of the nebulizable form of the drug has made this less of an issue. Given the increasing emphasis on the inflammatory component of asthma in children and the increased awareness of the effects of theophylline on behavior and cognitive function, DCG is likely to become more frequently prescribed.

Corticosteroids

Table 10-10 lists proposed mechanisms of glucocorticoid action in asthma. With the increasing recognition of the role of inflammation in asthma, early and more frequent use of corticosteroids has become the norm in pediatric practice. Multiple studies have shown the effectiveness of steroids in chronic asthma[91-96] and, in truth, probably all patients with chronic asthma would be treated with these drugs if not for their disastrous side effects. Unfortunately, the chronic use

Table 10-10. Mechanisms of Glucocorticoid Action in Asthma

Pathogenic Mechanism	Influence of Glucocorticoid
Production of IgE antibody to specific antigen	
IgE binds to Fc receptors on mast cells, basophils	Suppresses binding of IgE by Fc receptors
Antigen binds to IgE on cells	
Cells release mediators	Suppresses release of mediators
Mediators cause	
Inflammation	Suppresses inflammation
Constriction of airways	
Central	Suppresses response to constrictors
Peripheral	Potentiates response to dilators
Sensitization of airways	? Ca^{2+} entry; ? Receptor modification
Abnormal lung perfusion	Reduces pulmonary vascular resistance
Mucus secretion	Suppresses mucus secretion
Cells recruited during inflammation	
Produce other mediators	Suppresses formation of second-degree mediators
	Suppresses responses to mediators
Cause tissue injury	
Maintain inflammatory response	Anti-inflammatory effects
Maintain sensitization	
Sensitized airway hyperreactive to allergens, nonspecific stimuli, ? change in airway muscle	Suppresses hyperreactivity ? via suppression inflammation ? Effects on Ca^{2+} entry

(From Morris,[114] with permission.)

of steroids in children is associated with multiple adverse effects, the most serious of which are growth failure, adrenal suppression, posterior subcapsular cataracts, hypertension, and osteoporosis.

The effectiveness of steroids in acute asthma is less well established but has gained support from two recent studies in the pediatric literature. Storr et al.[97] demonstrated that use of steroids in the initial management of severe asthma in the emergency room significantly decreased rates of hospitalization relative to placebo control. Brunette et al.[98] showed that early treatment of severe asthmatics with corticosteroids during respiratory infections greatly diminished the number of days of wheezing, emergency room visits, and hospitalization. Earlier studies have shown improvement in measured pulmonary function and clinical parameters.[99,100] These data, coupled with the fact that short-term (less than 2 weeks) courses of steroids in non-steroid-dependent children has not been associated with significant adrenal suppression or other important side effects,[101] has lent support to their aggressive use early in severe asthmatic attacks. While there is no consensus, Ellis[78] and Stempel and Mellon,[102] in two recent reviews suggest that steroids be considered for any child who has been steroid dependent previously, required steroids in the past 6 months, or who is borderline in terms of the decision to hospitalize or send home after the initial therapy. Methylprednisolone (because of its minimal mineralocorticoid effect) 2 to 3 mg/kg/day IV in four divided doses is the usual starting dose. Changing to prednisone 1 to 2 mg/kg/day PO as soon as oral medication is tolerated and continuing 5 to 7 days with or without tapering is one suggested regimen.[78] Children treated with "bursts" of short-term, high-dose corticosteroids for acute exacerbations appear to have normal hypothalamic-pituitary-adrenal axis function provided these are limited to less than four such episodes per year.[101]

For many children inhaled steroids are effective and associated with little, if any, serious toxicity.[103,104] Specifically absent is growth and adrenal suppression. Furthermore, the problem of monilial or other oral fungal infections that plague adults so treated is rare in children.[105,106] Administration of eight puffs per day of beclomethazone via a metered (50-μg) inhaler produces an effect comparable to 7.5 mg of prednisone.[107] The drug is not effective in acute asthma, however.

Immunotherapy ("Desensitization")

Immunotherapy attempts by the repeated injection of a derivative of a presumed allergen to provoke the development of "blocking antibodies" of both IgE and IgA subclasses. These antibodies theoretically can neutralize the antigen after inhalation or ingestion and thereby reduce the rate of interaction with corresponding antibodies of the IgE class. The therapy is controversial and beyond the scope of this chapter. The reader is referred to Rosenthal and Lichtenstein's excellent review for further discussion of this issue.[108]

Physical Therapy

Despite the frequent prescription of physical therapy and breathing exercises, other than in the management of acute lobar collapse, there are no data to support or refute their effectiveness. It is reasonable to suggest that encouragement of physical activity—if coupled to good control of symptoms—is as important for asthmatic children as it is for children without asthma.

Psychotherapy

As previously discussed, severely asthmatic children often have psychological profiles similar to those of children with other chronic handicapping conditions.[20] Some of these children may indeed require skilled psychiatric care and manifest improvement with this type of intervention. Considerations in this regard should be the same as those for other children with chronic diseases.

TREATMENT OF STATUS ASTHMATICUS

Acute episodes of wheezing that fail to respond to the usually administered outpatient pharmacologic therapy and thus require hospitalization are considered status asthmaticus. The definition is a functional one as institutions differ in how aggressively they will treat asthmatics in the outpatient setting and there may be differences from patient to patient even in the same institution.

The initial evaluation of these children should include the usual complete history and physical examination, but with particular attention paid to previous episodes of asthma. One should ask specifically about previous steroid use or dependence and about respiratory failure requiring admission to the intensive care unit and/or mechanical ventilation. Children with previous episodes of respiratory failure are at great risk for repeat episodes with significant morbidity and mortality.[52] Signs of respiratory failure such as obvious fatigue, extreme restlessness, decline in the level of consciousness, or cyanosis should alert the clinician that the child cannot be left unattended.

The most critical laboratory data are the arterial blood gases. In any question of impending respiratory failure these should be assessed and repeated as often as needed. Placement of an arterial cannula is safe, easily accomplished, and spares the patient the trauma of repeated needle punctures. Hypocarbia and some degree of hypoxemia are the rule early in the acute attack. Normal or elevated $PaCO_2$ (>40 mmHg) implies respiratory failure and necessitates intensive therapy, ideally in an intensive care unit.

Initial therapy consisting of a β-agonist has generally been administered in the emergency room prior to admission but should be continued after admission. Frequent, repeated (or continuous) administration of $β_2$-agonists nebulized with oxygen appears to be safe,[109,110] and higher doses (albuterol 0.15 mg/kg) appear more effective than lower doses (0.05 mg/kg) without a significant increase in side-effects.[111] Cardiac monitoring while these drugs are administered should be routine. The addition of ipratropium 250 μg (1 ml) to the β-agonist may also be considered. In at least one study this produced significantly better bronchodilation than β-agonist alone without additional toxicity.[80] It is important to also administer oxygen concomitantly, as these agents may reverse hypoxic pulmonary vasoconstriction, thus worsening ventilation-perfusion matching in the lung, possibly leading to severe hypoxia. Oxygen should be administered early and continuously (e.g., while going to the radiology department or while drawing blood).

Initial fluid management is somewhat controversial. As shown by Stalcup and Mellins,[112] because of their high negative intrapulmonary pressure during inspiration, these children are prone to develop pulmonary interstitial edema. On the other hand, depending on the chronicity of their illness, these children may be dehydrated and hypovolemic on admission,[113] which can lead to acute hypotension when vasodilating $β_2$-agonists are given. The tendency in the past has been to overhydrate these patients to prevent inspissation of secretions. A rational compromise in the absence of definitive evidence would be to maintain normal hydration in these patients, avoiding either extremes of dehydration or overhydration.

Theophylline is routinely the second line of pharmacologic therapy. If the child is already taking a theophylline preparation, ideally a serum level should be checked before bolus administration. For the patient not taking theophylline, aminophylline 5 to 6 mg/kg administered over 15 to 30 minutes followed by an infusion of 1 mg/kg/hr is a reasonable starting dose. Maintenance infusions should be guided by measurements of serum levels. The toxicity of theophylline has been previously discussed, but one should keep in mind that mild signs of toxicity do not reliably precede signs of serious toxicity—including seizures and death.[58] Therapeutic serum levels are 10 to 20 μg/ml.

Steroids should, in my opinion, be started early in any child ill enough to require admission. There is a time lag before the onset of steroid action: most clinical effects begin 1 to 3 hours after steroid administration and become maximal in 4 to 8 hours.[114] It is probably wise to administer them in the emergency room for the child in significant distress to avoid the inevitable delay associated with admission procedures.

Impending respiratory failure—as heralded by a $PaCO_2$ greater than 40 mmHg, diminishing level of consciousness, or a rapidly tiring patient—requires more aggressive therapy and should be managed in an intensive care unit. Intravenous isoproterenol or intravenous albuterol administered as a continuous infusion have been shown to be effective in preventing the need for mechanical ventilation in the majority of patients,[70,115,116] and is the next step in therapy. Prior to beginning the infusion continuous electrocardiographic monitoring should be in place and, ideally, an arterial cannula placed for continuous blood pressure monitoring and frequent blood gas sampling. Pulse oximetry is also recommended. The infusion is begun at 0.1 μg/kg/min and increased by 0.1 μg/kg/min every 20 minutes until there is evidence of sustained clinical and arterial blood gas improvement or severe tachycardia or dysrhythmias develop.[102] Although albuterol for intravenous infusion has not been approved in this country, because of its more selective β_2-agonist effect we have preferred this drug and have found, as did Bohn et al.,[116] that it produces less tachycardia and dysrhythmias. We have used the sterile solution for nebulization (0.5 percent) and diluted it accordingly. There is some controversy regarding continuation of aminophylline infusions while administering isoproterenol or albuterol. Given the additive bronchodilating effects of a β-agonist used with aminophylline,[66,71] we have elected to continue both drugs under careful monitoring. Besides dysrhythmias and severe tachycardia, isoproterenol has been associated with myocardial necrosis in adults.[117] Inadvertent administration of boluses of the drug, inappropriate mixing, or other medication errors with this agent can precipitate severe dysrhythmias, so extreme care must be taken.

Mechanical ventilation is indicated when other measures fail. Generally PaCO2 greater than 60 mmHg or hypoxia despite maximal supplemental oxygen are considered criteria for intubation and ventilation but clinical judgment is important here. Intubation should be performed by skilled personnel, with thought given to the possibility that the child may have a full stomach and thus require prior evacuation via nasogastric tube and "rapid-sequence" induction with cricoid pressure to minimize chances of aspiration. Because of its bronchodilating effects and minimal cardiac depression,[118,119] ketamine may be preferred for anesthesia, although there is no specific contraindication to thiopental. Muscle relaxation is routinely accomplished with succinylcholine 1 to 2 mg/kg. Use of a volume ventilator is recommended because it will best compensate for rapid changes in compliance or resistance in the lung. In order to minimize high peak airway pressures, sedation and paralysis are normally used and bronchodilators continued until after the patient has been successfully extubated. Generally these patients can be weaned rapidly once their bronchospasm has resolved. Prior to extubation residual muscle relaxant effect should be reversed with atropine 0.02 mg/kg and neostigmine 0.07 mg/kg or edrophonium 0.5 to 1.0 mg/kg.

Despite the many advances in therapy, children continue to die of this disease. While no single factor can be identified, failure of either parent or physician to recognize the severity of the attack and institute appropriate therapy is the most common, preventable feature.[120,121] Other causes include aminophylline toxicity,[121] infection,[122] respiratory failure,[123] and acute pneumothorax with cardiac arrest.[124] This is particularly tragic in light of the fact that the natural history of childhood asthma is such that most indeed "grow out of" their asthma without residual effects.[125]

ANESTHETIZING THE CHILD WITH ASTHMA

Asthma affects 4 to 9 percent of children in the United States, so the anesthesiologist who frequently cares for children should expect to encounter this disease nearly daily. There is some comfort in the fact that most of the agents we use are bronchodilating or moderate airway reflexes to some degree. This, probably more than any other factor, accounts for the fact that it is rare for a child with asthma to have difficulty under anesthesia. Nonetheless, it is important for the anesthesiologist to understand how anesthetics affect the child with asthma and how to use these agents to their best advantage.

Preoperative Evaluation

From an anesthetic vantage point children with asthma generally separate into three categories: (1) asymptomatic children with a history of wheezing in the past but who take no medications, (2) children who require medications for symptom control but who are not wheezing currently, and (3) children who are actively wheezing at the time of evaluation.

Children who are asymptomatic and not receiving medication generally present no difficulties, although one should inquire in depth regarding allergic history, problems with wheezing with "colds" or exercise, and severity of episodes when they occur. In the absence of significant pathologic features further investigation other than the routine is unwarranted. Management should be geared toward using the technique and agents least likely to provoke bronchospasm, as is discussed later.

Children who are presently asymptomatic but require medications are more problematic. In addition to inquiring about what provokes the attacks, it is important to determine how severe these are when they occur. Specifically, one needs to know if the child has been hospitalized with the attacks (and how recently), if has he been admitted to the intensive care unit or ever been placed on mechanical ventilation because of asthma, or if he has required steroids or been steroid dependent. There is a wide range of severity covered here, from children who just require "prn" β-agonists to children who have experienced respiratory failure and/or have been steroid dependent. Even when asymptomatic, severe asthmatics have significantly diminished pulmonary function and are at risk for bronchospasm in the perioperative period. In addition to determining what medications have been prescribed, it is important to know if and how often the child actually takes them. It should be emphasized to the parents that medications should be continued the morning of surgery. Children who have been steroid dependent during the last 6 months, are taking systemic steroids, or are using inhaled steroids should be given intravenous steroids perioperatively (methylprednisolone 2 to 3 mg/kg/day). Assessment of the child's ventilatory status includes a comprehensive physical examination, focusing particularly on the respiratory system, and possibly spirometric measurement of the peak expiratory flow rate if the child has been followed with this measurement. In view of the tendency for asthmatic children to develop atelectasis,[56] a chest x-ray should be considered if there is a question of the child's current status. If the child is receiving chronic theophylline a recent serum level should be available. Additional laboratory studies should be guided by the history or physical examination.

The final group includes children who are actively wheezing at the time of preoperative evaluation. With the exception of the child who is never wheeze free and who is believed by the attending physician to be in optimal condition, wheezing is a cause to delay elective surgery. The small caliber of children's airways, their relatively smaller functional residual capacity, their higher oxygen consumption—to name but a few factors—conspire to predispose them to perioperative respiratory complications already. While no prospective studies exist, common sense would dictate avoidance of all but urgent surgery in the presence of bronchospasm. The reader is reminded that the "late phase" of the asthmatic response leads not only to inflammation and increased mucus production, but also increased airway reactivity. The placement of a foreign body (i.e., the endotracheal tube), the effects of inhalational agents on mucociliary clearance, and the possibility that pain and splinting may prevent adequate coughing may transform mild wheezing into respiratory failure. Should surgery be unavoidable all efforts should be made to optimize the child's pulmonary status, including therapeutic levels of theophylline and the addition of intravenous steroids in the event they are not already being given. These measures should be continued in the postoperative period as well.

One additional word of caution should be noted for all asthmatics. While there is some controversy regarding proceeding with anesthesia and surgery for the child with a viral respiratory infection (see Ch. 9), one should be particularly wary of the child with asthma and a "cold" or recent history of a viral respiratory tract infection. Most episodes of status asthmaticus in children are precipitated by a viral infection. The anesthesiologist should specifically inquire about recent viral infections and all but urgent surgery delayed if such a history is found.

Given the sophistication of current therapy for asthma adequate preoperative evaluation and therapy should allow all but the most refractory asthmatics to arrive in the operating room free of wheezing. It is the anesthesiologist's obligation to communicate with the child's primary physician and to seek his or her advice should a question arise. In the absence of a primary physician the anesthesiologist must assume (and surely can) that role and begin appropriate therapy, as outlined earlier in this chapter.

Premedication

As is true for the choice of premedication in children generally,[126] there is no agreement regarding the ideal agent for children with asthma. The issue is perhaps of greater importance here because emotional factors can precipitate or exacerbate wheezing. Thus a smooth, nontraumatic induction of anesthesia is optimal and is facilitated by having the child arrive calm in the operating room.

It is axiomatic that the most important "premedicant" is the preoperative interview itself. A calm, unhurried approach with a simple but complete explanation of what will happen from the child's perspective is important. The use of pharmacologic agents should be individualized. It is our strong bias to avoid intramuscular injections, as children report that "the shot" before surgery was the worst thing about the surgery.[127] So often an injection has exactly the opposite effect from what was intended, causing a previously calm child to arrive in the operating room screaming. A general discussion of premedication is found in Chapter 2. We have found that midazolam 0.5 mg/kg masked by a flavored syrup and given by mouth 30 to 40 minutes prior to arriving in the operating room has been well accepted and generally effective in achieving a calm (frequently happy!) but not overly sedated child. In asthmatics we would generally add atropine 0.02 mg/kg PO or glycopyrrolate 0.05 mg/kg given at the same time because of its potential bronchodilating effects.[37,38]

Anesthetic Approach

Where feasible, regional anesthesia is probably the anesthetic of choice in asthmatic patients because it avoids instrumentation of the airway and its attendant risk of bronchospasm.[128] Shnider and Papper showed a 1.9 percent incidence of wheezing during regional anesthesia as compared with a 1.6 percent incidence in nonintubated patients under general anesthesia and a 6.4 percent incidence in intubated patients under general anesthesia.[129] Unfortunately, regional anesthesia is not frequently an option in children but should be given consideration if the procedure and the patient are appropriate.

Induction of Anesthesia

Most induction agents either have little effect on bronchomotor tone or are bronchodilating. In contrast, instrumentation of the airway by placement of an endotracheal tube or oral airway, or aspiration of secretions or gastric contents, directly stimulates irritant receptors in the airway and can provoke bronchospasm. Thus the agent chosen is less important than how it is used.

As outlined in Chapter 2, consideration should be given to allowing the parents to accompany the child to the operating room and to remain during induction. The limitations and potential benefits of this approach have been discussed previously, but are mentioned here because it may be of particular relevance given the influence of the child's emotional state on bronchospasm.

All of the commonly employed induction agents have been used for patients with asthma. For intravenous induction, thiopental in the usually employed clinical doses does not appear to prevent reflex bronchospasm in response to instrumentation of the airway.[128] The use of adjunctive agents such as lidocaine or fentanyl or deepening anesthesia with a potent agent prior to intubation is suggested to blunt this reflex response. An anticholinergic such as glycopyrrolate in a large dose (0.01 mg/kg) may also be effective. Ketamine has been shown to both prevent bronchospasm during induction[119] and treat it once it occurs[118] and thus would appear an ideal agent, particularly in the actively wheezing child. This is likely an indirect effect of ketamine, via stimulation of catecholamine release rather than a direct effect on the tracheobronchial tree.[130]

The time-honored technique of inhalational induction of anesthesia using halothane remains probably the most common form of induction. Because of their pungent odor and an unacceptably high incidence of laryngospasm, enflurane and isoflurane are less desirable induction agents.[131] However, all three of these commonly used potent agents are equally effective in preventing[132] and reversing[133] bronchospasm and could theoretically be used.

Alternative approaches for induction include rectal methohexital 25 to 30 mg/kg,[134] rectal ketamine,[135] or intramuscular ketamine 3 mg/kg. We have used rectal methohexital extensively, and have found it to be reliable and safe; in addition, it has the advantage that the child can fall asleep in his parent's arms.

Regardless of the agent or technique chosen, the most important aspect of induction is to ensure a reasonable depth of anesthesia prior to inserting the endotracheal tube. Placement of an endotracheal tube is associated with significant elevation in airway resistance in normal individuals,[136] and can provoke profound bronchospasm in asthmatics. Adjunctive agents may be helpful in moderating this response. Intravenous lidocaine 1.5 mg/kg, although not intratracheal lidocaine,[137] has demonstrated efficacy and may be ideal because of its minimal effect on cardiac performance.

Muscle Relaxants

Succinylcholine is known to cause histamine release and has been associated with bronchospasm in at least two reports.[138,139] Despite these reports, clinically significant bronchospasm is rare, and succinylcholine is used routinely to achieve muscle relaxation in asthmatic individuals.

Of the nondepolarizing relaxants, *d*-tubocurarine has been associated with bronchospasm, undoubtedly related to its histamine-releasing properties,[140] and is thus generally avoided. Atracurium may have similar drawbacks.[141] Because of this, pancuronium, metocurine, and vecuronium are probably better choices should a muscle relaxant be required. Reversal of nondepolarizing blockade with cholinesterase inhibitors can potentially provoke bronchospasm, although this can be prevented by the additional use of glycopyrrolate or atropine.[142]

Maintenance of Anesthesia

The choice of a specific potent inhalational agent for maintenance of anesthesia is mildly controversial. Halothane has been chosen traditionally but Hirschman et al.[133] have shown enflurane and isoflurane to have equivalent bronchodilating properties. The dilemma has arisen because of the frequent use of theophylline preparations for control of asthma and the association of ventricular and other cardiac dysrhythmias when used concomitantly with halothane.[143,144] Halothane is well known to sensitize the myocardium to catecholamines,[145,146] and aminophylline causes catecholamine release from the adrenal medulla[60] as well as shares the property of catecholamines to increase cellular cyclic adenosine monophosphate.[147] Thus it is not surprising that the combination of the two agents may be dysrhythmogenic. Because of this problem, Stirt and Sternick[148] have suggested using enflurane or isoflurane in preference to halothane should the use of a theophylline preparation be anticipated. If dysrhythmias develop lidocaine has been reported effective in aminophylline-related dysrhythmias.[59]

The use of "balanced" or "nitrous-narcotic" techniques for maintenance of anesthesia in asthmatics has not been studied. It is probable that large doses of narcotics sufficient to block cardiovascular reflexes also suppress airway reflexes,[128] but this is unproven.

Treatment of Intraoperative Bronchospasm

Probably the most common cause of intraoperative bronchospasm is the presence of a foreign body (i.e., the endotracheal tube) during light anesthesia. Achieving an adequate level of anesthesia during intubation and extubating patients while they are deeply anesthetized (when appropriate!) should avoid many instances of bronchospasm. The adjunctive use of an anticholinergic and lidocaine during induction may be of further benefit.

Should bronchospasm occur deepening anesthesia with one of the commonly used potent agents has been shown, in studies by Hirschman et al.,[119,132,133] to be effective in reversing wheezing. Intravenous ketamine may also be helpful[118,119] and has the advantages of not generally causing cardiovascular depression and being rapid in onset. If an anticholinergic has not been previously administered, glycopyrrolate 0.01 mg/kg should be given. Should deepening the

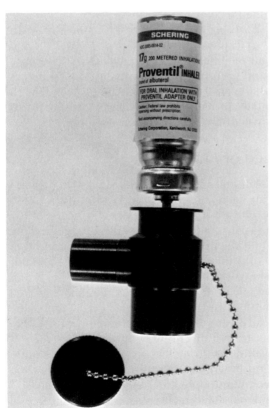

Fig. 10-3. Metered-dose manifold adapter (model #9056) for use in an anesthetic circuit. (Boehringer Laboratories, Wynnewood, PA.)

anesthetic be ineffective or contraindicated one is faced with a situation similar to that of the physician seeing the patient in the emergency room. A host of drugs is available and it is helpful to know what drugs the patient is currently taking and what has been required in the past. The first-line choice would be the β_2-agonists. Aerosolization into the airway is rapid and easily accomplished via adaptors that fit into the anesthetic circuit (Fig. 10-3). The preparations for aerosol administration have been listed previously in Table 10-7.

Aminophylline is a frequent choice in nonanesthetic practice if β-agonists are ineffective. The limitations of using this drug in the presence of halothane have been previously discussed. If aminophylline is to be used, it may be wise to obtain a serum level prior to administering a bolus if the patient is taking the drug chronically. A loading dose of 5 to 6 mg/kg followed by a continuous infusion of 1 mg/kg/hr should result in therapeutic levels (10 to 20 μg/ml), but serum levels should be followed both to optimize therapy and avoid toxicity.

Steroids are not bronchodilators and are thus not immediately effective. Nonetheless, they could be of great value in avoiding the late-phase response in the postoperative period and should be given consideration.

A further discussion of other potential therapeutic agents should these measures fail is given in the section on status asthmaticus.

REFERENCES

1. Dodge RR, Burrows B: The prevalence and incidence of asthma and asthma-like symptoms in a general population sample. Am Rev Respir Dis 122:567, 1980
2. Williams H, McNichol KN: Prevalence, natural history, and relationship of wheezing bronchitis and asthma in children. An epidemiological study. Br Med J 4:321, 1969
3. Kraemer R, Meister B, Schaad UB, Rossie E: Reversibility of lung function abnormalities in children with perennial asthma. J Pediatr 102(3):347, 1983
4. Young IH, Corte P, Schoeffel RE: Pattern and time course of ventilation-perfusion inequality in exercise-induced asthma. Am Rev Respir Dis 125:304, 1982
5. Friday GA, Fireman P: Morbidity and mortality of asthma. Pediatr Clin North Am 35(5):1149, 1988
6. Sly RM: Mortality from asthma in children 1979-1984. Ann Allergy 60:433, 1988
7. Mitchell EA: International trends in hospital admission rates for asthma. Arch Dis Child 60:637, 1985
8. Russell G, Jones SP: Selection of skin tests in childhood asthma. Br J Dis Chest 70:104, 1976
9. Adkinson NF: The radioallergosorbent test: Uses and abuses. J Allergy Clin Immunol 65:1, 1980
10. Bryant DH, Burns MW, Lazarus L: The correlation between skin tests, bronchial provocation tests, and the serum level of IgE specific for common allergens in patients with asthma. Clin Allergy 5:145, 1975
11. Cropp GJA: Exercise-induced asthma. Pediatr Clin North Am 22(1):63, 1975
12. Freed AN, Hirshman CA: Airflow-induced bronchoconstriction: A model of airway reactivity in humans. Anesthesiology 69:923, 1988
13. O'Byrne PM, Ryan G, Morris M, et al: Asthma induced by cold air and its relations

to nonspecific bronchial responsiveness to methacholine. Am Rev Respir Dis 125:281, 1982

14. McLaughlin FJ, Dazar AJ: Cold air inhalation challenge in the diagnosis of asthma in children. Pediatrics 72(4):503, 1983

15. Empey DW, Laitinen LA, Jacobs L, et al: Mechanisms of bronchial hyperreactivity in normal subjects after upper respiratory tract infections. Am Rev Respir Dis 113:131, 1976

16. Collier AM, Pimmel RL, Hasselblad V, et al: Spirometric changes in normal children with upper respiratory infections. Am Rev Respir Dis 117:47, 1978

17. Henderson FW, Clyde WA, Collier AM, et al: The etiologic and epidemiologic spectrum of bronchiolitis in a pediatric practice. J Pediatr 95(2):183, 1979

18. McIntosh K, Ellis EF, Hoffman LS, et al: The association of viral and bacterial respiratory infections with exacerbations of wheezing in young asthmatic patients. J Pediatr 82(4):578, 1973

19. Horton DJ, Suda WL, Kinsman RA, et al: Bronchoconstrictive suggestion in asthma: A role for airways hyperreactivity and emotions. Am Rev Respir Dis 117:1029, 1978

20. Neuhaus EC: A personality study of asthmatic and cardiac children. Psychosom Med 20:181, 1958

21. Lopez-Vidriero MT, Reid L: Pathological changes in asthma. In Clark TJH, Godfrey S (eds): Asthma. Chapman and Hall, London, 1983

22. Hossan S: Quantitative measurement of bronchial muscle in men with asthma. Am Rev Respir Dis 107:99, 1973

23. Houston JC, Navasquez S, Traunce JR: A clinical and pathological study of fatal cases of status asthmaticus. Thorax 8:207, 1953

24. Cutz E, Levison H, Cooper DM: Ultrastructure of airways of children with asthma. Histopathology 2:407, 1978

25. Leff A: Pathogenesis of asthma: Neurophysiology and pharmacology of asthma. Chest 81:224, 1982

26. Tattersfield AE: Autonomic bronchodilators. In Clark TJH, Godfrey S (eds): Asthma. Chapman and Hall, London, 1983

27. Richardson J, Beland J: Non-adrenergic inhibitory nervous system in human airways. J Appl Physiol 41:764, 1976

28. Leff AR, Munoz NM: Evidence for two subtypes of alpha-adrenergic receptors in canine airways. J Pharmacol Exp Ther 764, 1981

29. Barnes PJ, Wilson NM, Vickers H: Prazosin, an alpha-1 adrenoceptor antagonist, partially inhibits exercise-induced asthma. J Allergy Clin Immunol 68:411, 1981

30. Nergens HJ, Durverman EJ, Kerrbegn KF: Bronchial responsiveness in children. Pediatr Clin North Am 30:829, 1983

31. Hardy CC, Robinson C, Tattersfield AE, Hogate ST: The bronchoconstrictor effect of inhaled prostaglandin D2 in normal and asthmatic men. N Engl J Med 311:209, 1984

32. Gold WM, Kessler GF, Yu DYC: Role of vagus nerves in experimental asthma in allergic dogs. J Appl Physiol 33:719, 1972

33. Boushey HA, Holtzman MJ, Sheller JR, Nadel JA: Bronchial hyperreactivity. Am Rev Respir Dis 121:389, 1980

34. Takiyawa T, Thurlbeck WM: Muscle and mucous gland size in the major bronchi of patients with chronic bronchitis, asthma, and asthmatic bronchitis. Am Rev Respir Dis 104:331, 1971

35. Orehek J, Gaynard P, Smith AP, et al: Airway response to carbachol in normal and asthmatic subjects. Am Rev Respir Dis 115:937, 1977

36. Fish JE, Rosenthal RR, Batra G, et al: Airway responses to methacholine in allergic and non-allergic subjects. Am Rev Respir Dis 113:579, 1976
37. deTroyer A, Yernault JC, Rodenstein: Effects of vagal blockade on lung mechanics in normal man. J Appl Physiol 46:217, 1979
38. Cropp GJA: The role of the parasympathetic nervous system in the maintenance of chronic airway obstruction in asthmatic children. Am Rev Respir Dis 112:599, 1975
39. Golden JA, Nadel TA, Bouskey HA: Bronchial hyperreactivity in normal subjects after exposure to ozone. Am Rev Respir Dis 118:287, 1978
40. Glynn AA, Michaels L: Bronchial biopsy in chronic bronchitis and asthma. Thorax 15:142, 1960
41. Likura Y, Nagakura T, Walsh GM, et al: Role of chemical mediators after antigen and exercise challenge in children with asthma. J Allergy Clin Immunol 81:1050, 1988
42. Pinckard RN, Halonen M, Meng AL: Preferential expression of anti-bovine serum albumen IgE homocytotopic antibody synthesis and anaphylactic sensitivity in the neonatal rabbit. J Allergy Clin Immunol 49:301, 1972
43. Dolovich J, Zimmerman B, Hargreave: Allergy in asthma. In Clark TJH, Godfrey S (eds): Asthma. Chapman and Hall, London, 1983
44. Revilin J, Kuperman O, Freier S, Godfrey S: Suppressor T-lymphocyte activity in wheezing children with and without treatment by hyposensitization. Clin Allergy 11:353, 1981
45. Beer J, Osband ME, McCaffrey RP: Abnormal histamine-induced suppressor cell function in atopic subjects. N Engl J Med 306:454, 1982
46. Sly RM: Current theories of the pathogenesis of asthma. J Asthma 20(6):419, 1983
47. Dolovich J, Ruhno J, O'Byrne P, Hargreave FE: Early/late response model: Implications for control of asthma and chronic cough in children. Pediatr Clin North Am 35(5):969, 1988
48. Levison H, Collins-Williams C, Bryan AC, et al: Asthma: Current concepts. Pediatr Clin North Am 21(4):951, 1974
49. Bureau MA, Lipien L, Begin R: Neural drive and ventilatory strategy of breathing in normal children, and in patients with cystic fibrosis and asthma. Pediatrics 68:187, 1980
50. Kelsen SG, Altrose MD: The respiratory neuromuscular response to hypoxic, hypercarbia, and obstruction to outflow in asthma. Am Rev Respir Dis 120:517, 1979
51. Smith TF, Hudgel DW: Decreased ventilation response to hypoxia in children with asthma. J Pediatr 97(5):736, 1980
52. Newcomb RW, Akhter J: Respiratory failure from asthma. Am J Dis Child 142:1041, 1988
53. Galant SP, Grancy CE, Shaw KC: The value of pulsus paradoxus in assessing the child with status asthmaticus. Pediatrics 61:46, 1978
54. Berquist WE, et al: Gastroesophageal reflux-associated recurrent pneumonia and chronic asthma in children. Pediatrics 68:29, 1981
55. Simon G, Connolly N, Littlejohns DW, McAllen M: Radiologic abnormalities in children with asthma and their relation to clinical findings and some respiratory function tests. Thorax 28:115, 1973
56. Eggleson PA, Ward BH, Pierson WE, Bierman CW: Radiographic abnormalities in acute asthma in children. Pediatrics 54:442, 1974
57. American Academy of Pediatrics—Section on Allergy and Immunology: Management of asthma. Pediatrics 68:874, 1981

58. Weinberger M, Hendeles L, Abrens R: Clinical pharmacology of drugs used for asthma. Pediatr Clin North Am 28:47, 1981

59. Goldberg P, Leffert F, Gonyalez M, et al: Intravenous aminophylline therapy for asthma—a comparison of two methods of administration in children. Am J Dis Child 134:596, 1980

60. Atuk NO, Blaydes C, Westervelt FB, Wood JE: Effect of aminophylline on urinary excretion of epinephrine and norepinephrine in man. Circulation 35:745, 1967

61. Poisner AM: Direct stimulant effect of aminophylline on catecholamine release from the adrenal medulla. Biochem Pharmacol 22:469, 1973

62. Horobin DF, Manku MS, Franks DJ, et al: Methylxanthine phosphodiesterase inhibitors behave as prostaglandin antagonists in a perfused rat mesentery artery preparation. Prostaglandins 13:33, 1977

63. Furukawa CT, DuHamel TR, Weimer L, et al: Cognitive and behavioral findings in children taking theophylline. J. Allergy Clin Immunol 81:83, 1988

64. Weinberger M, Hendeles L: Use of theophylline for asthma. In Clark TJH, Godfrey S (eds): Asthma. Chapman and Hall, London, 1983

65. Zwillich CW, et al: Theophylline-induced seizures in adults. Ann Intern Med 82:784, 1975

66. Rossing TH, Fanta CH, McFadden ER, et al: A controlled trial of the use of single versus combined drug therapy in the treatment of acute episodes of asthma. Am Rev Respir Dis 123:190, 1981

67. Wolfe JD, Tashkin DP, Calouse B, et al: Bronchodilator effects of terbutaline and aminophylline alone and in combination in asthmatic patients. N Engl J Med 298:363, 1978

68. Wanner A: Clinical aspects of mucociliary clearance. Am Rev Respir Dis 116:73, 1977

69. Bourne HR, Lichtenstein LM, Henney CS, et al: Modulation of inflammation and immunity by cyclic AMP. Science 184:19, 1974

70. Galant SP: Current status of beta-adrenergic agonists in bronchial asthma. Pediatr Clin North Am 30:931, 1983

71. Ben-Zui Z, Lam C, Hoffman J, et al: An evaluation of the initial treatment of acute asthma. Pediatrics 70:348, 1982

72. Geumei AM, Miller WF: New oral bronchodilating drugs with relatively selective stimulation of beta-2 adrenergic receptors. Chest 72:267, 1977

73. Lee HS: Comparison of oral and aerosol adrenergic bronchodilators in asthma. J Pediatr 99:805, 1981

74. Becker AB, Nelson NA, Simms FE: Inhaled salbutamol versus injected epinephrine in the treatment of acute asthma in children. J Pediatr 102:465, 1983

75. Dusdielser L, Green M, Smith GD, et al: Comparison of orally administered metaproterenol and theophylline in the control of chronic asthma. J Pediatr 101:281, 1982

76. Rachelefsky GS, Katz RM, Milkey MR, et al: Metaproterenol and theophylline in asthmatic children. Ann Allergy 45:207, 1980

77. Kemp JP: Adrenergic bronchodilators, old and new. J Asthma 20(6):445, 1983

78. Ellis EF: Asthma: Current therapeutic approach. Pediatr Clin North Am 35(5):1041, 1988

79. Ruffin RE, Fitzgerald JD, Rebuck AS: A comparison of the bronchodilator activity of Sch 1000 and salbutamol. J Allergy Clin Immunol 59:136, 1977

80. Reisman J, Goldes-Sebalt M, Kazim F, et al: Frequent administration by inhalation of salbutamol and ipratropium bromide in the initial management of severe acute asthma in children. J Allergy Clin Immunol 81:16, 1988

81. Watson WTA, Becker AB, Simons FER: Comparison of ipratropium solution, fenoterol solution, and their combination administered by nebulizer and face mask to children with acute asthma. J Allergy Clin Immunol 82:1012, 1988

82. Storr J, Lenney W: Nebulized ipratropium and salbutamol in asthma. Arch Dis Child 61:602, 1986

83. Rayner RJ, Carlidge PHT, Upton CJ: Salbutamol and ipratropium in acute asthma. Arch Dis Child 62:840, 1987

84. Berman BA: Cromolyn: Past present, and future. Pediatr Clin North Am 30:915, 1983

85. Marshall R: Protective effects of disodium cromoglycate on rat peritoneal mast cells. Thorax 27:38, 1972

86. Breslin FJ, McFadden ER, Ingram RH: The effects of cromolyn sodium on the airway response to hyperpnea and cold air in asthma. Am Rev Respir Dis 122:11, 1980

87. Toogood JH: Multi-centre surveillance of long term safety of sodium cromoglycate. Acta Allergol (suppl 13) 32:44, 1977

88. Dickson W, Cole M: Severe asthma in children—a ten-year follow-up. In Pepys J, Edwards AM (eds): The Mast Cell—Its Role in Health Disease. Pitman Medical, London, 1979

89. Newth CJL, Newth CV, Turner JAP: Comparison of nebulized sodium cromoglycate and oral theophylline in controlling symptoms of chronic asthma in preschool children: A double blind study. Aust NZ J Med 12:232, 1982

90. Smith JM, Pezarro YA: Observations on the safety of disodium cromoglycate in long-term use in children. Clin Allergy 2:143, 1972

91. Aviado DM, Carrillo LR: Antiasthmatic action of corticosteroids: A review of the literature on their mechanism of action. J Clin Pharm 10:3, 1970

92. Clark TJH, McAllister WAC: Corticosteroids. In Clark TJH, Godfrey S (eds): Asthma. Chapman and Hall, London, 1983

93. Lefcoe NM: The effect of hydrocortisone hemisuccinate on the tracheal smooth muscle of the guinea pig and cat. J Allergy 27:353, 1956

94. Lalliers CJ, Bukatz R: Dexamethazone in childhood asthma. Ann Allergy 17:887, 1959

95. Langlands JHM, McNeill RS: Hydrocortisone by inhalation effects on lung function in bronchial asthma. Lancet 2:404, 1960

96. Ellul-Micallef, Fenech FF: Intravenous prednisolone in chronic bronchial asthma. Thorax 30:312, 1975

97. Storr J, Barrell E, Barry W, et al: Effect of a single oral dose of prednisolone in acute childhood asthma. Lancet 1:879, 1987

98. Brunnette MG, Lands L, Thibodeau L-P: Childhood asthma: Prevention of attacks with short-term corticosteroid treatment of upper respiratory tract infection. Pediatrics 81:624, 1988

99. Shapiro GG, Furukawa CT, Pierson WE, et al: A double-blind evaluation of methylprednisolone versus placebo for acute asthma episodes. Pediatrics 71:510, 1983

100. Fanta CH, Rossing TH, McFadden ER: Glucocorticoids in acute asthma—a critical controlled trial. Am J Med 74:845, 1983

101. Dolan LM, Kesarwala HH, Holroyde JC, Fischer TJ: Short-term, high dose, systemic steroids in children with asthma: The effect on the hypothalamic-pituitary-adrenal axis. J Allergy Clin Immunol 80:81, 1987

102. Stempel DA, Mellon M: Management of acute severe asthma. Pediatr Clin North Am 31(4):879, 1984

103. Godfrey S, Balfour-Lynn L, Tooley M: A three- to five-year follow-up of the use

of the aerosol steroid, beclomethazone dipropionate, in childhood asthma. J Allergy Clin Immunol 62(6):335, 1978

104. Kerrebign KF: Beclomethazone diproprionate in long term treatment of asthma in children. J Pediatr 89:821, 1976

105. McAllen MK, Kochanowski ST, Shaw KM: Steroid aerosols in asthma: An assessment of beclomethazone valerate and a 12 month study of patients on maintenance treatment. Br Med J 1:171, 1974

106. Godfrey S, Hambleton G, Konig P: Steroid aerosols candidiasis. Br Med J 2:387, 1974

107. Landau L: Outpatient evaluation and management of asthma. Pediatr Clin North Am 26:581, 1979

108. Rosenthal RR, Lichtenstein LM: The status of immunotherapy in asthma. In Weiss EB, Seigel MS (eds): Bronchial Asthma: Mechanisms and Therapeutics. Little Brown, Boston, 1976

109. Moler FW, Hurwitz ME, Custer JR: Improvement in clinical asthma score and $PaCO_2$ in children with severe asthma treated with continuously nebulized terbutaline. J Allergy Clin Immunol 81:1101, 1988

110. Portnoy J, Aggarwal J: Continuous terbutaline nebulization for the treatment of severe exacerbations of asthma in children. Ann Allergy 60:368, 1988

111. Schuk S, Parkin P, Rajan A, et al: High-verses low-dose frequently administered, nebulized albuterol in children with severe, acute asthma. Pediatrics 83:513, 1989

112. Stalcup SA, Mellins RB: Mechanical forces producing pulmonary edema in acute asthma. N Engl J Med 297:592, 1977

113. Straub PW, Buhlman AA, Rossier PH: Hypovolemia in status asthmaticus. Lancet 12:923, 1969

114. Morris HG: Mechanisms of glucocorticoid action in pulmonary disease. Chest 88:133s, 1985

115. Downes JJ, Wood DW, Harwood I, et al: Intravenous isoproterenol infusion in children with severe hypercapnia due to status asthmaticus. Effects on ventilation, circulation, and clinical score. Crit Care Med 1:63, 1973

116. Bohn D, Kalloghlian A, Jenkins J, et al: Intravenous salbutamol in the treatment of status asthmaticus in children. Crit Care Med 12:892, 1984

117. Lockett MF: Dangerous effects of isoprenaline in myocardial failure. Lancet 2:104, 1965

118. Corssen G, Gutierrez J, Reves JG, Huber FC: Ketamine in the anesthetic management of asthmatic patients. Anesth Analg 51:588, 1972

119. Hirshman CA, Downes H, Farbood A, et al: Ketamine block of bronchospasm in experimental canine asthma. Br J Anaesth 51:713, 1979

120. Buranakul B, Washington J, Hilman B, et al: Causes of death during acute asthma in children. Am J Dis Child 128:343, 1974

121. Kravis LP, Lecks HI, Wood DW, et al: Sudden death in childhood asthma. Advances in asthma/allergy and pulmonary disease 5:26, 1978

122. Richards W, Patrick JR: Death from asthma in children. Am J Dis Child 110:4, 1965

123. Downes JJ, Herser MS: Status asthmaticus in children. In Gregory GA (ed): Respiratory Failure in the Child. Churchill Livingstone, New York, 1981

124. Wood DW, Downs JJ, Lecks HI: The management of respiratory failure in childhood status asthmaticus. Experience with 30 episodes and evaluation of a technique. J Allergy 42:261, 1968

125. Blair H: Natural history of childhood asthma—20 year follow-up. Arch Dis Child 52:613, 1977

126. Steward DJ: Psychological preparation and premedication. p. 523. In Gregory GA (ed): Pediatric Anesthesia. 2nd Ed. Churchill Livingstone, New York, 1989

127. Eland J, Anderson J: The experience of pain in children. In Jacob AK (ed): A Sourcebook for Nurses and Other Health Professionals. Little Brown, Boston, 1977

128. Kingston HGG, Hirshman CA: Perioperative management of the patient with asthma. Anesth Analg 63:844, 1984

129. Shnider SM, Papper EM: Anesthesia for the asthmatic patient. Anesthesiology 22:886, 1961

130. Waltemath CL, Bergman NA: Effects of ketamine and halothane on increased respiratory resistance provoked by ultrasonic aerosols. Anesthesiology 41:473, 1974

131. Tresen RH, Lichtor JL: Cardiovascular effects of inhalation induction with isoflurane in infants. Anesth Analg 62:411, 1983

132. Hirshman CA, Bergman NA: Halothane and enflurane protect against bronchospasm in an asthma dog model. Anesth Analg 57:629, 1978

133. Hirshman CA, Edelstein G, Peetz S, et al: Mechanism of action of inhalational anesthesia on airways. Anesthesiology 56:107, 1982

134. Goresky GV, Steward DJ: Rectal methohexatone for induction of anaesthesia in children. Can Anaesth Soc J 26:213, 1979

135. Saint-Maurice C, Laquenie G, Cauturier C, et al: Rectal ketamine in paediatric anaesthesia. Br J Anaesth 51:573, 1979

136. Gal TJ: Pulmonary mechanics in normal subjects following endotracheal intubation. Anesthesiology 52:27, 1980

137. Downes H, Gerber N, Hirshman CA: IV lignocaine in reflex and allergic bronchoconstriction. Br J Anaesth 52:873, 1980

138. Eustace BR: Suxamethonium induced bronchospasm. Anaesthesia 22:638, 1967

139. Katz AM, Mullegan PG: Bronchospasm induced by suxamethonium. Br J Anaesth 44:1097, 1972

140. Landmesser CM: A study of the bronchoconstrictor and hypotensive actions of curarizing drugs. Anesthesiology 8:506, 1947

141. Payne JP, Hughs R: Evaluation of atracurium in anesthetized man. Br J Anaesth 53:45, 1981

142. Miller MM, Fish JE, Patterson R: Methacholine and physostigmine airway reactivity in asthmatic and non-asthmatic subjects. J Allergy Clin Immunol 60:116, 1977

143. Roizen MF, Stevens WC: Arrhythmogenecity of theophylline and halothane in combination. Anesth Analg 58:259, 1978

144. Stirt JA, Berger JM, Ricker SM, Sullivan SF: Arrhythmogenic effects of aminophylline during halothane anesthesia in experimental animals. Anesth Analg 59:410, 1980

145. Munson ES, Tucker WK: Doses of epinephrine causing arrhythmias during enflurane, methoxyflurane, and halothane anesthesia in dogs. Can Anaesth Soc J 22:495, 1975

146. Reisner LS, Lippman M: Ventricular arrhythmias: Epinephrine injection in enflurane and halothane anesthesia. Anesth Analg 54:468, 1975

147. Ueda I, Loehning RW, Ueyama H: Relationship between sympathomimetic amines and methylxanthines inducing cardiac arrhythmias. Anesthesiology 22:926, 1961

148. Stirt JA, Sternick CS: Aminophylline and anesthesia (Letter). Anesthesiology 57:252, 1982

149. Leff A: Pathophysiology of asthmatic bronchoconstriction. Chest (suppl) 82:135, 1982

150. Nelson HS: The beta adrenergic theory of bronchial asthma. Pediatr Clin North Am 22:53, 1975

151. Weng T, Levison H: Pulmonary function in children with asthma at acute attack and symptom-free status. Am Rev Respir Dis 99:719,1969
152. Weinberger M, Hendeles L, Bighley L: The relation of product formation to absorption of oral theophylline. N Engl J Med 229:852, 1978
153. Canny GJ, et al: Acute asthma: Observations regarding the management of a pediatric emergency room. Pediatrics 83:507, 1989
154. Boucher RC, Johnson J, Inoul S, et al: The effect of cigarette smoke on the permeability of guinea pig airways. Lab Invest 43:94, 1980

11

ACUTE PAIN MANAGEMENT IN CHILDREN: NEURAL BLOCKADE AND PATIENT-CONTROLLED ANALGESIA

Madelyn D. Kahana

Pain is perfect miserie, the worst
Of evils, and excessive, overturns
All patience.

Milton

The traditional responsibility of the anesthesiologist has been the management of the surgical patient's intraoperative awareness, pain, and muscle tone. This responsibility was initially expanded to include the management of the patient with chronic pain, and recently to the management of the patient with acute pain, regardless of etiology. In the setting of acute pain, the anesthesiologist can offer the affected patient a number of alternatives to limit the painful experience. This chapter discusses two of these options in children: the use of neural blockade and patient- or parent-controlled analgesia.

NEURAL BLOCKADE

The use of regional anesthetic techniques is not new in the pediatric population. In fact, the first reports of spinal anesthesia in the child appeared in the Medical Record in the early 1900s,[1-3] and there is extensive literature from the 1930s and 1940s describing the "kiddie caudal."[4] Nonetheless, these techniques were generally abandoned after 1960 in favor of inhalational general anesthesia because of the low morbidity associated with the newer general anesthetic agents.

There is now renewed interest in the pediatric application of regional anesthesia and analgesia. This is largely a result of the focus on pediatric pain management and the increasing demand for anesthesia in the child with debilitating disease. Regional techniques can be used as sole agents for intraoperative management, as adjuncts to general anesthesia, and/or for postoperative pain management. A thorough knowledge of pediatric regional analgesia and anesthesia will allow anesthesiologists involved in the care of children to optimize the intraoperative and postoperative course of their patients.

Local Anesthetic Pharmacology and Pharmacokinetics

Although the pharmacology of local anesthetics is similar in children and adults, there are a few important differences.[5,6] The use of regional anesthetic techniques in the child requires an understanding of these differences in order to avoid the dangers of local anesthetic toxicity.

Local anesthetic agents are tertiary amines of two classes: esters and amides. Ester-type local anesthetics are metabolized by plasma cholinesterase. Infants less than 6 months of age have markedly reduced levels of this enzyme. Clearance of ester anesthetics is therefore reduced. Because the duration of the ester local anesthetics remains quite short even in infants, this does not impact on clinical practice.

Amide local anesthetic agents undergo hepatic metabolism and are in significant quantity bound to plasma proteins. Infants less than 3 months old have immature hepatic enzyme systems and reduced levels of α_1-glycoproteins. This predisposes them to increased levels of unbound drug when repeated doses of amide agents are administered. A single dose of amide anesthetic, within the guidelines provided in Table 11-1, presents no greater risk of systemic toxicity than seen in the older patient. This may be explained by the balancing effect of

Table 11-1. Comparable Safe Doses of Local Anesthetics (mg/kg)[a]

Drugs	Peripheral Blocks[b]	Central Blocks[c] Plain	Central Blocks[c] With Epinephrine 1:200,000	Intercostal Blocks With Epinephrine 1:200,000[d]
2-Chloroprocaine	—	20	25	—
Procaine	—	14	18	—
Lidocaine	14	7	9	6
Etidocaine	6	4	4	4
Bupivacaine	3	2	2.5	2
Tetracaine	—	2	2	—

[a] Estimated to produce peak plasma levels that are less than half the plasma levels at which seizures could occur.

[b] Areas of low vascularity (i.e., axillary blocks using local anesthetic solutions containing epinephrine 1:200,000).

[c] Areas of moderate vascularity (i.e., caudal epidural blocks, interpleural blocks).

[d] Areas of high vascularity (i.e., intercostal blocks using local anesthetic solutions containing epinephrine 1:200,000).

Table 11-2. Pharmacokinetic Properties of Local Anesthetics

Drug	VDSS[a] (L/kg)	Plasma Protein Binding	$T_{1/2B}$ (Hours)
Lidocaine			
Neonate	1.4–4.9	25	3
Adult	0.2–1.0	55–65	1.6
Bupivacaine			
Neonate	—	50–70	9
Adult	0.8–1.6	85–95	2–3
Etidocaine			
Neonate	—	—	—
Adult	1.5–1.8	90–95	1–2

[a] Volume of distribution at steady state.

the larger volume of distribution for the local anesthetics in the small child (see Table 11-2).

An exception to this rule is the use of the amide agent prilocaine. A by-product of prilocaine biotransformation is 6-hydroxytoluidine, which can lead to severe methemoglobinemia in the young infant even when a single low dose of prilocaine is administered. Because of this risk, prilocaine is contraindicated in infants less than 6 months of age.

The clinical manifestations of local anesthetic toxicity in children are the same as those seen in the adult. Initial symptoms are generally confined to the central nervous system. Central nervous system toxicity culminates in generalized seizure activity. The symptoms that may precede the onset of such seizures include tinnitus, perioral numbness, slow speech, jerky movements, tremors, and hallucinations.[7] These warning symptoms are more commonly reported in those patients given lidocaine than those given bupivacaine. The treatment of these seizures consists primarily of preventing the detrimental effects of hypoxia.[8] Therefore, adequate ventilation with 100 percent oxygen must first be established. Suppression of the seizures can then be achieved using either thiopental or diazepam. Succinylcholine can also be used to facilitate adequate ventilation.

At higher blood concentrations, local anesthetics can have toxic effects on the human cardiorespiratory system.[9] Respiration first becomes shallow and rapid. As blood levels rise further, apnea occurs, dysrhythmias are seen, hypotension develops, and cardiovascular collapse ensues. This is a life-threatening emergency and immediate action to re-establish respiration and circulation must be taken. Prolonged cardiopulmonary resuscitation may be necessary when bupivacaine or etidocaine toxicity occurs.[9] It should be remembered that in the presence of a general anesthetic that masks the central nervous symptoms, cardiovascular dysfunction heralds local anesthetic toxicity.

Preparation for Neural Blockade

In most circumstances, the use of block techniques in children must be discussed with the parents in order to obtain informed consent. Parents should appreciate when a regional technique has been electively chosen, such as to

Table 11-3. Preoperative Sedative Agents

Drug	Suggested Dose (mg/kg)	Route	Preoperative Time Interval to Effect (min)	Duration
Methohexital[a]	30	PR	5–20	1–2 hrs
Chloralhydrate	50–100	PO, PR	30–60	4–6 hrs
Pentobarbital	1–4 (max. 120 mg)	IV	<5	2 hrs
Midazolam[a]	0.05–0.1	IV	<5	30 min
	0.1–0.2	IM	5–10	1 hr
	0.5–0.8	PO	5–15	30 min
Fentanyl	0.001–0.002	IV	<5	20 min
Ketamine	1–2	IV	<5	20 min
	3–4	IM	<5	30–60 min

[a] I recommend the use of rectal methohexital or oral midazolam.

reduce postoperative pain, and when it is more imperative, such as in the patient with chronic lung disease. In addition to providing the parents with an understanding of the methods and reasons for the anesthetic selection, the preoperative interview should also provide the anesthesiologist the opportunity to assess the ability of the child to cooperate in a regional anesthetic technique.

As a general rule, premedication with an opiate or sedative drug or both is very useful in helping the child to relax, and will facilitate the successful performance of the block. However, sedation of the high-risk premature nursery graduate for spinal anesthesia may result in postoperative apnea. Sedation can be achieved by drugs administered intravenously, rectally, intramuscularly, or orally (see Table 11-3). In addition, an intravenous infusion should be started prior to the performance of the block, to provide venous access for the treatment of any toxic reaction caused by a local anesthetic drug.

As stated previously, regional anesthetic techniques can be used as the sole anesthetic technique, as an adjunct to general anesthesia, and/or as a method of providing postoperative analgesia.[10] The selection of a local anesthetic drug and the concentration to be used will depend on factors such as the intended goal, the site of surgery, the duration of the procedure, and the ASA physical status of the patient. In general, higher concentrations of local anesthetics are associated with a more rapid onset of anesthesia, a greater intensity of motor blockade, and a longer duration of sensory blockade. In general, central neural blocks, such as spinal or epidural blocks, will have a shorter duration of action than major peripheral blocks, such as ilioinguinal nerve block, when similar drugs and drug concentrations are used (see Table 11-4).

Central Neural Blockade

Subarachnoid Block

Spinal (subarachnoid) blockade is one of the oldest forms of regional anesthesia. It is effective for surgical procedures on the lower extremities and on the abdomen below the umbilicus.[2] When performing a subarachnoid block in a

Table 11-4. Central Neural Blockade for Intraoperative Management

Block	Drug	Dose (mg/kg)	Duration (hrs)	Notes
Subarachnoid	0.5% Tetracaine	0.3−0.5	1	Minimum dose 1.0 mg. Use 0.5 mg/kg for neonates.
Lumbar epidural	1.5−2.0% Lidocaine	7−9	1−2	Motor block is more intense with 2% lidocaine and 0.5% bupivacaine
	0.25% Bupivacaine	1.5−2.5	2−3	
	0.5% Bupivacaine	1.5−2.5	2−3	
Caudal epidural	0.25% Bupivacaine	2−2.5	2−3	For abdominal procedures use large volume of 0.25% bupivacaine.
	0.5% Bupivacaine	2−2.5	2−3	For lower extremity procedures, 0.5% bupivacaine provides better muscle relaxation and may prevent the pain associated with muscle spasm.

child, it is important to remember that the spinal cord and dural sac extend farther down the vertebral canal in small children than in older children and adults. The tip of the spinal cord at birth is at the level of L2 or L3; by 1 year of age it has reached its permanent position at the L1 interspace. Ordinarily, the position of the lower end of the dural sac is independent of the tip of the spinal cord; it is at the S2-3 level in the newborn and retracts one interspace during the first year of life. A spinal anesthetic can therefore be administered safely to children of all ages at the L4-5 or L5-S1 interspace.

The technique for introducing a spinal anesthetic begins with sterile preparation of the field followed by the performance of a lumbar puncture with a 22- or 25-gauge 1½-inch short-bevel needle. Free flow of cerebrospinal fluid should be obtained prior to the injection of the local anesthetic of choice (see Table 11-4). Upon completion of the injection of the drug, a dermatomal level of anesthesia can be established by observing the level at which a grimace occurs with light pinching of the skin.

Spinal anesthesia has been used in a number of centers for routine anesthesia of the healthy child, as well as for the high-risk newborn or child with congenital anomalies.[11,12] The preanesthetic evaluation of the child for spinal anesthesia should include a clinical and/or a laboratory assessment of hydration. As in the adult, hypovolemia and the presence of a coagulopathy are contraindications to subarachnoid blockade.

The complications associated with subarachnoid block in children are few and mimic those seen in the adult. Hypotension secondary to the loss of sympathetic tone that accompanies spinal anesthesia, common in the adult, is rare in the child less than 5 years of age.[13] High spinal anesthesia in the infant may cause respiratory depression so that the initial finding may be a reduction in oxygen saturation.[14] Mild hypotension should be treated by a 5- to 10-ml/kg bolus of a balanced salt solution and the use of a moderate vasopressor such as ephedrine considered. In the event of severe hypotension, prompt treatment includes airway maintenance and assisted ventilation, a rapid infusion of a bolus (10 to 15 ml/kg) of a balanced salt solution, and the administration of epinephrine 3 to 5 µg/kg. The extension of a subarachnoid block to a level sufficient to produce respiratory depression also can occur and demands the vigilance of the anesthesiologist. Supportive care with attention to airway management and assisted ventilation may be necessary until the level of the block recedes. Finally, the possibility of permanent neuronal injury should be mentioned. This is exceedingly rare when proper technique and patient selection are followed.

Epidural Block: Lumbar and Caudal

Epidural anesthesia is also most commonly used for surgical procedures on the abdomen below the umbilicus and lower extremities (Figs. 11-1 and 11-2).[15] As in the adult, either a single dose or a continuous technique can be used. Continuous administration of anesthetic offers an advantage for the procedure that exceeds 90 minutes.

Lumbar epidural blockade in infants and children can be accomplished with the "loss of resistance" technique in a manner similar to that applied in adults. After sterile preparation of the field, a 22-gauge, short-bevel needle should be used for single-dose epidural anesthesia, and an 18- or 20-gauge Touhy needle that allows the introduction of a catheter should be used for a continuous epidural technique. The distance from the skin to the lumbar epidural space is considerably less in a child than in an adult. As an example, at the L3-4 interspace in the infant less than 1 year of age, there is a distance of approximately 1.5 cm between the skin and the epidural space, whereas at age 10, a distance of approximately 3 cm must be traversed before reaching the epidural space.[16] In the adult this distance ranges from 7 to 18 cm. Once the epidural space has been located, a local anesthetic can be introduced, with the drug chosen on the basis of the necessary duration of action and desired effect (see Table 11-4).

In the child less than 3 years of age, the difficulty of locating the lumbar epidural space and concern for the accidental total spinal block has led many clinicians to use the caudal approach.[17] Injection into the caudal epidural space can be accomplished with the child fully prone or in the lateral decubitus position. After sterile preparation of the skin over the sacrum, a 22-gauge short-bevel needle is introduced through the skin and the sacrococcygeal ligament at the sacral hiatus, which can be readily identified as the space between the sacral cornua. Once in the sacral hiatus, the needle should be minimally advanced (i.e., less than 3 mm), and a careful aspiration should be done for cerebrospinal fluid and blood. To avoid subarachnoid injection in the neonate, in whom the dural sac may end as low as the S3 level, it is essential that the needle not be advanced farther.

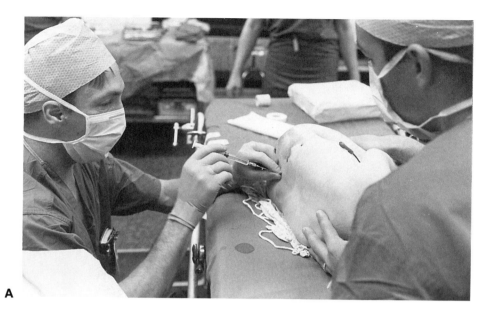

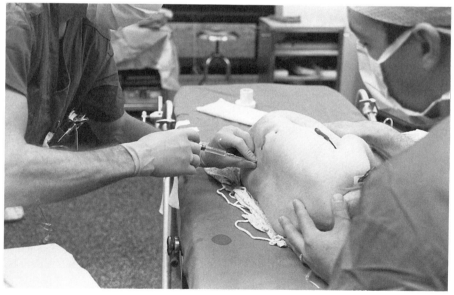

Fig. 11-1. **(A)** The pediatric epidural. After sterile preparation of the field, the lumbar epidural space is approached at the L3-4 level. **(B)** The epidural needle is advanced with constant pressure on a saline-filled syringe until the loss of resistance upon entry into the epidural space is noted.

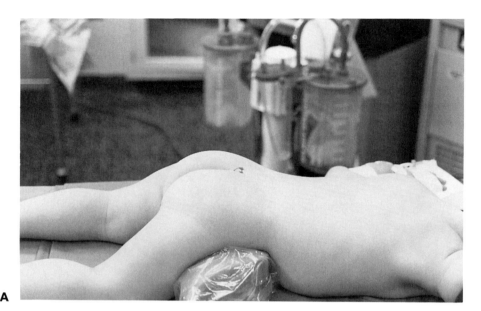

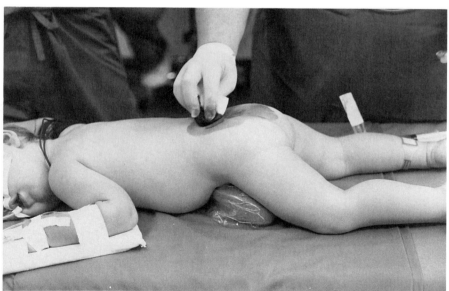

Fig. 11-2. (A) The pediatric caudal. The patient is positioned prone with support under the pelvis. The sacral cornua and sacrococcygeal ligament are outlined. **(B)** Sterile preparation of the field is performed.

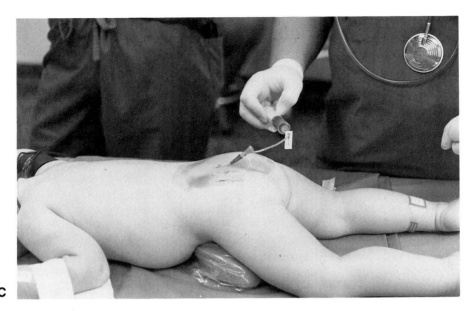

Fig. 11-2. (C) A short-bevel needle is placed into the caudal epidural space through the sacrococcygeal ligament.

For continuous caudal anesthesia, the sacrococcygeal ligament can be punctured with an intravenous catheter. For infants, a 24-gauge $\frac{3}{4}$-inch catheter is used; for older children, a 22- or 20-gauge $1\frac{1}{4}$-inch catheter is more appropriate. Alternatively, a Crawford epidural needle can be used to introduce a conventional epidural catheter into the caudal space. Caution in advancing the catheter is advised to avoid subdural and subarachnoid placement. Again the choice of local anesthetic agent will depend on the surgical site and desired duration of action.

Intrathecal and Epidural Narcotics and Epidural Infusions

As with the adult population, narcotics have been used either in the epidural space or in the subarachnoid space in the pediatric patient.[18–20] This route of administration produces prolonged effective analgesia. As in the older patient, urinary retention occurs uniformly, itching can be seen, and respiratory depression has been described.[21] The latter two side-effects respond to parenteral naloxone. The incidence of respiratory depression, particularly when morphine is used, necessitates monitoring of ventilation in these patients.

Intrathecal or epidural narcotics can be used alone or in combination with local anesthetics intraoperatively and/or postoperatively. Particularly effective for postoperative management is the use of an infusion of a low concentration of bupivacaine and fentanyl into the epidural space. The recommended doses for pediatric patients are found in Table 11-5.

Table 11-5. Central Neural Blockade for Postoperative Analgesia

| Block | Single Dose | | | Infusion | |
	Drug	Dose	Duration (hrs)	Drug Combinations	Starting Dose[c]
Lumbar or caudal epidural	0.125–0.25% Bupivacaine	1.0–2.5 mg/kg	6–12	0.1% bupivacaine + 2 µg/ml fentanyl	0.3 ml/kg/hr
	Morphine[a]	0.05–0.1 mg/kg Maximum 5.0 mg	8–24	0.125% bupivacaine	0.3 ml/kg/hr
	Fentanyl[b]	1–2 µg/kg	4–6		

[a] Use preservative-free morphine.
[b] Dilute fentanyl to a minimum volume of 0.3 ml/kg using preservative-free saline.
[c] When using an infusion, it is important to establish analgesia with an appropriate bolus dose before beginning the infusion. Adjust infusion to control pain while limiting the height of the block to a safe level.

For the postoperative patient, analgesia is achieved withminimal sedation, bowel function rapidly returns, and ambulation is speeded. In patients receiving epidural infusions of local anesthetic and narcotics, it is important to follow the level of neural blockade to prevent inadvertently producing a level above that required. In addition, should infusions be continued for several days, alteration in dose requirements is common.

Peripheral Neural Blockade

Brachial Plexus Block

As in the adult, the brachial plexus supplying the upper extremity can be anesthetized in the child using an axillary, interscalene, or supraclavicular approach. Because the utility of this block is somewhat limited in the small child and infant, a detailed description is provided elsewhere.[22]

Ilioinguinal/Iliohypogastric Block

Ilioinguinal/iliohypogastric nerve blocks are particularly effective in the intraoperative and postoperative management of the patient for inguinal herniorrhaphy irrespective of age (Fig. 11-3).[23] The iliohypogastric nerve is a derivative of T12-L1 spinal nerves; the ilioinguinal nerve originates from L1. These

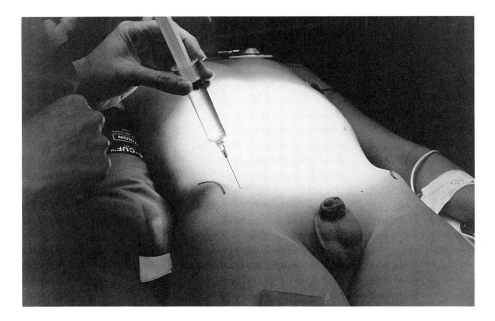

Fig. 11-3. Ilioinguinal/iliohypogastric block. The anterior superior iliac spine is outlined. The position for injection of local anesthetic is shown 1 to 2 cm medial to and 1 cm caudal to the anterior superior iliac spine. The injection is made into the muscle layers of the abdominal wall, *not* into the subcutaneous tissue.

nerves exit peripherally from the transversus abdominis muscle just medial to the anterior superior iliac spine. Local anesthetic is intentionally injected 1 to 2 cm medial to the anterior superior iliac spine between the transversus abdominis and internal oblique muscles to block the iliohypogastric nerve, and between the internal and external oblique muscles in order to block the ilioinguinal nerve. The use of a 22-gauge short-bevel needle will facilitate the location of these muscle planes. It is important to note that these nerves are *not* located in the subcutaneous space and therefore a subcutaneous wheal of anesthetic will *not* be effective. In the child less than 25 kg, the muscle layers are infiltrated with 1 mg/kg of 0.25 percent bupivacaine. In the child over 25 kg, 0.5 percent bupivacaine is used in the same dose (1 mg/kg per side) to a maximum of 10 ml.

Penile Block

Common surgical procedures in children include circumcision and the repair of hypospadias. The addition of a penile block to the primary anesthetic technique is another excellent example of the application of regional anesthesia in the pediatric patient (Fig. 11-4).[24,25]

The right and left dorsal nerves of the penis originate from the pudendal nerves. They enter the penile shaft after emerging from underneath the lower border of the symphysis pubis and course along the dorsal surface of the penis under a deep facial layer but superficial to the corpora cavernosa. From the main dorsal nerves, peripheral branches run in a circumferential pattern to the lateral and ventral aspects of the penis.

A penile nerve block can be performed at the site of exit of the dorsal nerves from the inferior border of the symphysis pubis. A 25- or 27-gauge, ¾- to 1-inch needle is inserted at approximately the 10 o'clock position of the dorsal penile shaft after aseptic cleansing of the area. The first pass of the needle should contact the lower border of the symphysis. The needle is then slightly withdrawn and redirected inferiorly to miss bony contact. A ''click'' may be appreciated as the needle pierces the deep fascia. After a negative aspiration for blood, 1 to 5 ml of 0.25 or 0.5 percent bupivacaine is injected, the volume being determined by the size and age of the patient (see Table 11-6). The procedure is repeated with the needle placed at approximately the 2 o'clock position of the penile shaft. Epinephrine should be omitted from the local anesthetic solution for penile block.

There are two alternative approaches to a penile block that are more easily performed. A ring of local anesthetic can be injected subcutaneously at the base of the penile shaft.[26] The other approach is to wrap the surgical site with local anesthetic-impregnated dressings.[32] Should local anesthetic be administered topically, care must be taken not to exceed toxic dose limits.

Intercostal/Interpleural Block

Intercostal nerve block, used as an adjunct to general anesthesia or as a means for decreasing postoperative pain, is a peripheral regional anesthetic technique that is useful whenever there is pain secondary to chest or abdominal wall

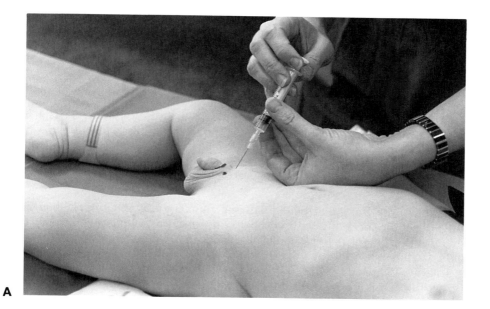

A

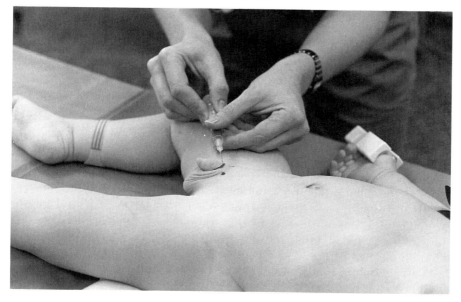

B

Fig. 11-4. The penile block. **(A)** Local anesthetic is injected at the 10 o'clock and 2 o'clock positions below the pubis in order to block the dorsal nerves to the penis. **(B)** The ring block is equally effective: a subcutaneous ring of local anesthetic is injected at the base of the penis.

Table 11-6. Dosage Guideline for Pediatric Penile Blocks

Patient Age (yrs)	Patient Weight (kg)	Dorsal Nerve Block	Ring Block
0–3	2–15	0.25% Bupivacaine 0.5–1 ml per side	0.25% Bupivacaine 2 ml
3–6	10–25	0.25% Bupivacaine 1–2 ml per side	0.25% Bupivacaine 4 ml
6–9	17–35	0.5% Bupivacaine 3–4 ml per side	0.5% Bupivacaine 4–6 ml
9–12	20–50	0.5% Bupivacaine 4 ml per side	0.5% Bupivacaine 5–7 ml
>12	>40	0.5% Bupivacaine 5 ml per side	0.5% Bupivacaine 6–8 ml

pathology. The incisional pain following thoracotomy and upper abdominal surgery can be markedly reduced by an intercostal nerve block. This decreases the need for potent narcotic medications and may improve postoperative pulmonary function.

The ribs are readily palpated in most pediatric patients. The intercostal nerves run in the costal groove with the intercostal vessels under their respective ribs. At the mid-axillary line, a lateral cutaneous branch of the intercostal nerve innervates the regional skin, and there are anterior cutaneous branches at the sternal termination of each nerve.

After the necessary levels for blockade are determined, the appropriate ribs are palpated. A 23- or 25-gauge, ¾- to 1-inch needle is inserted at a less than perpendicular angle to the skin from a spot slightly below the rib, and aimed to contact the lower costal border. Once bony contact is made, the needle tip is gently "walked" down and then under the rib until bony contact is lost. When aspiration for blood is negative, 1 to 3 ml of 1 to 1.5 percent lidocaine with 1:200,000 epinephrine or 0.25 to 0.5 percent bupivacaine with 1:200,000 epinephrine is injected. The procedure is repeated until all necessary intercostal nerves have been blocked.

It must be recalled that of all nerve blocks performed, intercostal nerve blocks result in the highest blood level of local anesthetic for a given dose injected,[28] and that strict adherence to the recommended maximal doses of local anesthetics is mandatory. The advantages of this technique—analgesia, decreased reflex muscle spasm, and an improved ability to cough and breathe deeply—are somewhat diminished by the need for multiple repeated injections.

As an alternative to intercostal blocks, the administration of interpleural local anesthesia was proposed by Reiestad and Stromskag in 1986.[29] After placement of an epidural catheter into the pleural space, local anesthetic can be repeatedly administered without the need for repeated needle punctures. This technique requires that an epidural catheter be placed in the posterior pleural space adjacent to the vertebral column either under direct vision or percutaneously.[30] Percutaneous catheter placement is best performed in the spontaneously ventilating patient by the "loss of resistance" technique. The patient is placed in a lateral decubitus position and the chest wall is prepped with sterile solution. A 17- or 20-gauge Touhy needle is "walked off" superior margin of the sixth or seventh rib along the posterior axillary line and directed toward the vertebral column. A lubricated glass syringe filled with 2 ml of air attached to the Touhy needle signals locations of the interpleural space by emptying during the patient's inhalation. An epidural catheter can then easily be passed into the interpleural space.[31] In the artificially ventilated patient, this technique can be modified to include slight pressure on the plunger of the glass syringe to ensure the syringe will empty upon entry into the correct location. A dose of 0.3 ml/kg of 0.25 percent or 0.5 percent bupivacaine can then be administered.

Local anesthetic can also be given through an existing chest tube. The tube is prepared with antiseptic solution as proximal to the chest wall as possible. Bupivacaine can then be injected through a 25-gauge needle introduced into the chest tube at an oblique angle. If the chest tube can be clamped for 10 minutes, analgesia will be enhanced.

Four to eight hours of analgesia can be expected using bupivacaine in the interpleural space. It is important to note that patient position significantly influences the successful production of analgesia using this technique. Should the patient stand or sit during the performance of the injection or afterward, analgesia may be reduced substantially, whereas the Trendelenburg position can result in Horner syndrome. Blood levels of local anesthetic are comparable to those seen in caudal epidural anesthesia, which makes this technique safer than multiple intercostal blocks.[31] Both techniques are associated with a small risk of pneumothorax. Interpleural administration of local anesthetics is contraindicated in the presence of inflammation of the pleural space, as under this circumstance, local anesthetic toxicity is common.

Femoral Nerve Block

The femoral nerve is located lateral to the femoral artery at the inguinal ligament. This nerve block is easily performed in the supine patient using the femoral artery as a landmark. Guided by the size of the patient, 1 mg/kg of 0.25 percent or 0.5 percent bupivacaine is infiltrated lateral to the artery at the approximate depth of the artery. For the child less than 10 kg, 0.25 percent bupivacaine is recommended. For the child greater than 10 kg, 0.5 percent bupivacaine should be used, with a maximum dose of 10 ml. This technique can be particularly effective in minimizing the pain associated with a fractured femur[32] or phantom limb.

PATIENT-CONTROLLED ANALGESIA

Over the last decade the use of self-administered narcotics has gained considerable popularity in the management of pain in the adult patient.[33] The concept is a simple one and requires a cooperative patient and an interactive pump that allows the physician to program the quantity of narcotic allowed per dose, a lockout interval when no additional doses are permitted, and a time-limited maximum dose. A number of these devices are now available.

Successful use of patient-controlled anesthesia (PCA) has now been reported in children older than 5 years of age by a variety of institutions.[34-36] With sufficient preoperative teaching, the small child can learn quickly the skills required for self-administration of narcotics. When compared with more conventional methods of narcotic administration, the total amount of drug used is significantly diminished and the child's pain control is often judged superior by the patient and parent.

Most PCA devices offer three modes of delivery: PCA, continuous infusion, and PCA plus continuous infusion. For the majority of children, PCA plus continuous infusion offers some advantages in the immediate postoperative setting to protect the child's sleeping hours. When the painful stimulus is modest, PCA alone is sufficient. For the child who cannot or will not activate the PCA device, the continuous mode can be employed. The advantage the PCA device offers over other pumps in the continuous mode is the time-limited maximum dose, which can protect the patient from accidental overdose.

There are a number of alternatives for dosage for PCA; that listed in Table 11-7 is only one such option.

Currently, recommendations for PCA use are limited to patient-activated devices. There are a number of centers investigating the parent's role in this therapy where *parent-controlled analgesia* more accurately describes the method of administration. The success and safety of this form of PCA is yet to be established. Therefore, although parental approval and guidance is mandatory for patient-controlled analgesia to be effective in the young child, the child must be capable of activating his or her own pump. For the very young child, conventional methods of narcotic administration and/or regional anesthetic techniques offer a better approach for pain management at this time.

PCA is recommended for any postoperative situation in which pain control is a problem and in which the patient is competent to participate in his own care. PCA is also useful in the nonsurgical patient with the problem of acute pain (e.g., a sickle cell crisis). With proper education and monitoring, PCA produces superior patient satisfaction, reduces the work of the nursing staff, and may speed the recovery process. Other advantages of this effective method of pain management are its safety[37] and the lack of special physician skills that are required.

Table 11–7. Suggested Orders for Patient-Controlled Anesthesia

Drug: Morphine 1 mg/ml
PCA dose: Morphine 10–20 μg/kg
Lockout interval: 5–10 minutes
Infusion: 10 μg/kg/hr
4-Hour maximum dose: 0.25 mg/kg every 4 hours

CONCLUSION

It is recommended that all infants and children be considered for local infiltration field blocks or specific nerve blocks to minimize postoperative pain.[38] With the concomitant administration of a general anesthetic, this simple practice will allow the child to awaken from that anesthetic with minimal pain and discomfort. This will reduce the excitement and agitation caused by pain that commonly occur when the child awakens from general anesthesia. In the postoperative period, either continuation of the regional technique should be considered (i.e., continuous infusion epidural) or sufficient narcotics administered. When available and appropriate, the delivery of narcotics via the PCA device will enhance their efficacy.

In this era of modern medicine, in order to provide the best patient care, one can only expect ever-expanding applications of these and other creative techniques to eliminate pain in the pediatric population.

REFERENCES

1. Bainbridge WS: Analgesia in children by spinal injection. Med Record Dec. 15, 1900
2. Gray HT: A study of spinal anaesthesia in children and infants. Lancet 2:913, 1909
3. Gray HT: Further study of spinal anaesthesia in children and infants. Lancet 1:1611, 1910
4. Campbell MF: Caudal anesthesia in children. J Urol 30:245, 1933
5. Meffin P, Long GJ, Thomas J: Clearance and metabolism of mepivacaine in the human neonate. Clin Pharmacol Ther 14:218, 1973
6. Blankenbaker WL, DiFazio CA, Berry FA: Lidocaine and its metabolites in the newborn. Anesthesiology 42:325, 1975
7. Wagman IH, deJong RH, Prince DA: Effect of lidocaine on the central nervous system. Anesthesiology 28:155, 1967
8. Moore DC: Administer oxygen first in the treatment of local anesthetic-induced convulsions. Anesthesiology 53:346, 1980
9. Albright GA: Cardiac arrest following regional anesthesia with etidocaine or bupivacaine (Editorial). Anesthesiology 51:285, 1979
10. Melman E, Pennelas J, Maruffo J: Regional anesthesia in children. Anesth Analg 54:387, 1975
11. Berkowitz S, Greene BA: Spinal anesthesia in children: Report based on 350 patients under 13 years of age. Anesthesiology 12:376, 1951
12. Abajian JC, Melish P, Browne AF, et al: Spinal anesthesia for surgery in the high risk infant. Anesth Analg 63:359, 1984
13. Dohi S, Naito H, Takahasi T: Age-related changes in blood pressure and duration of motor block in spinal anesthesia. Anesthesiology 50:319, 1979
14. Baily A, Valley R, Bigler R: High spinal anesthesia in an infant. Anesthesiology 70:560, 1989
15. Dalens B, Tanguy A, Haberer J: Lumbar epidural anesthesia for operative and postoperative pain relief in infants and young children. Anesth Analg 65:1069, 1986
16. Kosaka Y, Sato I, Kawaguchi R: Distance from skin to epidural space in children. Jpn J Anesthesiol 23:874, 1974

17. Dalens B, Hasnaoui A: Caudal anesthesia in pediatric surgery. Anesth Analg 68:83, 1989
18. Krane EJ, et al: Caudal morphine for postoperative analgesia in children. Anesth Analg 66:647, 1987
19. Rosen KR, Rosen DA: Caudal epidural morphine for control of pain following open heart surgery in children. Anesthesiology 70:418, 1989
20. Shapiro L, Jedeikin R, Shalev D, Hoffman S: Epidural morphine analgesia in children. Anesthesiology 61:210, 1984
21. Krane EJ: Delayed respiratory depression in a child after caudal morphine. Anesth Analg 67:79, 1988
22. Yaster M, Maxwell L: Pediatric regional anesthesia. Anesthesiology 70:324, 1989
23. Shandling B, Steward DJ: Regional anesthesia for postoperative pain in pediatric outpatient surgery. J Pediatr Surg 15:477, 1980
24. Kirya C: Neonatal circumcision and penile dorsal nerve block. J Pediatr 92:998, 1978
25. Soliman MG, Tremblay NA: Nerve blocks of the penis for postoperative pain relief in children. Anesth Analg 57:495, 1978
26. Broadman L, Hannallah RS, Belman B, et al: Post-circumcision analgesia—a prospective evaluation of subcutaneous ring block of the penis. Anesthesiology 67:399, 1987
27. Tree-Trakarn T, Pirayavaraporn S: Postoperative pain relief for circumcision in children: Comparison among morphine, nerve block and topical analgesia. Anesthesiology 62:519, 1985
28. Rothstein P, Arthur GR, Feldman H, et al: Pharmacokinetics of bupivacaine in children following intercostal block. Anesthesiology 57:A426, 1982
29. Reiestad F, Stromskag K: Interpleural catheter in the management of postoperative pain. Reg Anaesth 11:89, 1986
30. Covino B: Interpleural regional anesthesia. Anesth Analg 67:427, 1988
31. McIlvaine W, Knox R, Fennesey P, Goldstein M: Continuous infusion of bupivacaine via intrapleural catheter for analgesia after thoracotomy in children. Anesthesiology 69:261, 1988
32. Berry FR: Analgesia in patients with fractured shaft of femur. Anaesthesia 32:576, 1977
33. White P: Patient-controlled analgesia: A new approach to the management of postoperative pain. Semin Anesth 4, No. 3:255, 1985
34. Rodgers B, Webb C, Stergios D, Newman B: Patient-controlled analgesia in pediatric surgery. J Pediatr Surg 23:259, 1988
35. Broadman L, Brown R, Rice L, et al: Patient controlled analgesia in children and adolescents: A report of postoperative pain management in 150 patients. Anesthesiology 71:A1170, 1989
36. Dodd E, Wang J, Rauck R: Patient controlled analgesia for post-surgical pediatric patients ages 6-16 years. Anesthesiology 69:A372, 1988
37. Thomas DW, Owen H: Patient-controlled analgesia—the need for caution. Anaesthesia 43:770, 1988
38. Dalens B: Regional anesthesia in children. Anesth Analg 68:654, 1989

12

PEDIATRIC NEUROANESTHESIA

Mark M. Harris

Pediatric neuroanesthesia covers a wide variety of complex clinical challenges, ranging from emergency management of intracranial catastrophes to elective neuroradiographic imaging. The anesthesiologist may first encounter the patient in an emergency room or preoperatively the night before elective surgery. Intracranial catastrophes mandate delivery of basic life support: airway, ventilation, and circulation, before the anesthesiologist can turn to the traditional challenges of neuroanesthesia: intracranial compliance, intracranial pressure (ICP) and cerebral blood flow (CBF). The elective pediatric patient is evaluated preoperatively for alteration in intracranial compliance, abnormalities in neurologic function, and associated medical conditions; the pathophysiology of the lesion is reviewed, the anesthetic is planned, and induction techniques are discussed with the child and parent. Whether the child presents with acute neurologic disaster or with elective revision of a congenital or acquired lesion, the goal of the anesthesiologist is to preserve vital function and maintain neural integrity. Brain ischemia, brain herniation, and at times, brain death result from failure to control ICP, reduce CBF, lower CO_2 tension, drain excess cerebrospinal fluid (CSF), deliver adequate oxygen, or select the right anesthetic drugs and induction techniques. Successful outcome in pediatric neurosurgery—whether emergency or elective—requires teamwork between surgeon and anesthesiologist and a basic understanding of neurophysiology, neuropathology, and neuroanesthesia in the child. (The reader is referred to the recent book by Sperry et al.[1] for a more comprehensive discussion of neuroanesthesia.)

Pediatric neurosurgery differs from neurosurgery in adults in many ways. Children have different psychological needs, and different types and locations of lesions. They react differently to anesthetic agents and they require anesthesia services for virtually every neuroradiographic procedure requiring prolonged immobilization, involving pain or discomfort, or demanding absolute cooperation. This means that the Department of Anesthesiology is commonly asked to provide services for procedures undertaken in locations far removed from the operating room (e.g., nuclear magnetic resonance imaging [MRI], angiography, myelography, computed tomography [CT], and radioneurosurgery [Gamma Knife or linear accelerators]). Currently, transportation and maintenance of anesthesia in these locations requires the same vigilance that is normally expected in operating room environments. How to optimally monitor physiological function, support CNS function, and deliver anesthesia in remote locations is a significant challenge to hospital administrators, neurosurgeons, radiologists, and anesthesiologists. What support personnel should be available in these areas? What monitors should be available and who should purchase and maintain the equipment? How should staffing and other cases be scheduled to arrange this care? Unless anesthesia services are planned rationally, neuroradiology and other locations for administering anesthesia outside of the operating rooms will remain hostile environments associated with the potential for additional anesthetic risk.

BASIC ELEMENTS OF NEUROANESTHESIA
Developmental Neuroanatomy

The developing brain and central neural axis grow faster than the remainder of the body. The term neonatal brain weighs about 335 g, comprises 15 to 20 percent of total body weight, and more than doubles in weight during the first year. By age 2 years, it has reached 80 percent of adult weight. During childhood, growth of the neural axis slows and body mass catches up, and by adolescence, the brain weighs less than 1 percent of body weight.[2,3] The neonatal brain is covered by dura, cranial plates, subcutaneous tissue, and scalp. During the first months of life, the individual cranial plates fuse to produce the infant skull. The cranial plates remain distinct bones with the potential for expansion along the fibrous cranial sutures until adolescence.[4] The infant skull has two temporary open defects, the anterior and posterior fontanelles, which act as volume buffers to decompress sudden increases in intracranial volume and as "windows" for noninvasive ICP measurement. The posterior fontanelle closes at 2 to 3 months but the anterior fontanelle may remain open until the 19th month.[5] Chronic intracranial hypertension in the neonate leads to expansion of the dura, skin, and individual cranial plates; in the child it results in opening of the sutures.

Intracranial Compliance

The adult brain is surrounded by a rigid skull of fixed finite dimension and is completely filled by brain parenchyma (80 percent), cerebral blood (10 percent), and CSF (10 percent). Any increase in one of those components must be met by a corresponding decrease in the volume of the others if ICP is to remain unchanged. The child can absorb additional intracranial volume, such as from hemorrhage or tumor, by decompressing ICP through the fontanelles or by increasing head circumference. Since spinal fluid is the brain's principal volume "shock-absorber," it must be able to flow freely through the ventricular and subarachnoid channels. Pathologic conditions that impede flow result in ventricular dilatation, hydrocephalus, and elevated ICP, and if unchecked, will lead to brain ischemia, brain herniation, and death. The relationship between ICP and intracranial volume is defined in terms of intracranial compliance, and is described in the familiar hyperbolic function known as the *intracranial pressure-volume curve*. The infant's skull is more compliant than the adult's: open fontanelles, incomplete cranial shell, and fibrous suture lines explain the differences, yet in spite of the anatomic and functional differences, neonates and infants will develop acute intracranial hypertension in response to noxious stimulation. For example, awake endotracheal intubation in normal neonates and infants results in acute intracranial hypertension.[6,7] This results because the dura functions as the adult skull: it is noncompliant, although more compliant than the bony skull.[8] By analogy, if one wants to conceive of the adult skull as a rigid box, then the infant's immature skull is a "leather bag." Figure 12-1 describes hypothetical compliance curves for three subjects: a neonate, an infant with open fontanelles, and an adult. The neonate, with the smallest total intracranial volume and the slowest rise in ICP above the "knee" of the curve, is contrasted with the adult, which has the largest total volume but most rapid rise in the steep portion of the curve.

Cerebral Blood Flow and Cerebral Perfusion Pressure

Cerebral blood flow is lower in the infant and young child than in the adult; blood flow is reported to be 50 ml/100 g/min in the adult, 12 ml/100 g/min in the premature infant, and 23 to 40 ml/100 g/min in the term neonate.[9-12] Under physiologic conditions, cerebral metabolism of oxygen ($CMRO_2$) is closely coupled to CBF by a mechanism involving metabolic byproducts (such as adenosine) to produce local vasodilatation. Since delivery of metabolic substrate is dependent on metabolic need and independent of mean arterial pressure (MAP), cerebral vasculature tone must vary to deliver constant flow at different driving pressures. This is referred to as *cerebral autoregulation* and in the normotensive adult, it occurs at a MAP between 50 and 150 mmHg. In hypertensive adults, the range is shifted to higher pressures, while in infants and children, it is shifted to lower pressures. For example, in canine puppy models, autoregulation occurs at 40 to 100 mmHg; in the adult dog it is shifted to 70 to 150 mmHg[13,14] (Fig. 12-2). Exceeding the upper limits of autoregulation results in excessive brain blood flow (luxury perfusion), whereas reducing pressure below the lower limit risks cerebral ischemia. Because the brain is encased in a supporting skull, cerebral perfusion is often defined in terms of cerebral perfusion pressure (CPP) and written: CPP = MAP − ICP. Since the pressure-volume relationships change during growth and development, CPP is also reported to change with age. It is approximately 25 mmHg in neonates, 40 mmHg in toddlers, 50 mmHg in older children,[15] and 80 to 90 mmHg in adults.

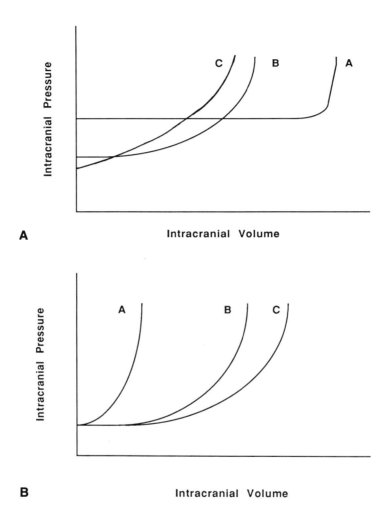

A   Intracranial Volume

B   Intracranial Volume

Fig. 12-1. (A) These curves represent the familiar hyperbolic intracranial pressure-volume relationship in two hypothetical children and an adult. The larger total volume (1,300 ml) of the adult skull is enclosed in a noncompliant skull, *A*, which can accommodate additional volume before reaching the knee of the curve. Curve *B* describes the compliant smaller infant skull (650 ml and open fontanelles), and *C* depicts the neonatal compartment (335 ml) before cranial plate fusion. Small volume changes in *C* produce changes in ICP relatively sooner in neonates, however, the slope of the rise is flattened. **(B)** The pressure-volume relationships from Fig. A are normalized for total intracranial volume. The neonatal (*C*) cranial compartment is significantly more compliant than that of the infant (*B*) or adult (*A*). (Redrawn from Shapiro et al.,[8] with permission.)

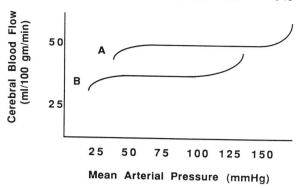

Fig. 12-2. Adult (*A*) cerebral autoregulation displaces CBF above and to the right of CBF in the infant (*B*). The infant can maintain normal CBF at lower arterial pressures than the adult but may develop cerebral hyperemia from relatively modest increases in MAP. (Data from Hernandez et al.[11])

Normal Intracranial Pressure in Childhood

Total ICP is the sum of the individual pressures within the brain (i.e., neural tissue, CSF, and blood volume). In the immediate postpartum period, the neonate undergoes an obligate diuresis, which reduces birth weight approximately 10 percent, shrinks head circumference,[16] and reduces measured ICP to near zero.[17] In one study, direct lumbar puncture pressures in neonates was reported to be 2.8 ± 1.4 mmHg with a range of 0 to 5.7 mmHg,[18] whereas in a different study neonatal anterior fontanelle pressures were reported to range from 8.3 to 9.1 mmHg.[19] In general, directly measured ICP is believed to be age related and is reported to be between 5.8 and 10.9 mmHg in toddlers and between 13 and 14.5 mmHg in older children and adolescents.[15]

Measurement and Control of Intracranial Pressure

Although the preoperative assessment is an inexact guide to intracranial compliance and ICP, it will suggest whether the child is at risk for intracranial hypertension. Any history of alterations in behavior, sleeping or feeding disturbances, abnormal breathing patterns, and nausea or vomiting may be important clues to the presence of intracranial hypertension. Abnormal pupillary responses, gaze paralysis, papilledema, bulging fontanelles, "sunset" eyes, and the Cushing triad (hypertension, bradycardia, and intracranial hypertension) may be seen on physical examination. CT or MRI scans may reveal enlarged ventricles, brain edema, or midline shifts, suggesting dramatically altered intracranial compliance. A "copper-beaten" appearance to the skull or separated cranial sutures on plain films of the head suggests the presence of chronically elevated ICP.

Preoperative confirmation of suspected intracranial hypertension is rarely available in the child outside of the intensive care setting. Ventricular reservoirs may be tapped and lumbar punctures can be performed to confirm the presence of intracranial hypertension or to drain CSF. This is difficult in the majority of elective neurosurgical patients. Alternatively, infant ICP may be monitored by means of noninvasive transducers secured to the skin overlying the anterior fontanelle. Their accuracy varies with position, the length of monitoring, the presence of edema or injury, and type of sensor,[20] and in spite of their short-comings, newer fontanelle monitors are highly reliable in the physiologic range. Anterior fontanelle transducers may be placed in intensive care units or on the floor. If this is not possible, manual fontanelle palpation will reliably differentiate shrunken, firm, and bulging fontanelles.

Aspiration of CSF through a percutaneous ventriculostomy or indwelling ventricular drain is a rapid way to reduce ICP in some settings, but should only be performed with knowledge of the intracranial dynamics. Either excessive or inadequate volume of CSF may lead to displacement of brain tissue, compression of vital structures, disruption of arterial supply, and brain death. Herniation across the midline or caudad displacement into the brain stem will usually result in death.[21] Less commonly, upward transtentorial herniation of a posterior fossa mass will cause brain death.[4] Conventional therapy for elevated ICP includes administration of mannitol 0.25 to 2 g/kg, which dehydrates brain parenchyma and reduces intracranial volume, but also alters red cell rheology and scavenges free radicles. Intravenous administration of mannitol results in a transient rise in cardiac output, a fall in serum sodium and potassium, and a reduction in ICP.[22] It may be administered with furosemide 0.5 to 1 mg/kg and dexamethasone 1 to 3 mg/kg/day. Elevation of the head, positioning the neck, and reducing sympathetic stimulation are other important strategies to control intracranial hypertension.

Hyperventilation is the first line of therapy for intracranial hypertension. It acts by causing vasoconstriction and reducing CBV.[23] Under normal physiologic conditions CBF in the adult is reduced 1.8 to 2.5 ml/100 g/min for every 1-mmHg reduction in $PaCO_2$. Carbon dioxide reactivity is attenuated in both injury[24] and immaturity, and the infant's CO_2 response ranges between 0.58 and 1.74 ml/100 g/min/mmHg.[25,26] This suggests that extreme hyperventilation may be required for clinical control of elevated ICP in infants (Fig. 12-3).

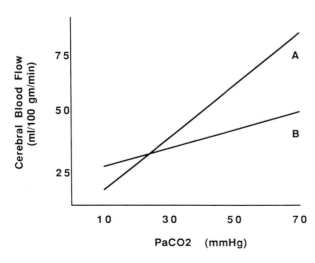

Fig. 12-3. The adult CO_2 response curve (*A*) is considerably steeper than the curve of the neonate (*B*). The immature cerebral vasculature cannot vasoconstrict or vasodilate as effectively as the adult's. Extreme hyperventilation may be better tolerated in the neonate and infant. (Data from Reivich et al.[25] and Bruce[37].)

General Anesthesia and Intracranial Hypertension

Volatile anesthetics are potent cerebral vasodilators that increase cerebral blood volume, alter CSF dynamics, and attenuate the CO_2 response. Halothane causes the greatest increase in ICP,[27] but the increase can be blunted by prior induction of hypocapnia.[28] Isoflurane maintains coupling between blood flow and metabolic activity better than other agents and tends to preserve CO_2 response.[29] Nonetheless, isoflurane can lead to increased ICP in settings of severely reduced intracranial compliance.[30] Virtually all studies of volatile anesthetics and brain function are derived from animal experimentation or clinical investigations in adults and their direct applicability in pediatric neuroanesthesia is unclear. In acute pediatric ventricular shunt malfunction, isoflurane 1.5 percent and modest hyperventilation results in a 25 percent drop of CPP and a 4- to 8-mmHg increase in ICP.[31,32] In a similar clinical setting, halothane 1.0 to 1.5 percent inspired concentration increased ICP 25 percent in the presence of modest intracranial hypertension (20 to 25 mmHg) but no change was observed if ICP exceeded 40 mmHg (Harris MM: unpublished data). In general, at 1 to 1.5 MAC anesthesia, hyperventilation will control ICP in most clinical situations and the choice of volatile agent is relatively unimportant.

Intravenous anesthetics, such as thiopental, lidocaine (in therapeutic doses), benzodiazepines, droperidol, and propofol reduce CBF, $CMRO_2$, and ICP and preserve coupling, whereas ketamine increases CBF and ICP. In general, narcotics have modest effects on CBF and cerebral metabolism: fentanyl decreases CBV and lowers resistance to CSF reabsorption[33]; sufentanil will increase ICP in selected patients with supratentorial tumors[34]; and narcotic-induced rigidity increases ICP.[35] In adults with supratentorial brain tumors, administration of succinylcholine increases ICP, but this can be prevented by pretreatment with metocurine.[36] Without pretreatment, succinylcholine 1.5 mg/kg increases ICP 50 percent in hydrocephalic infants with moderate intracranial hypertension (20 to 25 mmHg) and increases it more than 75 percent if administered in the presence of severe intracranial hypertension (Harris MM: unpublished data). Neuromuscular relaxants that increase cardiac output, such as pancuronium, may also increase CBF and worsen intracranial hypertension.

Anesthetic techniques for children who are at risk for intracranial hypertension should emphasize cardiovascular and central nervous system stability. Patients with severely reduced intracranial compliance will not tolerate even small increases in CBF brought about by induction of general anesthesia, or by struggling and crying. The optimal induction technique in pediatric neurosurgery includes a secure intravenous catheter, preoxygenation when possible, intravenous induction agents such as thiopental and lidocaine, hyperventilation (keeping in mind that the optimal $PaCO_2$ in children with immature cerebral vasculature is speculative but probably is below the comparable value for adults[37]), and neuromuscular relaxation with nondepolarizing relaxants not possessing sympathomimetic properties or with succinylcholine and pretreatment. Rectal methohexital is a satisfactory alternative in the child who does not have an intravenous catheter, but care must be taken to prevent airway obstruction, hypercarbia, and emesis. Conventional mask inhalational induction with halothane risks intracranial hypertension, although this risk is mitigated by open cranial sutures and prior hyperventilation. Substituting isoflurane for halothane by mask increases the risks of breathholding, coughing, and laryngospasm, all of which are poorly tolerated in children with intracranial lesions.

Traumatic Head Injury

Severe head trauma is a human tragedy of immense proportions that burdens the family and the medical system with months of acute intensive care and, often, years of chronic custodial care. Head trauma may be defined as any injury to the scalp or cranial vault or its contents, and may be classified as severe or trivial. Ironically, forceful concussive or penetrating injuries in children may leave little neurologic residual if vital centers are spared and secondary brain injury is avoided, whereas relatively trivial-appearing head trauma may lead to delayed clinical deterioration and death.[38]

Trauma accounts for more than half of the deaths in children each year[39] and the vast majority of traumatic episodes involve severe head injury.[40] In spite of these statistics, the outcome of severe pediatric head injury is significantly better than that of similar head trauma in adults.[41] This improved outcome may be due to differences in brain function and anatomy, the salutary effects of pediatric life support and intensive management, or of other strategies designed to minimize secondary brain injury. The damaged brain suffers vasoparalysis, which attenuates cerebral autoregulation, hypoxic response, and CO_2 reactivity and increases the brain's susceptibility to respiratory embarrassment and to hemorrhagic hypotension.[42,43] Hemorrhagic hypotension will reduce CBF and cause cerebral ischemia unless rapidly corrected by volume infusion, however, there appear to be few significant differences among resuscitation fluids as long as hypotonic solutions and glucose are avoided.[44,45] In a large proportion of children (41 percent) and in a few adults, severe head trauma is accompanied by increased CBF, general cerebral hyperemia, and diffuse swelling.[46]

The incidence of cervical spine injury is reported to be 17.5 percent following motor vehicle accidents,[47] 1.7 percent after blunt head trauma,[48] and 1 percent in general multiple trauma.[49] In children sustaining severe head injury (Glasgow Coma Scale < 7) following motor vehicle accidents, 16 percent will have cervical spine injuries.[50] Because of its unique mechanical and elastic properties, the immature cervical spine is especially susceptible to high cervical spine injury such as fractures of the odontoid and subluxations at the atlanto-occipital, atlantoaxial, and C2-3 levels. In contrast, children over 8 years of age display an adult-type injury pattern characterized by fractures anywhere along the length of the cervical spine.[51]

The severity of neurologic injury in children is graded by means of a modified Glasgow Coma Scale (GCS), which evaluates eye opening, motor function, and to a lesser degree, verbal skills (Table 12-1).[52] In general, GCS < 8, fluctuating neurologic function, or progressive decrease in consciousness necessitates endotracheal intubation and ventilation. In these settings, the physician must rap-

Table 12-1. Modified Coma Score for Infants

Activity	Best Response	Score
Eye opening	Spontaneous	4
	To speech	3
	To pain	2
	None	1
Verbal	Coos and babbles	5
	Irritable cries	4
	Cries to pain	3
	Moans to pain	2
	None	1
Motor	Normal spontaneous movements	6
	Withdraws to touch	5
	Withdraws to pain	4
	Abnormal flexion	3
	Abnormal extension	2
	None	1

(From Davis et al.,[52] with permission.)

idly evaluate and manage the airway while minimizing regurgitation and aspiration and avoiding injury to the cervical spine without increasing ICP. Although there are many different strategies for securing the airway in the suspected cervical spine injury, we believe the optimal approach is to maintain the neck in the neutral position with manual inline axial traction and cricoid pressure while the patient is oxygenated, ventilated, and intubated orally.[53,54] The availability of back-up support and equipment, the associated injuries, cardiovascular status, and personal experience will influence the choice of awake or rapid-sequence intubation technique. Topical lidocaine, transtracheal lidocaine, and nerve blocks may block the stress response to endotracheal intubation but will also depress protective airway reflexes. In contrast, the glossopharyngeal nerve block appears to be effective without blocking airway reflexes.[55] Nasotracheal intubation offers some advantages in neurologically compromised patients, but it risks bacteremia, hemorrhage, sinusitis,[56] and possibly meningitis. In the presence of direct facial or airway trauma, use of fiberoptic bronchoscopy, light wands, or other airway aids is an alternative to direct surgical cricothyroidotomy.

NEURODIAGNOSTIC PROCEDURES

Transportation and Monitoring

Managing children for neurodiagnostic imaging demands special vigilance and attention because unexpected neurologic deterioration, oversedation, airway obstruction, drug reactions, and respiratory arrest are common in this setting. Preparation, mobility, and flexibility are the best guarantees of successful outcome. Supplemental oxygen and gas delivery systems, suction, airway equipment, physiologic monitoring equipment, including blood pressure monitor, electrocardiograph, temperature monitor, and pulse oximeter, should be available before beginning anesthesia services. In general, body temperature does not change appreciably during radiologic procedures, but temperature monitoring should be available for all anesthetized patients. Capnography is especially valuable in neuroradiology when the anesthesiologist is physically remote from the patient. However, dispensing with some or all of these physiologic monitors may be done at the discretion of the anesthesiologist.

Sedation for Neuroradiology

The healthy child may require little more than simple reassurance from the physician or nearby parent. Other children, especially those involved in protracted or uncomfortable procedures, will require sedation or general anesthesia. *Sedation* implies that the patient is comfortable, cooperative, and arousable, and the selection of sedatives is often a matter of personal or institutional bias. Chloral hydrate 25 to 75 mg/kg PO, pentobarbital 4 to 6 mg/kg PO, IM, or PR, narcotics, and lytic cocktails (demerol cocktail or DPT (Demerol, Phenergan, Thorazine) 1 ml/15 kg with a maximum dose of 2 ml) are commonly used,[57] although demerol compound has a high incidence of serious respiratory side effects.[58] Midazolam 0.5 to 0.75 mg/kg PO and anesthesia induction agents such as methohexital 25 to 30 mg/kg PR or ketamine 3 mg/kg IM (a 23-gauge needle combines minimal insertion pain with rapid injection capability) should be reserved for physicians skilled in pediatric resuscitation. It is worth remembering that children with significant neuropathology may respond unpredictably to sedatives.

General Anesthesia for Neuroradiology

Infants, toddlers, uncooperative, or retarded older children undergoing even relatively short neuroradiographic imaging will usually require general anesthesia. In older cooperative children, pain, prolonged procedures, and absolute immobility may be other indications for general anesthesia. General anesthesia may be preferable in the child with significant underlying medical or neurologic conditions.

Parents usually accompany their children to the radiology department and wish to be present during induction of anesthesia. This parent-child interaction should be encouraged by construction of appropriate radiologic induction facilities, adoption of pediatric-oriented induction techniques, and recovery from anesthesia in "child-friendly" recovery rooms. Common induction agents can be safely used in neurologically normal children who are otherwise free of medical problems, but children with significant neuropathology require careful preoperative evaluation to assess ICP, airway reflexes and patency, ventilatory drive, drug interactions, altered response to neuromuscular relaxants, seizures, fluid and electrolyte disturbances, nausea, vomiting, and delayed gastric emptying. Children receiving phenobarbital for control of seizure disorders often require large doses of methohexital (30 to 40 mg/kg) and chronic phenytoin therapy may antagonize neuromuscular blockade.[59] Fluid and electrolyte disturbances can occur in the child with nausea or vomiting, or after externalization of a shunt. (Externalized shunts can drain 150 to 200 ml/day.)

Most pediatric neuroradiology is performed on an outpatient basis, therefore medical records should clearly detail the patient's current neurologic condition and previous anesthetic experience. The scheduling physician will usually not appreciate the risks of anesthesia and may overlook the significance of cranial nerve palsies, nausea, alterations of behavior, or other findings associated with intracranial hypertension. If ICP is elevated, percutaneous ventriculostomy, lumbar puncture, or needle aspiration of the ventricular reservoir may reduce ICP prior to induction of general anesthesia. Intravenous induction techniques are preferred in children with elevated ICP; unfortunately, few infants and children will come with their own IV and repeated unsuccessful cannulation attempts result in a hysterical child and anxious family. When you cannot secure an intravenous catheter, rectal methohexital or a gentle mask induction with hyperventilation, nitrous oxide, or volatile anesthetic agent will induce anesthesia and allow intravenous catheter placement. Ketamine is useful in the very uncooperative child and vigorous hyperventilation will usually control any increase in ICP. Most children will be discharged home following recovery and their preoperative neurologic status should be communicated to the recovery room staff, for without this history, it may be difficult to determine whether the child has returned to baseline neurologic status.

Computed Tomography Scan

Computed tomography (CT) scans are either relatively painless or completely painless for the majority of children. However, it may be difficult to convince infants and children between the ages of 6 months and 4 to 5 years that they need to lie still. In addition, some children in this age group are difficult to sedate with the usual medications. Therefore, the anesthesiologist is called to manage the anesthetic for the CT scan. If there is evidence of increased ICP, the anesthetic technique is tailored toward management of ICP using the techniques already described. If there is no increase in ICP, the usual anesthetic technique is rectal methohexital 30 mg/kg. If the scan is unenhanced, this is usually sufficient to perform the entire scan. If contrast material is necessary, an IV is started with local anesthesia. If an IV is in place, additional anesthetic agents such as lidocaine 1 mg/kg, thiopental 1 mg/kg, or ketamine 0.5 to 1 mg/kg can be administered to attain satisfactory anesthesia. If the child arrives on the scene with an IV in place, then an intravenous anesthetic can be accomplished with titrating doses of thiopental, ketamine, and lidocaine. Except in unusual circumstances, these patients do not need intubation.

Neuroangiography

Cerebral angiography is a powerful diagnostic and therapeutic tool for intracranial tumors and vascular lesions. It is usually performed by means of a femoral artery puncture and requires immobility for variable periods of time. The puncture and injection of contrast material or adhesive polymers are the only stimulating portions of the procedure. As with all radiographic procedures, older children do well with small amounts of sedation and younger children or infants often require general anesthesia.

Arteriovenous malformations (AVMs) are the most common vascular lesions in childhood and can be treated using embolization with detachable balloons, Silastic pellets, or quick-setting acrylic glue. Complications include hemorrhage, catheter failure, and neurologic catastrophe resulting either from alteration of blood flow or injection into the wrong vessel. High-flow AVMs in neonates, such as vein of Galen malformations, are associated with high operative mortality, diffuse cerebral ischemia, congestive heart failure, hemorrhagic infarction, mass effect, and hydrocephalus.[60] Because excessive flow through these AVMs reduces the success rate of embolization, nitroprusside 0.5 to 1 μg/kg or esmolol 1 to 2 mg/kg may be indicated to reduce flow. Intravenous or inhalational inductions are safe in children without recent hemorrhage or congestive heart failure, but when intracranial compliance is reduced, barbiturates and hyperventilation are prudent options and congestive heart failure should be controlled before embolization. Solid tumors can be embolized preoperatively to reduce vascularity and intraoperative hemorrhage.

Myelography

Both monitored anesthesia care and general anesthesia are appropriate options for pediatric myelography or combined myelography/CT scan. The goal of the anesthesiologist is to keep the child still during lumbar puncture, injection of contrast material, and the subsequent radiographic imaging. Newer contrast media are relatively nontoxic and pose little danger to the patient.[61] The anesthetic principles are similar to those for other imaging techniques; we use either a ketamine or a methohexital induction followed by intravenous sedation with combinations of ketamine, barbiturates, narcotics, and lidocaine. These agents minimize the discomfort of lumbar puncture, after which the patient can be positioned easily on the myelography table while maintaining control of his or her own airway and ventilation. After completion of the myelogram, the patient is transported to the CT scanner; additional thiopental 1 to 2 mg/kg, ketamine 1 mg/kg, alfentanyl 10 to 20 μg/kg, and fentanyl 1 to 2 μg/kg can be given if needed.

Nuclear Magnetic Resonance Imaging

Nuclear magnetic resonance imaging (MRI) is a special anesthetic challenge for several reasons. First, the child is positioned in a remote, noisy location where communication is all but impossible. Second, ferrous metals are attracted to the magnet and cannot be used. Third, certain radio frequencies from unshielded sources will distort the MRI. Fourth, people within the magnetic field may experience electromagnetic-induced body temperature elevations. To overcome some of these problems, a variety of innovative anesthetic delivery and monitoring systems have been introduced for MRI, and the reader is referred to the work of Rao et al.[62] and Boutros and Pavlicek[63] for descriptions of MRI compatible equipment.

Monitored anesthesia care with intravenous agents is effective at producing calm, cooperative children in nearly every radiographic location and there is no particular combination of medications that appears preferable in MRI. The key to effective and safe delivery of anesthetic services is to maintain contact with the patient by way of direct observation or by use of remote cameras and monitors. The unprotected airway is always a risk in MRI, but general endotracheal anesthesia eliminates the problem. Inhalational anesthesia can be delivered from the relative safety of beyond the magnetic field by employing long breathing hoses or by use of nonferrous equipment. Intravenous anesthesia with fixed agents (propofol or methohexital) administered by constant infusion or intermittent bolus is a relatively simple and effective alternative to inhalational anesthesia.

Radiotherapy and Radiosurgery

Radiotherapy and radiosurgery are linked because they require absolute immobility in a setting of ionizing radiation exposure. Physicians and parents are excluded from the immediate treatment area and both the physiologic monitoring and the conduct of the anesthetic are directed from a remote location. Patient exposure to ionizing radiation during cancer therapy may last only a few minutes, but is often repeated daily for several weeks. Heparin locks and central access facilitate administration of fixed agents such as ketamine 1 to 2 mg/kg that cause immobility with good airway control for relatively short periods of time. Children can develop tolerance to repeated administration of ketamine or they may be bothered by sleep and personality disorders. Combining ketamine with thiopental 1 to 2 mg/kg IV or midazolam 0.1 mg/kg IV will help to manage both of these problems. Inhalational general anesthesia by mask has been reported as an alternative to endotracheal intubation,[64] but it should be remembered that the patient will be monitored from behind a radiation-proof lead-lined door and access will be delayed in any emergency.

Radiosurgery, the paradox of "noninvasive neurosurgery," uses high-energy particle beams or gamma radiation to destroy intracranial lesions such as AVMs, acoustic neuromas, and selective tumors. It can be done either in linear accelerators or in a radioactive cobalt source known as a "Gamma Knife."[65] The latter is used exclusively in radiosurgery and is available in only a few centers; linear accelerators have diverse applications in the field of cancer radiotherapy. A single Gamma Knife treatment lasts 10 to 40 minutes, but is preceded by hours of radiographic localization and complex treatment planning. The case begins with a CT scan or cerebral angiography, after which the anesthetized child is transported to the radiation facility. Virtually all children require general anesthesia for radiosurgery because of the duration, discomfort, and immobility. Once positioned on the Gamma Knife gantry, the room is evacuated, and the child is moved approximately 5 feet into the unit. Airway disconnection and accidental extubation can occur. We maintain general anesthesia with spontaneous ventilation, a volatile agent, and 100 percent oxygen; monitoring is with remote cameras and direct observation is through a leaded window.

Transport oxygen, delivery systems, and airway and intubating equipment should be available for the trip to the recovery room. If the trip is short, monitoring may be minimal. In general, monitoring will vary with the physical condition of the patient and distance to be traveled; the healthy patient can be moved safely with a pulse oximeter and a finger on the pulse. Oxygen tank-driven portable suction devices are valuable and should be available for longer transports.

ANESTHETIC MANAGEMENT IN NEUROSURGERY

Brain Tumors

Brain tumors are the second most common pediatric neoplasm and occur with an incidence of between 2 and 5 per 100,000.[66] In the United States, the most common tumors are brain stem gliomas, cerebellar astrocytomas, and medulloblastomas; meningiomas, pituitary adenomas, and glioblastomas are more common in adults.[4] A large percentage of pediatric tumors arise in the posterior fossa near the fourth ventricle, the brain stem, and other midline structures, whereas 70 percent of adult brain tumors lie above the tentorium.[4] This midline location explains why many pediatric tumors block the flow of CSF and patients first present with hydrocephalus. In the absence of hydrocephalus, pediatric brain tumors can grow relatively large because of the child's tremendous compensating ability and the tendency to disregard minor neurologic findings in children.[67] Posterior fossa masses can compress the brain stem or displace the tentorium upward into the cerebral hemispheres. Impending upward transtentorial herniation can be diagnosed on CT scan by compression of the quadrigeminal cistern or by flattening of the posterior portion of the third ventricle.[68] In theory, transtentorial herniation can occur during hyperventilation[69] if cerebral volume were reduced significantly, but in practice it happens infrequently and requires drainage of large quantities of CSF.[70]

The preanesthetic assessment of the child with a brain tumor should address intracranial compliance and elevated ICP. Do the child's signs and symptoms refer to tumor invasion, direct compression, or distant pressure effects? Headache, gait disturbance, vomiting, and ocular findings are relatively nonspecific but clinical evaluation, discussion with the neurosurgeon, and review of the radiographic findings may suggest whether ICP is elevated. Sometimes it is impossible to rule out compartmental increases in ICP and, in general, we take "ICP precautions" in all children with intracranial tumors—supratentorial or infratentorial—whether the fontanelles are open or closed. We do not premedicate these children, but administer benzodiazepines, barbiturates, or narcotics as needed under close observation in the induction room. Ideally, these children will arrive in the operating room with an intravenous catheter in place, permitting rapid-sequence intravenous induction of anesthesia using short-acting narcotics such as fentanyl 3 to 10 μg/kg or alfentanil 20 to 100 μg/kg, thiopental 3 to 5 mg/kg, lidocaine, neuromuscular relaxants, cricoid pressure, hyperventilation, and 100 percent oxygen. If the child arrives without an intravenous catheter, placement can be accomplished in any manner that is appropriate and arterial and central venous catheters may be inserted after induction.

Positioning the head for access to the tumor is essential in neurosurgery. Most supratentorial lesions can be reached with the patient in the supine position and the head turned to one side or the other, but occasionally turning the head will obstruct jugular venous drainage and lead to a marked increase in ICP. Care should be taken to minimize neck rotation and venous obstruction. Normally, the prone position requires bilateral pelvic girdle and clavicle support and special protection for the legs, arms, and groin, although the modified prone position minimizes some of these problems by using a beanbag mattress and neck hyperextension. This technique gives access to the entire calvarium from the supraorbital ridges to the posterior rim of the foramen magnum.[71] The seated position may offer some surgical advantages[72] but is associated with an increased risk of venous air embolism, venous pooling, hemodynamic instability, pressure injuries, and massive swelling of the tongue.[73] As an alternative to the sitting position, we use the modified prone, the supine position with extreme neck flexion, or the lateral position.

Venous air embolism (VAE) has been documented during 6 to 45 percent of seated craniectomies[74,75] and in a lesser number of supine, lateral, and prone craniotomies. The incident of Doppler-detected VAE during seated pediatric craniectomy is 33 percent,[76] whereas use of echocardiography increases the rate of detection to 66 percent.[77] Venous air embolism is caused by a Venturi effect from returning venous blood, and usually air enters as a stream of tiny bubbles, passes quickly into the pulmonary circulation, and is excreted by the lung without hemodynamic or pulmonary consequences. Larger quantities of air cause pulmonary vasoconstriction, increase pulmonary artery pressure, and lead to right-sided cardiac failure or complete heart block.[78] Elevated right-sided pressure may force air across septal defects into the left heart, causing paradoxical air embolism.[79] Treatment of VAE includes discontinuing nitrous oxide, flooding the surgical field, lowering the head, covering open bone, supporting the circulation, aspirating air directly from the central circulation, and turning the patient into the left lateral position. The left lateral position displaces air away from the right ventricular outflow tract. Both positive end-expiratory pressure (PEEP) and jugular venous compression increase cerebral venous back pressure and reduce the Venturi effect. In adults, less than 10 cmH$_2$O of PEEP will not produce paradoxical VAE,[80] however, there are no similar data for children. We use Doppler ultrasonic probes during pediatric craniotomy and follow end-tidal nitrogen and carbon dioxide levels, but reserve insertion of central lines for major cases in which we believe there to be significant blood loss or hemodynamic instability. In our hands, the yield during aspiration of a central line for presumed VAE is negligible.

Brain stem and cranial nerve injury frequently accompanies posterior fossa exploration and may result in intraoperative cardiovascular or respiratory instability.[81,82] Cardiac dysrhythmias or changes in blood pressure should be relayed promptly to the neurosurgeons so that they can identify nearby vital brain stem centers. If the brain stem is involved at surgery, the patient should be left intubated and observed carefully in the intensive care unit for altered respiratory drive or airway reflexes. Patients with isolated posterior fossa lesions, little preoperative symptomatology, and a benign intraoperative course can be weaned and extubated at the end of the procedure.

Craniofacial Surgery

Craniofacial repair involves the cosmetic restoration of congenital or acquired bony anomalies of the skull and face. Although both neurosurgeons and plastic surgeons work in this field, their emphases, operative techniques, and outcomes may differ significantly. The surgery varies in length and in complexity; a isolated sagittal craniosynostosis repair may last 45 minutes and cause the loss of 20 ml of blood whereas a repeat hypertelorism repair can take 24 hours and result in the loss of several blood volumes. Anesthetic considerations for craniofacial surgery (i.e., hypertelorism, craniofacial dysostoses, and facial clefts or asymmetries) include hemorrhage, elevated ICP, airway difficulties, hypothermia, and coagulopathies. Close cooperation among the craniofacial team is important to anticipate intraoperative needs such as elective tracheostomy, availability of blood products, and postoperative care. Airway complications are common: intubations may be difficult because of mandibular hypoplasia or scar tissue, and once the patient is intubated, accidental intraoperative extubation occurs often. This results from the large number of surgeons, their close proximity to the endotracheal tube, and the frequent movement of head and face. Nasal intubation fixes the tube but may not prevent extubation if the maxilla is involved at surgery. Sewing the endotracheal tube around the teeth has proven to be successful in our hands but it does not guarantee against inadvertent extubation or endotracheal tube obstruction. Maintaining normothermia in the face of massive hemorrhage and radical cranial exposure is nearly impossible in spite of the use of warming lamps, blood warmers, and blankets,[83,84] but we have found that wrapping the infant in cast padding or cellophane minimizes heat loss.

Massive hemorrhage during craniofacial surgery is the single greatest intraoperative challenge. Blood loss in excess of one blood volume is common, even when hypotensive anesthetic techniques are used. Blood loss is continuous throughout surgery but is especially brisk during the cranial osteotomy. It is very difficult to play "catch up" with replacement blood volume, therefore we routinely administer warmed balanced salt solution 75 to 100 ml/kg prior to the surgical incision, maintain hypervolemic hemodilution in the early hours of surgery, and then transfuse with blood products to maintain hematocrits in the mid 20s. In general, massive blood replacement is complicated by dilutional thrombocytopenia, coagulopathy,[85,86] and calcium-mediated hypotension.[87] Minor increases in serum potassium have been reported during transfusion of packed red cells in craniofacial surgery[88] and frequent hematocrits and electrolytes and ionized calcium levels are routine.

Craniosynostosis is the premature closure of the cranial sutures. It occurs with a frequency of 0.6 per 1,000, and most commonly involves the metopic, sagittal, and coronal sutures.[89] Several sutures may be involved simultaneously and craniosynostosis may occur together with other facial anomalies. Blood loss during repair of isolated sagittal and coronal synostosis is approximately 22 percent of the estimated blood volume (EBV), whereas loss during surgery for metopic and bicoronal synostosis is approximately 50 percent of the EBV.[90] Preoperative evaluation of all children with premature closure of cranial sutures should include an assessment of ICP. Intracranial hypertension is common in multiple craniosynostosis (41 percent) and should be expected in a smaller percentage of isolated lesions.[91]

Meningomyelocele and Arnold-Chiari Malformation

Meningomyelocele is a spinal cord disorder of unknown etiology characterized by failure of the neural tube to close during embryogenesis. It is reported to occur with an incidence of approximately 20 per 100,000[92] and may be seen anywhere along the spinal cord, giving rise to a variety of neurologic deficits in the lower extremity, bowel, and bladder. At birth, the open defective spinal cord is covered by only a thin layer of meninges, and infection, fluid loss, electrolyte imbalance, and hypothermia will follow unless the defect is closed. After stabilization in the neonatal intensive care unit, the defect is covered with a moist, sterile drape and the infant is transferred to the operating room. Positioning for induction of general anesthesia may be difficult if the lesion is large, however, a "donut" can be constructed of towels to accommodate the child. Anesthesia may be induced with either a volatile inhalation agent or with intravenous administration of thiopental and a neuromuscular relaxant. Administration of succinylcholine will not result in hyperkalemia.[93]

Following repair of the primary defect, the child with meningomyelocele may require later surgery because of abnormalities in the cervical spine and brain stem. Virtually all children with meningomyelocele possess an Arnold-Chiari malformation, which is characterized by caudal displacement of lower portions of the brain stem. This malformation results in frequent brain stem compression and complete obstruction of the foramina of Luschka and Magendie. The latter leads to progressive hydrocephalus and dilatation of the cervical central canal (hydromyelia). Brain stem abnormalities in Arnold-Chiari malformation result in respiratory obstruction, vocal cord paralysis, abnormal respiratory drive, autonomic instability, and spasticity.[94–96] Decompressive posterior fossa craniectomy relieves some, but not all of these symptoms.[97]

Hydrocephalus

Hydrocephalus results from decreased reabsorption or excess secretion of CSF. The anesthetic implications include intracranial hypertension and, to a lesser extent, head positioning during induction of anesthesia. Intracranial hypertension is a function of the time course of the disorder and of the volume buffering capacity of the brain. CT scanning will usually diagnose the etiology. Communicating hydrocephalus follows intraventricular hemorrhage or bacterial meningitis; noncommunicating hydrocephalus results from tumor or congenital obstruction. Ventricular shunts that drain CSF into the pleural cavity and central venous system can result in hydrothorax or VAE.[98] Ventriculoperitoneal shunts are most common, but they can be complicated by infection, obstruction, extravasation of CSF, overshunting (slit ventricle syndrome), as well as undershunting.

Surgical revision of a malfunctioning shunt may be limited to replacing the valve or the shunt tubing, or both. If the valve is defective, the surgical field will be limited to the head; if the tubing is to be replaced, both the abdomen and head will be involved. As mentioned previously, anesthesia for acute shunt malfunction associated with intracranial hypertension should commence with intravenous access, preoxygenation, cricoid pressure, intravenous barbiturate, and hyperventilation. The adverse effects of volatile anesthetics and succinylcholine are mitigated by prior hyperventilation and by pretreatment with nondepolarizing muscle relaxants. Following induction of general anesthesia, most neonates will become hypothermic during the "head to pubis" surgical preparation unless they are actively warmed with heating blankets and warming lights. Accidental extubation can occur if the surgeon moves the head during placement of the shunt tubing; extreme flexion can kink the endotracheal tube or position it in the mainstem bronchus. The anesthetic goal is to awaken the child after surgery, assess neurologic function, and extubate. Failure to awaken quickly suggests perioperative neurologic insult. Those children should be transported to the intensive care unit or to the recovery room for further evaluation.

REFERENCES

1. Sperry RJ, Stirt JA, Stone DJ (eds): Manual of Neuroanesthesia. BC Decker, Toronto, 1989
2. Amiel-Tison C, Larroche JC: Brain development and neurological survey during the neonatal period. p. 245. In Stern L, Vert P (eds): Neonatal Medicine. Masson, New York, 1987
3. Hoffman HJ, Hendrick EB, Munro I: Craniosynostosis and craniofacial surgery. p. 121. In Section of Pediatric Neurosurgery of the American Academy of Neurological Surgeons (eds): Pediatric Neurosurgery: Surgery of the Developing Nervous System. Grune & Stratton, Orlando, FL, 1982
4. Milhort TA: Pediatric Neurosurgery. FA Davis, Philadelphia, 1978
5. Aisenson MR: Closing of the anterior fontanelle. Pediatrics 6:223, 1950
6. Friesen RH, Honda AT, Thieme RE: Changes in anterior fontanelle pressure in preterm neonates during tracheal intubation. Anesth Analg 66:874, 1987
7. Raju TNK, Vidyasagar D, Torres C, et al: Intracranial pressure during intubation and anesthesia in infants. J Pediatr 96:860, 1980
8. Shapiro K, Fried A, Takei F, et al: Effect of the skull and dura on neural axis pressure-volume relationships and CSF hydrodynamics. J Neurosurg 63:76, 1985
9. Greisen G: Cerebral blood flow in preterm infants during the first week of life. Acta Paediatr Scand 75:43, 1986

10. Friis-Hansen B: Perinatal brain injury and cerebral blood flow in newborn infants. Acta Paediatr Scand 74:323, 1985
11. Hernandez MJ, Bernan RW, Vannacci RC, et al: Cerebral blood flow and oxygen consumption in the newborn dog. Am J Physiol 234:R210, 1978
12. Brennan RW, Patterson RH, Kessler J: Cerebral blood flow and metabolism during cardiopulmonary bypass: Evidence of microembolic encephalopathy. Neurology 21:665, 1971
13. Hernandez MJ, Brennan RW, Bowman GS: Autoregulation of cerebral blood flow in the newborn dog. Brain Res 184:199, 1980
14. Haggendal E, Johansson B: Effects of arterial carbon dioxide tension and oxygen saturation on cerebral blood flow autoregulation in dogs. Acta Physiol Scand (Suppl) 258; 66:27, 1965
15. Newton RW: Intracranial pressure and its monitoring in childhood: A review. J R Soc Med 80:566, 1987
16. Williams J, Hirsch NJ, Corbet AJS, et al: Postnatal head shrinkage in small infants. Pediatrics 59:619, 1977
17. Welch K: The intracranial pressure in infants. J Neurosurg 52:693, 1980
18. Kaiser AM, Whitelaw AGL: Normal cerebrospinal fluid pressure in the newborn. Neuropediatrics 17:100, 1986
19. Philip AGS, Long JG, Bonn SM: Intracranial pressure. Am J Dis Child 135:521, 1981
20. Bunegin L, Albin MS: Pitfalls encountered in relating anterior fontanelle pressure to intracranial pressure. Anesth Analg 66:1196, 1987
21. Fishman RA: Brain edema. N Engl J Med 293:706, 1975
22. Manninen PH, Lam AM, Gelb AW, et al: The effect of high-dose mannitol on serum and urine electrolytes and osmolality in neurosurgical patients. Can J Anaesth 34:442, 1987
23. Mitchenfelder JD: Anesthesia and the Brain. Churchill Livingstone, New York, 1988
24. Saunders ML, Miller JD, Stablein D, et al: The effects of graded experimental trauma on cerebral blood flow and responsiveness to CO_2. J Neurosurg 51:18, 1979
25. Reivich M, Brann AW, Shapiro H, et al: Reactivity of cerebral vessels to CO_2 in the newborn rhesus monkey. Eur Neurol 6:132, 1971
26. Levine MI, Shortland D, Gibson N, et al: Carbon dioxide reactivity of the cerebral circulation in extremely premature infants: Effects of postnatal age and indomethacin. Pediatr Res 24:175, 1988
27. Jennett WB, Barker J, Fitch W, et al: Effect of anesthesia on intracranial pressure in patients with space-occupying lesions. Lancet 1:61, 1969
28. Adams RW, Gronert GA, Sundt TM, et al: Halothane, hypocapnia and cerebral fluid pressure in neurosurgery. Anesthesiology 37:510, 1972
29. Drummond JC, Todd MM: The response of the feline cerebral circulation to $PaCO_2$ during anesthesia with isoflurane and halothane and during sedation with nitrous oxide. Anesthesiology 62:268, 1985
30. Grosslight K, Foster R, Colohan AR, et al: Isoflurane for neuroanesthesia: Risk factors of increases in intracranial pressure. Anesthesiology 63:533, 1985
31. Aloy A, Dirnberger H, Kalinowsky R, et al: Characteristics of isoflurane in hydrocephalic children with ventricular shunt malfunction. Anesthesiology 63:A348, 1985
32. Lundar T, Lindegaard KF, Refsum L, et al: Cerebrovascular effects of isoflurane in man. Br J Anaesth 59:1208, 1987
33. Artru AA: Relationship between cerebral blood volume and CSF pressure during anesthesia with isoflurane and fentanyl in dogs. Anesthesiology 60:575, 1984
34. Marx W, Shah N, Long C, et al: Sufentanil, alfentanil and fentanyl: Impact on CSF pressure in patients with brain tumors. Anesthesiology 69:A627, 1988

35. Benthuysen JL, Kien ND, Quam DD: Intracranial pressure increases during alfentanil-induced rigidity. Anesthesiology 68:438, 1988
36. Minton MD, Grosslight KR, Stirt JA: Increases in intracranial pressure from succinylcholine. Prevention by prior non-depolarizing blockade. Anesthesiology 65:165, 1986
37. Bruce DA: Treatment of intracranial hypertension. p. 245. In Section of Pediatric Neurosurgery of the American Association of Neurological Surgeons (eds): Pediatric Neurosurgery. 2nd Ed. WB Saunders, Philadelphia, 1989
38. Snoek JW, Minderhoud JM, Wilmink JT: Delayed deterioration following mild head injury in children. Brain 107:15, 1984
39. Haller JA: Pediatric trauma: The no. 1 killer of children. JAMA 249:47, 1983
40. Mayer T, Walker ML, Johnson DG, et al: Causes of morbidity and mortality in severe pediatric trauma. JAMA 245:719, 1981
41. Luerssen TG, Klauber MR, Marshall LF: Outcome from head injury related to patient's age. J Neurosurg 68:409, 1988
42. Lewelt W, Jenkins LW, Miller JD: Effects of experimental fluid-percussion injury of the brain on cerebrovascular reactivity to hypoxia and to hypercapnia. J Neurosurg 56:332, 1982
43. Ishige N, Pitts LH, Berry I: The effects of hypovolemic hypotension on high-energy phosphate metabolism of traumatized brain in rats. J Neurosurg 68:129, 1988
44. Zornow MH, Scheller MS, Todd MM, et al: Acute cerebral effects of isotonic crystalloid and colloid solutions following cryogenic brain injury in the rabbit. Anesthesiology 69:180, 1988
45. Lanier WL, Stangland KJ, Scheithauer BW: The effects of dextrose infusion and head position on neurologic outcome after complete cerebral ischemia in primates: Examination of a model. Anesthesiology 66:39, 1987
46. Bruce DA, Alavi A, Bilaniuk L, et al: Diffuse cerebral swelling following head injuries in children: The syndrome of "malignant brain edema." J Neurosurg 54:170, 1981
47. Mackenzie CF, Shin B, Fisher R, et al: Four year mortality of trauma victims admitted directly from the accident by helicopter. Anesthesiology 57:A96, 1982
48. Bayless P, Ray VG: Incidence of cervical spine injuries in association with blunt head trauma. Am J Emerg Med 7:139, 1989
49. Grande CM, Barton CR, Stene JK: Appropriate techniques for airway management of emergency patients with suspected spinal cord injury. Anesth Analg 67:714, 1988
50. Bohn D, Swan P, Sides C, et al: High cervical spine injuries associated with severe head injury in children: An unrecognized cause of cardiorespiratory arrest. Crit Care Med 17:S117, 1989
51. Hill SA, Miller CA, Kosnik EJ, et al: Pediatric neck injuries. J Neurosurg 60:700, 1984
52. Davis RJ, Dean M, Goldberg AL, et al: Head and spinal cord injury. p. 649. In Rogers MC (ed): Textbook of Pediatric Intensive Care. Williams & Wilkins, Baltimore, 1987
53. Yearly DM, Cantees KK, Verdile VP, et al: Emergency airway management in trauma patients with suspected cervical spine injury. Anesth Analg 68:415, 1989
54. Crande CM, Barton CR, Stene JK: In response. Anesth Analg 68:416, 1989
55. Woods AM, Lander CJ: Abolition of gagging and the hemodynamic response to awake laryngoscopy. Anesthesiology 67:A220, 1987
56. Hansen M, Poulsen MR, Bendixen DK, et al: Incidence of sinusitis in patients with nasotracheal intubation. Br J Anaesth 61:231, 1988
57. Sander JE, Lo W: Computed tomographic premedication in children. JAMA 249:2639, 1983

58. Mitchell AA, Louik C, Lacouture P, et al: Risks to children from computed tomographic scan premedication. JAMA 247:2385, 1982
59. Ornstein E, Matteo RS, Silverberg PA, et al: Chronic phenytoin therapy and non-depolarizing muscular blockade. Anesthesiology 63:A331, 1985
60. Wisoff JH, Berenstein A, Epstein, FJ: Vein of Galen aneurysms. Combined treatment of embolization and surgery. Presented at the Pediatric Neurosurgery Section, American Academy of Neurological Surgeons Meeting, December 1984
61. Junck L, Marshall WH: Neurotoxicity of radiological contrast agents. Ann Neurol 13:469, 1983
62. Rao CC, McNiece WL, Emhardt J: Modification of an anesthesia machine for use during magnetic resonance imaging. Anesthesiology 68:640, 1988
63. Boutros A, Pavlicek W: Anesthesia for magnetic resonance imaging. Anesth Analg 66:367, 1987
64. Glauber DT, Audenaert SM: Anesthesia for children undergoing craniospinal radiotherapy. Anesthesiology 67:801, 1987
65. Steiner L, Lindquist C, Steiner: Radiosurgery with focused gamma-beam irradiation in children. In Edwards MSB, Hoffman HJ (eds): Cerebral Vascular Disease in Children and Adolescents. Williams & Wilkins, Baltimore, 1989
66. Rorke LB, Schut L: Introductory survey of pediatric brain tumors. In Section of Pediatric Neurosurgery of the American Association of Neurological Surgeons (eds): Pediatric Neurosurgery. 2nd Ed. WB Saunders, Philadelphia, 1989 p 335
67. Bruno L, Schut, L, Bruce DA: Cerebellar astrocytoma. p. 367. In Section of Pediatric Neurosurgery of the American Association of Neurological Surgeons (eds): Pediatric Neurosurgery. Grune & Stratton, Orlando, FL, 1982
68. Osborn AG, Heaston DK, Wing SD: Diagnosis of ascending transtentorial herniation by cranial computed tomography. AJR 130:755, 1978
69. Swedlow DB: Anesthesia for neurosurgical procedures. p. 961. In Gregory GA (ed): Pediatric Anesthesia. 2nd Ed. Churchill Livingstone, New York, 1989
70. Eisenberg HM, Sarwar M: Ventriculographic features of ascending transtentorial herniation. Acta Neurochir (Wein) 42:225, 1978
71. Park TS, Broadous WC, Harris MM: Vacuum-stiffened bean-bag for cranial remodeling procedures in modified prone position. J Neurosurg 71:623, 1989
72. Young ML, Smith DS, Murtagh F, et al: Comparison of surgical and anesthetic complications in neurosurgical patients experiencing venous air embolism in the sitting position: Neurosurgery 18:157, 1986
73. Mayhew JF, Miner M, Katz J: Macroglossia in a 16 month child after a craniotomy. Anesthesiology 62:683, 1985
74. Standefer M, Bay JW, Trusso R: The sitting position in neurosurgery: A retrospective analysis of 488 cases. Neurosurgery 14:649, 1984
75. Albin MS, Carroll RG, Maroon JC: Clinical considerations concerning detection of venous air embolism. Neurosurgery 3:380, 1978
76. Cucchiara RF, Bowers B: Air embolism in children undergoing suboccipital craniotomy. Anesthesiology 57:338, 1982
77. Harris MM, Yeman TA, Davidson A, et al: Venous embolism during craniectomy in supine infants. Anesthesiology 67:816, 1987
78. English JB, Westenskow D, Hodges MR, et al: Comparison of venous air embolism monitoring methods in supine dogs. Anesthesiology 48:425, 1978
79. Gronert GA, Messick JM, Cucchiara RF, et al: Paradoxical air embolism from a patent foramen ovale. Anesthesiology 50:548, 1979
80. Zasslow MA, Pearl RG, Larson CP: PEEP does not affect left atrial-right atrial pressure differences in neurosurgical patients. Anesthesiology 68:760, 1988

81. Artru AA, Cucchiara RF, Messick JM: Cardiorespiratory and cranial-nerve sequelae of surgical procedures involving the posterior fossa. Anesthesiology 52:83, 1980

82. Drummond JC, Todd MM: Acute sinus arrhythmia during surgery in the fourth ventricle: An indicator of brain-stem irritation. Anesthesiology 60:232, 1984

83. Finucane BT, Brown RG, O'Brien MS: Anesthesia for craniofacial reconstructive surgery. Anesth Rev 7:39, 1980

84. Whitaker LA, Munro IR, Salyer KE, et al: Combined report of problems and complications in 793 craniofacial operations. Plast Reconstr Surg 64:198, 1979

85. Cote CJ, Liu LM, Szyfelbein SK, et al: Changes in serial platelet counts following massive blood transfusion in pediatric patients. Anesthesiology 62:197, 1985

86. Hewson JR, Neame PB, Kumar N, et al: Coagulopathy related to dilution and hypotension during massive transfusion. Crit Care Med 13:387, 1985

87. Cote CJ, Drop LJ, Hoaglin DC, et al: Ionized hypocalcemia after fresh frozen plasma administration to thermally injured children. Anesth Analg 67:152, 1988

88. Brown K, Bissonnette B, Poon AO: Hyperkalemia during paediatric craniofacial surgery. Can J Anaesth 36:S99, 1989

89. Shuper A, Merlob P, Grunebaum M, et al: The incidence of isolated craniosynostosis in the newborn infant. Am J Dis Child 139:85, 1985

90. Kearney RA, Rosales JK, Howes WJ: Craniosynostosis: An assessment of blood loss and transfusion practices. Can J Anaesth 36:473, 1989

91. Shillito J, Matson DD: Craniosynostosis: A review of 519 surgical patients. Pediatrics 41:829, 1968

92. Stein SC, Feldman JG, Freidlander M: Is myelomeningocele a disappearing disease? Pediatrics 69:511, 1982

93. Dierdorf SF, McNiece WL, Chalapathi CR, et al: Failure of succinylcholine to alter plasma potassium in children with myelomeningocele. Anesthesiology 64:272, 1986

94. Ishak BA, McLone D, Seleny FL: Intraoperative autonomic dysfunction associated with Arnold-Chiari malformation. Childs Brain 7:146, 1980

95. Oren J, Kelly DH, Todres ID, et al: Respiratory complications in patients with myelodysplasia and Arnold-Chiari malformation. Am J Dis Child 140:221, 1986

96. Park TS, Cail WS, Maggio WM, et al: Progressive spasticity and scoliosis in children with myelomeningocele. J Neurosurg 62:367, 1985

97. Park TS, Hoffman HJ, Hendrick EB: Experience with surgical decompression of the Arnold-Chiari malformation in young infants with myelomeningocele. Neurosurgery 13:147, 1983

98. Nehls DG, Carter LP: Air embolism through a ventriculoatrial shunt during posterior fossa operation: Case report. Neurosurgery 16:83, 1985

13

POSTOBSTRUCTIVE PULMONARY EDEMA

Raeford E. Brown, Jr.

Pulmonary edema has been reported for many years as an infrequent sequela of airway obstruction.[1] The true incidence of this phenomenon is unknown, although recent reports suggest that it may be relatively common.[2]

Pulmonary edema has been described after laryngospasm, epiglottis, croup, and hanging, and concurrent with chronic airway obstruction.[3-6] Most patients in these clinical settings are healthy, and there is no indication that superimposed medical disease is important in the etiology of this problem. Likewise, inappropriate fluid management has not been thought to be problematic in any case. The onset of pulmonary edema was usually noted on relief of airway obstruction, hence the name "postobstructive pulmonary edema." Occasionally, as in children with epiglottitis, clinical deterioration and diagnosis of pulmonary edema came minutes to hours after re-establishing the airway. Many episodes were suspected after the appearance of frothy, pink-tinged sputum from the endotracheal tube. In some children the condition was suspected on the basis of cough and tachypnea following an operative procedure in which intubation was difficult and associated with laryngospasm, obstruction, and hypoxia. Many patients present in the recovery room with low O_2 saturation as the only indication of difficulty. Some patients were noted to have radiologic signs or symptoms of respiratory distress. All patients in the cases reviewed responded well to conservative management and were discharged without further complications.

This chapter describes two episodes of our experience with postobstructive pulmonary edema. These case reports are compared with the experience of others. Possible mechanisms for the development of postobstructive pulmonary edema are reviewed, as well as approaches to its therapy and prevention.

363

CASE REPORTS

Case Report 1

A healthy, 65-kg, 17-year-old boy was admitted for repair of his left shoulder subsequent to multiple dislocations. His history and physical examination were unremarkable. No premedication was given. After an intravenous induction, the airway was maintained with ease and the patient was intubated after direct laryngoscopy with a 7-mm interior diameter endotracheal tube. Maintenance anesthesia was established with 70 percent nitrous oxide in oxygen and halothane. Morphine 3 mg was administered during the operative procedure in anticipation of postoperative pain. During 1 hour in the operating room, 1,500 ml of crystalloid was administered.

At the conclusion of the case, the patient was extubated while spontaneously breathing 1 percent halothane and oxygen. Within seconds the patient developed airway obstruction unresponsive to positive pressure, and had marked retraction during inspiratory efforts. After several minutes, succinylcholine 10 mg was given after a presumptive diagnosis of laryngospasm was made. Subsequently, the airway obstruction resolved, spontaneous ventilation resumed, and the patient was taken to the recovery room.

Initial vital signs in the recovery room were blood pressure 138/70, pulse 104, and respirations 22. Within 15 minutes of admission to the recovery room the patient was tachypneic and complained of shortness of breath. He developed a cough productive of blood-tinged sputum. A chest x-ray (Fig. 13-1) was obtained that revealed bilateral fluffy alveolar infiltrates, and a diagnosis of postobstructive pulmonary edema was made. Oxygen by mask

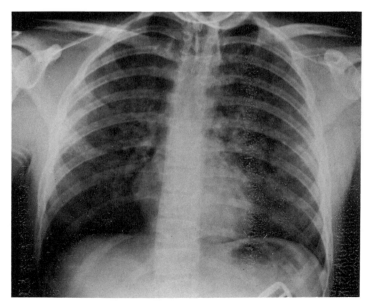

Fig. 13-1. Chest x-ray with findings consistent with pulmonary edema after airway obstruction.

was continued and furosemide was administered. The patient improved rapidly but was admitted to the surgical intensive care unit for overnight observation. He was discharged early the next morning in good condition. No sequelae were noted in a follow-up.

Case Report 2

A 5-year-old boy with Goldenhar syndrome was scheduled for ear surgery. Goldenhar syndrome, or oculoauriculovertebral syndrome, is characterized by malar hypoplasia, macrostomia, and micrognathia, as well as fusion of the cervical spine. In this case, endotracheal intubation was difficult. A number of techniques were attempted prior to successful intubation, all under deep general anesthesia with the patient breathing spontaneously. Fifty minutes were required to intubate this patient, and during that time multiple episodes of complete airway obstruction and hypoxia were encountered.

During the 2-hour surgical procedure, the patient was allowed to breath spontaneously. His vital signs were stable throughout the operative course with no evidence of respiratory compromise, and he was taken to the recovery room with an endotracheal tube in place. Shortly after his arrival, large amounts of pink, frothy secretions were suctioned from the endotracheal tube. A chest x-ray (Fig. 13-2) revealed bilateral infiltrates consistent with pulmonary edema. An arterial blood gas sample was drawn and revealed a PaO_2 of 55 mmHg and a $PaCO_2$ of 45 mmHg on room air. A presumptive diagnosis of postobstructive pulmonary edema was made on the basis of the clinical course, and the child was placed on continuous positive airway pressure (CPAP). Within 1 hour, his chest was clear and a repeat chest x-ray was obtained (Fig. 13-3). The child was extubated and observed

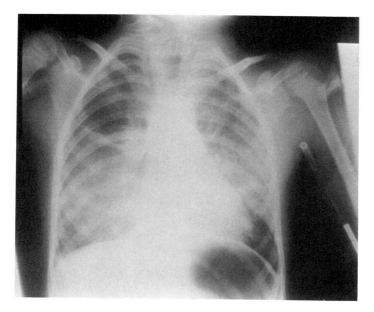

Fig. 13-2. Chest x-ray with bilateral infiltrates consistent with pulmonary edema after airway obstruction.

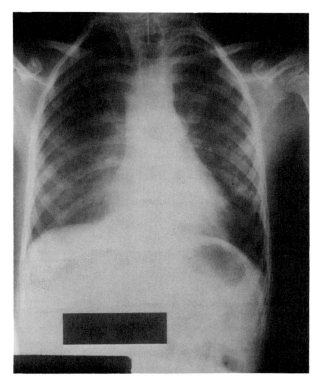

Fig. 13-3. Clearing chest x-ray obtained within 1 hour of application of endotracheal CPAP. Previous film had shown bilateral infiltrates consistent with pulmonary edema.

for 1 hour. He was returned to his room in stable condition. No postoperative sequelae were noted.

CASE REVIEWS

Case reports of pulmonary edema following airway obstruction in the pediatric, anesthesia, and pulmonary literature undoubtedly have increased because of heightened awareness of the problem. Oswalt et al.,[1] in 1977, were the first to associate pulmonary edema with acute airway obstruction, though others had previously entertained the possibility on theoretical grounds. They described three patients with obstruction secondary to laryngeal tumors, strangulation, and hanging. All of the patients developed pulmonary edema soon after the airway was re-established. Each patient was treated with steroids, diuretics, and positive-pressure ventilation. All recovered, although one patient was left with chronically reduced pulmonary compliance.

Cazanitis et al.[6] reported acute pulmonary edema due to laryngospasm in a 14-year-old undergoing simple mastectomy. Laryngospasm developed immediately on extubation, and the patient was reintubated. Pink secretions were immediately noted. This patient was treated with digoxin, furosemide, and naloxone, was subsequently extubated, and was observed overnight. His condition was satisfactory by the next morning.

Lee and Downes[2] described two cases of pulmonary edema following laryngospasm in children. The first case involved a 3-month-old male infant admitted for the repair of bilateral inguinal hernia. The infant was healthy at the time of surgery. An inhalational induction with nitrous oxide and halothane was unremarkable, and the patient was paralyzed with pancuronium and intubated. The surgical procedure and maintenance anesthesia were uncomplicated. Muscle relaxants were reversed at the end of the surgery. Subsequently the infant was able to flex his arms and legs and was believed to be awake. He was extubated and immediately developed laryngospasm. Cyanosis and bradycardia followed the unsuccessful attempts to ventilate with positive pressure. Succinylcholine was administered and adequate ventilation resumed. The trachea was reintubated and pink secretions were immediately noted. Following this, furosemide was given, a chest x-ray demonstrated a right middle lobe haze, and a blood gas sample on an FiO_2 of 1.0 revealed a PaO_2 of 201 mmHg and a $PaCO_2$ of 54 mmHg. The infant was subsequently treated with CPAP, observed overnight, and was discharged from the hospital on the second postoperative day.

In the second case reported by Lee and Downes, a 10-year-old boy was admitted for elective orchiopexy. The induction of anesthesia was uneventful and he was maintained with 70 percent nitrous oxide and halothane by mask. On awakening the patient developed severe laryngospasm that was unresponsive to positive-pressure ventilation. Succinylcholine was administered, followed by positive-pressure ventilation by mask. The child was intubated and pink secretions were suctioned from the endotracheal tube. He was subsequently managed with oxygen alone and rapidly improved. He was discharged from the hospital on the second postoperative day.

Soliman and Richter have reported several cases of pulmonary edema following epiglottitis.[4] In one case, a 19-month-old girl presented to the emergency room with an airway obstruction. She was intubated after an inhalational induction with halothane, and a diagnosis of epiglottitis was made. The child did well until transferred to the intensive care unit, where her condition deteriorated. Pink secretions were noted in her endotracheal tube and the findings on chest x-ray were consistent with pulmonary edema. The child was mechanically ventilated for 10 hours but had no other therapy. She was subsequently discharged from the hospital after an otherwise uneventful course.

In the adult literature, postobstructive pulmonary edema has been reported after strangulation, epiglottitis, laryngospasm, tracheal tear, arytenoid edema, and a malpositioned endotracheal tube.[7] In these adult patients, the time to onset ranged from less than 20 minutes to more than 6 hours after the initial insult. The time to resolution in these patients ranged from less than 6 hours to more than 36 hours, with a few isolated cases requiring 3 days for complete resolution of abnormal pulmonary compliance. As might have been expected in many of the adult patients, hemodynamic parameters were measured. In no

Table 13-1. Clinical Settings of Postobstructive Pulmonary Edema

Postlaryngospasm
Epiglottitis
Croup
Foreign body
Asthma
Chronic airway obstruction secondary to enlarged tonsils or adenoids

patient in whom intracardiac filling pressures were measured were these values found to be abnormal.

A review of these and similar cases leads us to believe that the presentation of pulmonary edema after airway obstruction is variable and that it may often be confused with other clinical entities such as aspiration pneumonia or fluid overload (Table 13-1). There are common features in these reports. In some earlier reports, pulmonary edema was first suggested by cyanosis and frothy secretions from a recently extubated patient who developed airway obstruction, usually from laryngospasm. In others, mild dyspnea and a cough, rales on auscultation, or an abnormal chest x-ray were suggestive of the diagnosis. In recent reports the diagnosis is suggested by an abnormal O_2 saturation discovered postoperatively or in the recovery room. In most cases, pulmonary edema was noted soon after or concurrent with re-establishment of the airway. In a few patients, such as those with epiglottitis, several hours passed after intubation before a diagnosis was made.

Although fluid overload is often considered to be one of the primary causes of postoperative pulmonary edema, there was no indication of inappropriate fluid management in any pediatric or adult case. Additionally, all but one of the patients in the cases reviewed were noted to have normal cardiac function. In the one patient a subendocardial infarction occurred subsequent to airway obstruction.[8]

HYPOXIA AND POSTOBSTRUCTIVE PULMONARY EDEMA

Recent work has brought to light the critical role that hypoxia plays in the production of pulmonary edema with airway obstruction. Hypoxia is considered to be the major etiologic factor in the development of postobstructive pulmonary edema. Fishman and others have suggested that hypoxia may incite regional or global vasoconstriction within the lung.[9] Constriction of pulmonary veins in response to hypoxia has been demonstrated. Reductions in pulmonary venous outflow during hypoxia favors transcapillary filtration, according to the Starling equation. In fact, Hansen et al. have demonstrated that lowering pleural pressure at a constant lung volume does not affect lung fluid balance, which suggests that edema formation subsequent to airway obstruction is the result of alveolar hypoxia.[10] In their studies in lambs, in which a graded resistance was applied to the airway, hypoxemia was prevented. These investigators note the previous demonstration of an increase in transvascular filtration of fluid in the lung subsequent to alveolar hypoxia alone[11] and speculate that hypoxia-induced increases in microvascular pressure may be an important determinant of pulmonary edema formation in syndromes of upper airway obstruction.

Lorch and Sahn have suggested a multifactorial mechanism for the production of postobstructive pulmonary edema.[12] In their view, negative intrathoracic pressure and hypoxia occur concurrently in this syndrome. During the course of the acute obstruction, negative intrathoracic pressure produces increased pulmonary blood volume and increased pulmonary arterial pressure, with subsequent transudation of fluid into pulmonary alveoli. Concurrently, hypoxemia produces pulmonary arterial constriction and pulmonary capillary damage, which increases capillary permeability and raises pulmonary arterial pressures. This produces subsequent transudation of fluid into alveoli.

DIFFERENTIAL DIAGNOSIS

The patient who presents with low O_2 saturation or cough, tachypnea, an abnormal chest x-ray, or an abnormal blood gas reading subsequent to airway obstruction may or may not have pulmonary edema. This clinical presentation, although strongly suggestive after acute airway obstruction, is consistent with several other entities.

Aspiration pneumonitis resulting from silent regurgitation after airway obstruction has been well described. These patients may present with dyspnea and an increasing oxygen requirement in the recovery room. The time course of the onset of symptoms depends on the severity of the aspiration. It may become manifest in a matter of minutes or may require several hours. The clinical course is usually more protracted and severe.

Primary pulmonary edema may present incidentally after mild airway obstruction, and may be unrelated to it. Fluid overload, the injection of naxolone,[13] heroin overdose, and exposure to high altitudes have been implicated in some reports. At particular risk for primary pulmonary edema with marginal airway management is the graduate of the neonatal intensive care unit, who often has a history of bronchopulmonary dysplasia.

Each of these conditions must be considered in the patient who appears to have pulmonary edema following an airway obstruction.

TREATMENT

A variety of therapies have been suggested for postobstructive pulmonary edema. Earlier reports suggested steroids, oxygen, ventilation with positive end-expiratory pressure (PEEP), aminophylline, and digoxin as treatments.[1] Most recent case reports suggest conservative management, as found in Table 13-2. Oxygen therapy sufficient to produce normal arterial oxygen levels may be all

Table 13-2. Treatment of Postobstructive Pulmonary Edema

1. Re-establish airway
2. Oxygen therapy
3. Positive pressure as needed
   a) Facial CPAP
   b) Endotracheal CPAP
   c) PEEP
4. Morphine 0.05 mg/kg as indicated for sedation. Titrate as needed.

that is required. Failing this, positive pressure in the form of facial or endotracheal CPAP or PEEP may be necessary.

Patients who develop pink, frothy sputum while intubated and subsequent to airway obstruction require immediate supportive therapy. Such therapy can often be adequately provided by attaching an anesthesia reservoir bag to the endotracheal tube while awaiting the results of chest x-ray and arterial blood gas measurement. Mild CPAP may be applied as a high FiO_2 is administered. Endotracheal suctioning should not be performed, since it will only intensify the outpouring of edema fluid while reducing functional residual capacity. Intravenous sedation in the form of morphine 0.05 mg/kg may be needed. Rarely, a diuretic such as furosemide 1 mg/kg may be helpful in individual patients. Drugs such as digoxin and steroids are not indicated when the pulmonary edema is secondary to airway obstruction. As has been previously noted in this clinical setting, filling pressures are not elevated. Myocardial dysfunction associated with this condition is transient if the heart was previously healthy. Digoxin has very little, if any, effect on a healthy heart. There is thus far no evidence that this syndrome is due to a cytotoxic mechanism that might be amenable to steroid therapy.

As the major differential is between aspiration and postobstructive pulmonary edema, several hours may be required to make a diagnosis. Even after a diagnosis is made, aspiration may respond in much the same way as primary or secondary edema. If the clinical condition improves and the chest is clear on auscultation and on chest x-ray, and if O_2 saturation permits, consideration should be given to extubation with close observation for several hours and perhaps overnight in an intensive care unit.

Needless to say, the best treatment for edema secondary to airway obstruction is prevention. Most reported cases of postobstructive pulmonary edema follow laryngospasm prior to intubation or after extubation. Laryngospasm can be avoided if the child is either sufficiently awake to have normal glottic reflexes or sufficiently anesthetized to suppress the response to foreign matter in and around the larynx. It has been suggested that the child with open eyes and mobile extremities is at low risk for the development of the laryngospasm at the time of extubation.[2] Although laryngospasm has been reported in the awake patient, this rule seems to apply in most cases. In those children with reactive airways or with copious secretions, such as in upper respiratory tract infection, the judicious use of drying agents such as glycopyrrolate, as well as lidocaine 1.5 mg/kg IV at the time of extubation, may prevent the development of laryngospasm. In the child who has developed laryngospasm, similar doses of intravenous lidocaine, given while administering positive-pressure (5 to 10 cmH_2O) oxygen by mask, may terminate the spasm. The total dose of lidocaine should be 3 mg/kg over a 5-minute period and 6 mg/kg over a 1-hour period. If laryngospasm continues, paralysis with succinylcholine and intubation and/ or ventilation are indicated before severe arterial desaturation occurs.

REFERENCES

1. Oswalt CE, Gates GA, Holmstrom MG: Pulmonary edema as a complication of acute airway obstruction. JAMA 238:1833, 1977
2. Lee KW, Downes JJ: Pulmonary edema secondary to laryngospasm in children. Anesthesiology 59:347, 1983
3. Travis KW, Todres ID, Shannon DC: Pulmonary edema associated with croup and epiglottitis. Pediatrics 59:695, 1977
4. Soliman MG, Richter P: Epiglottitis and pulmonary oedema in children. Can Anaesth Soc J 25:270, 1978
5. Luke MJ, Mehrizi A, Folger GM Jr, Rowe RD: Chronic nasopharyngeal obstruction as a cause of cardiomegaly, cor pulmonale, and pulmonary edema. Pediatrics 37:762, 1966
6. Cazanitis DA, Leijala M, Pasonen E, Zaki HA: Acute pulmonary oedema due to laryngeal spasm. Anaesthesia 37:1198, 1982
7. Willms D, Shure D: Pulmonary edema due to upper airway obstruction in adults. Chest 94:1090, 1988
8. Younker D, Meadors C, Coveler L: Postobstruction pulmonary edema. Chest 95:687, 1989
9. Fishman AP: Hypoxia on the pulmonary circulation: How and where it acts. Circ Res 38:221, 1976
10. Hansen TN, Gest AL, Landers S: Inspiratory airway obstruction does not affect lung fluid balance in lambs. J Appl Physiol 58(4):1314, 1985
11. Bressack MA, Bland RD: Alveolar hypoxia increases lung fluid filtration in unanesthetized newborn lambs. Circ Res 46:111, 1980
12. Lorch DG, Sahn AS: Post extubation pulmonary edema following anesthesia induced by upper airway obstruction. Are certain patients at increased risk? Chest 90:802, 1986
13. Prough DS, Roy R, Bumgarner J, Shannon G: Acute pulmonary edema in healthy teenagers following conservative doses of intravenous naloxone. Anesthesiology 60:485, 1984

14

ANESTHESIA FOR THE STEROID-DEPENDENT CHILD

Fred Koch

The anesthesiologist needs to understand the practical aspects of the physiology and pharmacology of the hypothalamic-pituitary-adrenal axis (HPA) in order to determine which children are or should be considered steroid dependent, and to develop an anesthetic management plan that specifically considers the need for steroid supplementation and supportive care. Unfortunately, the scientific underpinnings for this approach are not clear, and therefore recommendations and guidelines based on it cannot be rigid. The important clinical point is awareness of the potential problem and a therapeutic approach to its treatment. The patient who is or has recently been treated with suppressive doses of steroids is considered potentially steroid dependent, and may be at risk for developing varying degrees of adrenal insufficiency in the perioperative period. The anesthesiologist needs to know the suppressive doses of steroids, how long the HPA remains suppressed after cessation of therapy, and how to evaluate and manage these patients. The remainder of this discussion focuses on these issues.

BACKGROUND

The importance of the adrenal glands gained attention through Addison's work in the nineteenth century and became of further interest in the 1930s with the work of Selye. In this latter period, the importance of the adrenal cortex in allowing the organism to cope with "fight or flight" stress was particularly recognized. The role of adrenocorticotropic hormone (ACTH) as secreted by the anterior pituitary gland in stimulating the release of corticosteroids was also appreciated at this time.[1] The recognition in the early 1950s of the therapeutic role of glucocortical steroids in inflammatory and allergic conditions resulted in their widespread clinical use. Accompanying this usage were the first case reports implicating these drugs in intra- or postoperative cardiovascular collapse in patients who had been undergoing corticosteroid therapy, who did not respond to such maneuvers as volume replacement for hypotension, and who were ultimately found to have adrenal atrophy after death. These reports, coupled with the knowledge that exogenous corticosteroid use could indeed result in adrenal atrophy, led to concern among anesthesiologists that their patients currently or previously undergoing such therapy were at markedly increased risk when under operative stress.[2-6]

How real is this risk? That there is such an entity as adrenocortical insufficiency with an impaired stress response is not at issue here. Rather, the matter is to ascertain the risk that pertains for a specific patient currently or previously on a steroid regimen and about to undergo a surgical operation. The anesthesiologist must take into account a wide variety of variables, such as the type of corticosteroid, its dosage and regimen of administration, the nature of the initial clinical problem, and the interval since discontinuation of the drug in order to have a sense of the patient's steroid dependence. But melding all these factors together can be difficult, and results in a therapeutic approach more empiric than precise. As Christy put it: "The heterogeneity of patients, treatments, and testing methods precludes useful interpretation. Indeed, the literature might most charitably be described as a quagmire."[7]

Although adrenocortical extracts were first used to treat Addison's disease in the 1930s, it was soon discovered that many steroids could be isolated from these preparations. These corticosteroids have been classified into the two categories of mineralocorticoids and glucocorticoids, depending on whether their effect is predominantly but not exclusively that of sodium retention or liver glycogen deposition. Cortisol is the main glucocorticoid. The healthy adult male secretes about 25 mg/day in a circadian pattern, with the highest levels in the early morning hours and the lowest around midnight.[1] Cortisol as a glucocorticoid, aldosterone as a mineralocorticoid, and other androgens and estrogens are all biosynthesized in various layers of the adrenal gland from cholesterol as a common precursor. The corticosteroids are not stored but rather are synthesized and secreted on demand. Cortisol is more dependent on ACTH as a stimulus than is aldosterone, which is more responsive to renin from the kidney.[1]

When cortisol is released into the circulation, a high percentage—perhaps 95 percent—is bound to plasma proteins.[8] Particularly important in this regard are transcortin, a highly specific but relatively low-capacity binding agent for cortisol, and albumin, which is much less specific but has a greater potential binding capacity. Important to note is that synthetic analogues of cortisol do not bind well to transcortin, and hence may more completely diffuse into the tissues. Accordingly, the plasma half-life of these agents can be much shorter than the duration of their biologic effects. Because the major activity of cortisol derives from the 11β hydroxyl group, any synthetic analogue, such as prednisone, which is an 11-keto compound, must be converted within the liver in order to realize glucocorticoid activity.[8]

REGULATION OF ENDOGENOUS CORTICOSTEROIDS

The functional control of the adrenal cortex, and hence the release of cortisol, is by ACTH. This hormone is released continuously, also in a circadian pattern.[1] It is stored in the anterior pituitary gland as part of a larger precursor molecule, which includes amino acid sequences of some of the endogenous opioid peptides. When released in larger quantities due to stress, ACTH interacts with receptor sites in the adrenal cortex, giving rise to an increased generation of cyclic adenosine monophosphate and the initiation of the synthesis of cortisol and other corticosteroids from cholesterol. Relative to cortisol, ACTH has a much shorter plasma half-life, being quickly enzymatically degraded.[1] Though it is clear that ACTH plays an important role in the adrenal release of cortisol, the regulation of ACTH itself is less lucid. That the hypothalamus has so-called corticotropin releasing factor (CRF) became evident when extracts of hypothalamic tissue were found to promote pituitary ACTH release. However, the exact chemical nature of CRF remains unknown, and it may indeed be more than one compound. It also appears evident that blood corticosteroid levels play a role in regulating ACTH release via a negative feedback mechanism. Whether the primary influence of corticosteroid levels on ACTH release is via the hypothalamus or the pituitary gland remains debatable, and may depend on the degree of stress.[1]

EFFECTS OF CORTICOSTEROIDS

It appears that corticosteroids exert their effect throughout the body on a wide variety of metabolic pathways. They do so primarily via a superfamily of proteins, all of which regulate gene transcription. These receptor proteins display three characteristics. They have a domain for binding to the steroid ligand, another for binding to specific DNA sequences, and they thus modify the transcriptional activity of specific genes.

These receptors appear to be present in both the cytoplasm and nucleus, the distribution being dependent on the degree of steroid binding. They are labile, being sensitive to both heating and proteases. A present working model suggests a pair of receptor proteins combined with a so-called heat shock protein to form a receptor-protein complex. The heat shock protein may protect the DNA binding locus.

Hence, one mechanism is as follows. The steroid ligand enters the cell and binds to the steroid domains of a pair of receptor proteins. Binding of the steroid causes the heat shock protein to be released. This event allows the steroid-receptor complex to enter the nucleus and bind to the DNA. The receptor DNA domain binds to the double helix via two "zinc fingers," special structures that contain zinc molecules, cysteine, and histidine, and which correctly position the receptor protein in the major groove of the DNA double helix.

The manifestation of genomic activity in response to steroids can be categorized either as a quick response or as a response that occurs only after several hours. The quick response is not blocked by the inhibition of protein synthesis, as is the case with the slower response. Accordingly, the quick-responding genes appear to be producing proteins that regulate the activity of the slower-responding genes. Hence, while steroids may activate or deactivate many genes, they seem to do so only through the mediation of a few "trigger" genes of the first category.[9] This might explain how some mechanisms of steroid action may be more permissive than causal.[1] Cortisol, for instance, may enhance the efficacy of norepinephrine on the vasculature at the level of the arterioles, as well as stimulate β-receptor synthesis.[10–12]

EFFECTS OF ANESTHESIA ON CORTICOSTEROIDS

The increase in corticosteroid level occurring in response to anesthesia and surgery is but one of many endocrine changes. The plasma cortisol level can, depending on the anesthetic agent and its manner of use, rise after induction and stay elevated intra- and postoperatively. This increase is associated with increased levels of ACTH, and is also related to the magnitude of surgical stress. For the anesthesiologist, important considerations of this increase are the possible relationship between glucocorticoids and catecholamine synthesis and the cardiovascular responses to catecholamines. However, the relationships remain unclear, as the cortisol increase can be blocked in either peridural or high-dose narcotic anesthesia without there necessarily occurring an impaired cardiovascular response to stress. On the other hand, some have advocated that the most appropriate anesthetic technique would prevent the cortisol increase in response to operative stress.[13–15] This issue is far from being settled.

SUPPRESSION OF ADRENAL FUNCTION

Though impaired adrenal function has many etiologies, the anesthesiologist is most apt to encounter it as a secondary condition; at present, the use of exogenous corticosteroids is probably, via the HPA, the most common cause of suppression of the secretion of ACTH and the resultant adrenal cortical depression. Table 14-1 gives the various steroids and their dosages. Whatever its cause, the anesthesiologist confronting the patient with varying degrees of adrenocortical insufficiency may be contending with the problems of hyponatremia, hyperkalemia, hypovolemia, hypotension, weakness, and hypoglycemia. Thus, in addition to impaired cardiovascular reactivity, there may be changes in blood volume and composition. These conditions do not present themselves in a florid manner in most patients receiving corticosteroids. The most common dilemma facing the anesthesiologist is likely to be presented by the individual coming to surgery for a procedure unrelated to steroid usage as, for instance, the child undergoing intermittent steroid therapy for asthma who appears for a tonsillectomy and adenoidectomy. Hence, the most common question will frequently center on the risk and preoperative preparation of the patient who was or is undergoing exogenous steroid therapy. Other conditions that present problems

Table 14-1. Commonly Used Glucocorticoids

Duration of Action	Equivalent		
	Gluco-corticoid Potency	Gluco-corticoid Dose (mg)	Mineralo-corticoid Activity
Short-acting			
Hydrocortisone (cortisol)	1	20	Yes
Methylprednisolone	5	4	No
Prednisone	4	5	No
Long-acting			
Dexamethasone	30	0.75	No
Betamethasone	25	0.60	No

include rheumatoid disease, the nephrotic syndrome, inflammatory bowel disease, and steroid-treated malignancies.

When the problem of postoperative cardiovascular collapse in patients receiving steroids first gained attention, steroid therapy was empirically designed to provide as supplementation that dose of corticosteroid believed to be maximally secreted under extreme stress. However, the initial reports in the 1950s of cardiovascular collapse in patients undergoing steroid therapy implicated this class of drugs only circumstantially; no blood samples were taken for the measurement of cortisol levels during a given crisis; rather, adrenal atrophy would be found at autopsy. In fact, it was not until the early 1960s that perioperative hypotension in a patient receiving steroids was shown to be associated with low plasma cortisol levels.[16,17] This lack of a demonstrated association resulted in the belief among some that etiologies other than adrenocortical insufficiency might better explain many reports of perioperative collapse. This skepticism, coupled with studies demonstrating that the lack of increase in cortisol levels in response to operative stress did not necessarily correlate with the development of hypotension, lent credence to the notion that the incidence of such collapse was not as great as had been believed.[18,19]

SURGERY AND SERUM CORTISOL LEVELS

Addressing the issue of operative risk for patients receiving corticosteroids, Kehlet and Binder studied 104 patients (ages not given) taking prednisone or equivalent drugs (specific equivalents whose half-lives were not given) whose steroid treatment was stopped 36 hours before operation.[20] The daily dosage of prednisone or its equivalent was 5 to 80 mg for periods ranging from 2 weeks to over 10 years. Of these patients, 74 had "major surgery." Plasma corticosteroid samples were taken at intervals from the time of incision until 24 hours later in order to measure "stress response." The study is interesting for two reasons. First, hypotension (systolic pressure less than 80 mmHg) was observed in 18 of the 74 patients. Of these 18, 11 had hypotension ascribed to causes such as bleeding, sepsis, or anaphylactic reaction. The adrenocortical function was normal in 8 of the 11, and "only slightly impaired" in the other 3. "Slightly impaired" meant that an increase in the cortisol level was present, but not in the same degree as found for other patients not receiving steroids and undergoing operative stress.[19,21] The remaining 7 patients had hypotension without a readily evident explanation. Of these 7, 4 had normal and 3 had "only slightly impaired" adrenocortical function. The hypotension was reversed in all 18 either spontaneously or by treating presumed hypovolemia. Hence, although adrenocortical insufficiency could not be ruled out as a source of hypotension in 6 patients, it was deemed unlikely to be so because the hypotension was corrected without glucocorticoid administration. Second, and equally interesting, was the finding that 33 patients in this study who did not have hypotension had "relatively reduced" adrenocortical function as reflected by low serum cortisol levels. In brief, the presence of low plasma corticosteroid levels was not necessarily associated with hypotension. In the study as a whole, only 6 patients with "impaired" adrenocortical function had hypotension, but in all of these either there were other, more probable causes for the hypotension or it was corrected without steroid therapy. This study did not contend that hypotension secondary to adrenocortical insufficiency did not occur, but only that it was uncommon. And though the possibility of the tissue levels of prednisone or equivalent drugs being sufficient when plasma cortisol levels were low was not addressed, it was argued that the plasma level of cortisol was not a major determinant of blood pressure intra- or postoperatively in patients receiving corticosteroids. Hence, while a rise in the plasma cortisol level in response to surgical stress is indicative of an intact HPA, it does not follow that the lack of such a rise is necessarily associated with hypotension as a manifestation of adrenal inadequacy.

RECOVERY OF THE HPA AFTER CESSATION OF STEROID THERAPY

Although Kehlet and Binder[20] concluded that acute adrenal insufficiency must be rare in the context of steroid-treated patients going to surgery after the abrupt termination of such therapy, they did not contend that it never happens. Consequently, it remains useful to have a sense of when the HPA exhibits a biochemical manifestation of a return to normal function. For children, the study of Lightner et al. gives some guidance.[22] They noted that several investigators showed that patients who could respond to insulin-induced hypoglycemia with a normal cortisol increase displayed no manifestation of adrenal insufficiency during surgery. They also noted that a return of fasting morning cortisol levels to normal after the cessation of steroid therapy correlated well with the ability of the HPA to respond to insulin-induced hypoglycemic stress. They studied children who had been undergoing high-dose daily corticosteroid therapy for 1 month out of every 4 for acute leukemia. In all 13 children so studied, the morning serum cortisol concentrations returned to normal within 9 days of discontinuing prednisone. None of the children reportedly displayed signs or symptoms of adrenal insufficiency.

Morris and Jorgensen studied children given daily prednisone dosages sufficient to cause unmeasurable morning cortisol levels.[23] These children had previously been receiving daily steroids for asthma for periods from 6 months to 5 years. When entered into the study, all were given prednisone 10 to 15 mg daily for at least 1 month, and the daily dose was then tapered off in 2.5-mg increments every 10 to 14 days until the drug was completely stopped. Morris and Jorgensen found that the initial degree of HPA depression correlated with the size of the prednisone dose. Two to 4 weeks after the therapy was stopped, all of the children had plasma cortical responses to induced hypoglycemia that were similar to those of a control group who had not received steroid therapy for at least 1 year. Both these studies were notable in that the patients had a rapid return of the HPA to normal whether they had been on long-term or high-dose steroid therapy. Adrenocortical suppression was found even at low dosages of steroids, but a rapid return came despite prednisone being given in daily and sometimes divided dosages.

The studies cited above lend support to the notion that adrenocortical insufficiency during surgery is rare, and that in children at least, the return to normalcy of the HPA is more rapid than in adults. But it must be emphasized that while intraoperative adrenal insufficiency may be rare, one must not rush to the conclusion that it will never occur. Unfortunately there is no rapid, inexpensive, and unequivocal way to test the HPA. Thus, if the patient is thought to be steroid dependent, supplementation should be considered in the perioperative period.

STEROID SUPPLEMENTATION

What should be the manner of steroid supplementation? In a small study, Symreng et al. attempted to avoid some of the possible adverse effects of high-dose steroids, including decreased glucose tolerance, impaired wound healing, and greater susceptibility to infection.[24] Through a low-dose hydrocortisone substitution system proposed by Kehlet to mimic a normal adrenocortical stress response, patients taking preoperative corticosteroids were separated according to the responses of their HPA to a synthetic ACTH.[25] Those who responded normally underwent surgery without steroid coverage; those who did not respond received the hydrocortisone coverage. All of the groups studied, including the control group, did well, without exhibiting hypotension. Hence, if the practice of providing glucocorticoid coverage comparable to that in the normal stress response is adopted for children, the anesthesiologist might at least start by matching that amount of cortisol secreted daily (6.3 to 16.5 mg/m^2/day) with hydrocortisone or its equivalent.[26] For convenience, this is rounded off to 20 mg/m^2/day.

GUIDELINES FOR EVALUATING THE POTENTIALLY STEROID-DEPENDENT PATIENT

For the anesthesiologist faced with caring for the patient who is potentially steroid dependent and about to undergo surgery, the following thoughts and guidelines are offered until such time that we have a more precise understanding and the ability to delineate the HPA status of our patients.

Acute adrenal insufficiency intraoperatively is rare among patients receiving steroids preoperatively, even when they display a subnormal response to HPA provocation tests. Given the number of patients treated with supraphysiologic doses of steroids, adrenocortical insufficiency syndromes documented biochemically are rare.[27] No test exists to pinpoint the individual who will unequivocally need steroid supplementation intraoperatively. In general, the longer an individual has received steroids, the higher the dosages, and the shorter the interval between discontinuation of the drugs and surgery, the greater the probability that the HPA will be depressed. Alternate-day steroid coverage is no guarantee that HPA depression will not be present. Full-strength, sodium-containing intravenous solutions, such as lactated Ringer's solution or normal saline, can be given to prevent hypotension secondary to any ongoing sodium and volume deficit, which is one of the main consequences of mineralocorticoid insufficiency.

In the face of incomplete knowledge, then, what might be practical and prudent recommendations for perioperative management of the patient who is potentially steroid dependent? First, it must be determined which patients are potentially steroid dependent. There are two groups of patients to consider: those currently taking steroids, and those who have recently been taking steroids. The patient who is taking steroids up until the time of operation needs to have that same dosage regimen continued perioperatively for treatment of the underlying condition and to meet his or her basic steroid needs. The patient's usual morning dose can be given orally with a sip of water. If the child is unable to take later doses orally, then intravenous supplementation in a dose of 20 mg/m^2 of cortisone acetate every 6 to 8 hours is suggested. Excessive doses may be associated with sodium retention and hypertension.

The more nebulous condition occurs in the patient who has recently discontinued steroids. Since the studies cited above indicate that children regain their HPA function within 2 to 4 weeks, providing low-dose coverage during that period seems quite conservative. Beyond that time it seems reasonable not to administer steroids indiscriminately, but rather to remain watchful and treat only as warranted. If the anesthesiologist is nevertheless uncomfortable with recent steroid termination and yet is insistent on biochemical documentation of returned HPA function, perhaps the most practical way would be to obtain an early morning cortisol level along with an ACTH stimulation test.[28]

Perioperative cardiovascular collapse secondary to steroid-induced HPA suppression is a rare phenomenon. But because of the impracticality or inability to ascertain that it will not occur, it is common practice to give supplemental steroids. In effect, it is seeking to prevent the uncommon from occurring by medication with a high therapeutic index. This is treatment with a low cost:benefit ratio. Nevertheless, it is important that one not be conditioned to impugn too quickly a suppressed HPA axis for intraoperative hypotension but to look readily for other causes such as inadequate or inappropriate volume repletion with hypotonic solutions.

Perioperative fluid management is extremely important in these patients, as lack of mineralocorticoids will result in sodium loss, hyponatremia, and hypovolemia. For that reason, regardless of the type of surgery, full-strength saline or lactated Ringer's solution with appropriate amounts of glucose are the perioperative fluids of choice.

REFERENCES

1. Hodges JR: The hypothalamo-pituitary-adrenocortical system. Br J Anaesth 56:701, 1984
2. Lewis L, Robinson RF, Yee J, et al: Case report: Fatal adrenal cortical insufficiency precipitated by surgery during prolonged continuous cortisone treatment. Ann Intern Med 39:116, 1953
3. Salassa RM, Bennett WA, Keating FR Jr: Postoperative adrenal cortical insufficiency. JAMA 152:1509, 1953
4. Slaney G, Brooke BN: Postoperative collapse due to adrenal insufficiency following cortisone therapy. Lancet 1:1167, 1957
5. Bayliss RIS: Surgical collapse during and after corticosteroid therapy. Br Med J 2:935, 1958
6. Fraser CG, Preuss FS, Bigford WD: Adrenal atrophy and irreversible shock associated with cortisone therapy. JAMA 149:1542, 1952
7. Christy NP: HPA failure and glucocorticoid therapy. Hosp Pract 19:77, July 1984
8. Kehrl JH, Fauci AS: The clinical use of glucocorticoids. Ann Allergy 50:2, 1983
9. Harrison RW, Lippman SS: How steroid hormones work. Hosp Pract 24:63, 1989
10. Langer SZ, Hicks PE: Physiology of the sympathetic nerve ending. Br J Anaesth 56:689, 1984
11. Shapiro GG: Corticosteroids in the treatment of allergic disease: Principles and practice. Pediatr Clin North Am 30:955, 1983
12. Ellis EF: Corticosteroid regimens in pediatric practice. Hosp Pract 19:143, May 1984
13. Traynor C, Hall GM: Endocrine and metabolic changes during surgery: Anaesthetic implications. Br J Anaesth 53:153, 1981
14. Gordon NH, Scott DB, Percy Robb IW: Modification of plasma corticosteroid concentrations during and after surgery by epidural blockade. Br Med J 1:581, 1973
15. Engquist A, Brandt MR, Fernandes A, et al: The blocking effect of epidural analgesia on the adrenocortical and hyperglycemic responses to surgery. Acta Anaesthesiol Scand 21:330, 1977
16. Sampson PA, Brooke BM, Winstone NE: Biochemical confirmation of collapse due to adrenal failure. Lancet 1:1377, 1961
17. Sampson PA, Winstone NE, Brooke BM: Adrenal function in surgical patients after steroid therapy. Lancet 2:2322, 1962
18. Cope CL: The adrenal cortex in internal medicine: Part 1. Br Med J 2:847, 1966
19. Plumpton FS, Besser GM, Cole PV: Corticosteroid treatment and surgery. Anaesthesia 24:3, 1969
20. Kehlet H, Binder C: Adrenocortical function and clinical course during and after

surgery in unsupplemented glucocorticoid-treated patients. Br J Anaesth 45:1043, 1973

21. Kehlet H, Binder C, Engbak C: Imitation of the adreno-cortical response to surgery by intravenous infusion of synthetic human ACTH. Acta Endocrinol 72:75, 1973

22. Lightner ES, Johnson H, Corrigan JJ: Rapid adrenocortical recovery after short-term glucocorticoid therapy. Am J Dis Child 135:790, 1981

23. Morris HG, Jorgensen JR: Recovery of endogenous pituitary-adrenal function in corticosteroid-treated children. Pediatr Pharmacol Ther 79:480, 1971

24. Symreng T, Karlberg BE, Kagedal B, et al: Physiological cortisol substitution of long-term steroid-treated patients undergoing major surgery. Br J Anaesth 53:949, 1981

25. Kehlet H: A rational approach to dosage and preparation of parenteral glucocorticoid substitution therapy during surgical procedures. Acta Anaesthesiol Scand 19:260, 1975

26. Chamberlin P, Meyer WJ III: Management of pituitary-adrenal suppression secondary to corticosteroid therapy. Pediatrics 67:245, 1981

27. Truhan AP, Ahmed AR: Corticosteroids: A review with emphasis on complications of prolonged systemic therapy. Ann Allergy 62:375, 1989

28. Seale JP, Compton MR: Side-effects of corticosteroid agents. Med J Austral 144:139, 1986

15

MALIGNANT HYPERTHERMIA SYNDROME: IDENTIFICATION AND MANAGEMENT

Charles G. Durbin, Jr.

Since the report by Denborough and Lovell in 1960 of the occurrence of accelerated metabolism under anesthesia, the syndrome of malignant hyperthermia (MH) has been widely identified.[1] The original case involved a 21-year-old student with a fractured leg who was quite concerned with the risk of general anesthesia since 10 of his relatives had died under ether anesthesia. He was anesthetized with halothane and developed MH, but, fortunately, survived the episode. Since this case, the familial nature of this anesthetic-related disorder has become apparent, as has the high mortality rate when MH goes untreated.

Clinically, an episode of MH may be triggered by any of a large list of drugs (see Table 15-10), many of which are used in anesthesia. All of the potent volatile anesthetic vapors are known precipitating agents. Depolarizing muscle relaxants, especially in conjunction with volatile agents, are potent precipitating agents. There is also some weak evidence that the syndrome may occur spontaneously in susceptible individuals.

Patients who develop MH exhibit the signs of hypermetabolism, which include tachycardia, tachypnea, acidosis, and fever. Muscle rigidity may occur. The rise in temperature for which the syndrome is named is a late finding; and if the fever is not aggressively controlled it will lead to brain damage and death. Other findings are generalized or localized muscle rigidity and a rise in the serum creatine phosphokinase (CPK) and myoglobin concentrations.

The high mortality rate of the MH syndrome (at least 25 percent if untreated) and its nonspecific presenting findings have led to the search for a preoperative predictive test to identify patients at risk. Unfortunately, a reliable noninvasive screening test has not been found. A family history of an episode compatible with MH and a high degree of suspicion are the main ways of preoperatively identifying patients at risk for the syndrome. The confirmation of such susceptibility requires a muscle biopsy and in vitro halothane and caffeine contracture studies, which can only be performed reliably at a research center. The muscle must be tested within several hours of biopsy and thus the patient must be sent to the specialized center. Even with this invasive technique, however, the detection rate is only 90 percent, with false-positive and more significantly, false-negative results.[2] There is hope that new test methods (including genetic cloning) will improve the accuracy of preoperative diagnosis.

Malignant hyperthermia has been reported worldwide in both sexes and at all ages. Its incidence is not known, but it is estimated to occur in from 1 in 15,000 anesthetic administrations in children to 1 in 50,000 anesthetic administrations in adults. With increasing awareness and detection, this rate will probably increase.

There is a higher incidence of MH in children and young adults. Whether this is due to greater anesthetic exposure in children, associated muscular abnormalities, or a difference in susceptibility is not known. Some investigators believe that the frequency in children may be as high as 1 in 500 to 1 in 1,000 anesthetic administrations.

An investigation of the familial occurrence of MH (in the 1960s) suggested that susceptibility to this condition was inherited through an autosomal-dominant gene with incomplete penetrance and variable expression.[3] More recent research suggests that perhaps several genetic defects may lead to the syndrome of MH and thus more than one gene locus may be involved.[4,5] It is likely that there are different inheritance patterns in different families, and related members should be presumed at risk regardless of the assumed inheritance pattern. A family history of anesthetic difficulty or the presence of a muscle abnormality is found in approximately 30 percent of patients who develop MH.[6]

The specific cause of susceptibility to MH is not known but undoubtedly involves a defect in muscle calcium metabolism. Although most MH-susceptible persons and their families appear totally normal physically, muscular abnormalities may be associated with MH susceptibility. Many patients are described as having a "muscular" build, but claim to be weak or to fatigue easily. Muscle cramps and high fevers with viral syndromes have been reported in patients with MH. Ptosis, congenital hernias, and kyphoscoliosis may be present in a high number of susceptible patients.[7] Patients with muscular dystrophies may also have a higher incidence of MH susceptibility.[8] The diagnostic tests used to confirm MH susceptibility in some cases have been called into question, however, the risk of succinylcholine in this group is a significant problem.[9] A distinctive dysmorphic clinical picture, the King syndrome (or King-Denborough syndrome), is associated with MH reactions under anesthesia.[10] Children with this syndrome are short of stature, have pectus carnatum, kyphosis, undescended testicles, slowly progressive myopathy, and characteristic facies, with small chin, low-set ears, and antemongoloid palpebral fissures.

This chapter discusses the pathophysiology of MH, the perioperative treatment of a clinical episode of MH, the workup and treatment of families believed to be at risk for the syndrome, the anesthetic management of persons who are MH susceptible, and areas of controversy. A similar clinical syndrome occurs in several animal species. Investigation of the porcine stress syndrome (PSS) has provided a good deal of our current understanding of the pathophysiology and the management of the human MH syndrome.

In inbred strains of pig (Poland China, Pietrain) developed for large muscle mass, some individual animals develop a stress-induced condition (often when being loaded for market, during coitus, or during heat stress) in which the animal becomes spontaneously hot and rigid, and often dies. The meat has a boggy white appearance and is not suitable for market. A great deal of economic attention has been focused on this condition. Dantrolene was found to prevent this syndrome. These susceptible pigs also develop the syndrome on exposure to succinylcholine and anesthetic vapors. This animal model has been extensively studied and the similarity to human MH has led to much of what is believed to be true in humans. Many other animals, including horses, ponies, cats, and dogs, also have similar muscular syndromes.

The sympathetic nervous system is an important trigger and propagating component in the PSS, however, in humans, it is less involved. α-Stimulation causes the syndrome in pigs, and α-blockade prevents it. This is certainly not true in humans. Other differences also exist, and caution should be used in extrapolating findings from animal models directly to humans.

PATHOPHYSIOLOGY OF MALIGNANT HYPERTHERMIA

Many theories have been suggested to explain the cause of MH. Early investigators found that the elevated CPK in patients with episodes of MH primarily comprised the isoenzyme from the central nervous system (CPK-BB).[11] This suggested that MH was a neurologic disease. In pigs susceptible to PSS, activation of the sympathetic nervous system often precipitates the syndrome of MH. Sympathetic blockade (in pigs but not in humans) will ameliorate or prevent it. Later investigators, using better assay techniques, have failed to confirm this initial finding. The CPK in MH is from muscle (CPK-MM), and MH is a disorder of muscle metabolism in man and pig.

Routine and special fixation techniques have been used to microscopically examine biopsy samples from MH-susceptible muscles. Many abnormalities have been identified. These include "motheaten" fibers, an abnormal distribution of type I (fast) and type II (slow) fibers, an abnormally wide distribution of fiber diameters, the degeneration of fibers, and, occasionally, "central cores," which are muscle fibers with a round, clear (less dense) center. Electron microscopy has demonstrated Z-band slurring and other intracellular abnormalities in MH-susceptible muscles. None of the abnormalities seen in biopsy specimens represent a unique finding for MH; all are seen in other types of myopathies. That MH is a myopathy seems clear from the pathologic findings, but a unique pathologic change diagnostic of MH does not occur. A possible exception may be the occurrence of central cores. "Central core disease" is a recognized clinical entity with characteristic pathologic manifestations, which have been seen in a few patients with MH.[12] It is not clear whether central core disease is a form of

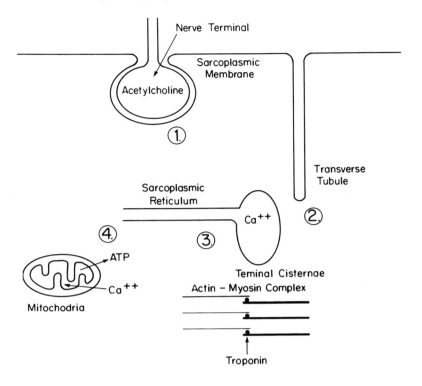

1. Depolarization
2. Excitation – Contraction Coupling
3. Calcium Release
4. Calcium Reuptake

Fig. 15-1. Schematic outline of normal muscle contraction and relaxation processes. See text for details.

MH, but patients with this diagnosis or whose biopsy specimens show central cores should be treated as being susceptible to MH.[13]

The abnormality in MH is within the muscle cell. The most widely accepted hypothesis is that the condition is a disorder of intracellular calcium regulation. To discuss the possible sites of this defect, a general review of normal muscle contraction is necessary.

The schematic representation in Figure 15-1 outlines the major components of the normal muscle contractile process. Several mechanisms have been identified that carefully regulate the intracellular free levels of calcium (Ca^{2+}). Ionized intracellular Ca^{2+} initiates and maintains muscle contraction. The primary storage site of Ca^{2+} in skeletal muscle are the terminal cisternae of the sarcoplasmic reticulum (SR). On nervous discharge the muscle endplate is depolarized (number 1 in Figure 15-1), primarily by acetylcholine binding to postjunctional receptors and opening sodium channels. The electrical depolarization wave is propagated through the sarcolemmal invaginations, termed *transverse tubules* (T-tubules), and then, through a not yet elucidated mechanism, causes the release of the stored Ca^{2+} from the terminal cisternae of the SR (numbers 2 and 3 in Figure 15-1). This process is termed *excitation-contraction coupling* (EC coupling).

As intracellular Ca^{2+} rises, changes in the configuration of several regulatory proteins occur. When the intracellular Ca^{2+} concentration rises from resting levels of about $10^{-6}M$, Ca^{2+} binding to troponin occurs. With this binding, a shape change of troponin occurs, and actin and myosin are free to interact. Adenosine triphosphate (ATP) is dephosphorylated, providing the energy to enable the short and long fibers to move. There is consequential shortening of the fiber bundles, and muscle contraction occurs.

Muscle relaxation is also a complicated process involving active Ca^{2+} transport. The SR is the primary organelle that actively sequesters Ca^{2+}, although in some circumstances mitochondria may also sequester the Ca^{2+} (number 3 and 4 in Figure 15-1). The sarcoplasmic Ca^{2+} concentration falls to its resting level and troponin returns to its inhibitory conformation. Both the normal contraction process and the relaxation process are energy dependent.

Undoubtedly, sarcoplasmic Ca^{2+} concentration remains elevated during an episode of MH. If high enough, this Ca^{2+} causes a sustained contraction called a *contracture*. A high sarcoplasmic Ca^{2+} causes the uncoupling of oxidative phosphorylation, thereby requiring muscle metabolic needs to be met by the inefficient glucose-to-lactate pathway. Large amounts of lactate are produced as the muscle cell uses ATP in an attempt to reduce the intracellular Ca^{2+} levels. The metabolic rate may rise 8- to 10-fold. Heat is produced as a by-product in the muscle and in the liver, where gluconeogenesis takes place and continued lactate metabolism occurs. A generalized stress reaction ensues, with elevations of epinephrine and norepinephrine, further increasing the metabolic rate and heat production.

The site of the defect in calcium regulation in MH-susceptible muscles has not been identified. Possible sites are listed in Table 15-1. It has been suggested that extracellular Ca^{2+} is the source of the Ca^{2+} elevation, and that an abnormally large Ca^{2+} flux across the cell membrane is responsible for elevating the

Table 15-1. Possible Sources of Elevated Sarcoplasmic Calcium in Malignant Hyperthermia

Site	Possible Defect
Extracellular	Increased sarcolemmic Ca^{2+} flux
Intracellular	
Terminal cisternae	Enhanced release of Ca^{2+}
Sarcoplasmic reticulum	Decreased reuptake Ca^{2+}
Excitation-contraction coupling	Enhanced release of Ca^{2+} from terminal cisternae
Mitochondrion	Decreased uptake of Ca^{2+} Uncoupling of oxidative phosphorylation
Membrane lipids	Multiple defects

sarcoplasmic Ca^{2+} levels. This abnormality would be of the so-called slow calcium channels. Halothane is known to increase this flux in normal as well as MH-susceptible muscles. Against this theory is the fact that even in a Ca^{2+}-free bath, halothane produces contractures in MH-susceptible muscle fibers. Also, slow calcium channel blockers have no therapeutic use in the management of clinical cases of MH (in humans), and in vitro do not effect caffeine-induced contractures in susceptible muscles; thus making the sarcolemmic Ca^{2+} channels an unlikely source of the defect.

The source of the sarcoplasmic Ca^{2+} in MH-susceptible muscles is the SR. A defect in uptake, release, or both could result in an elevated Ca^{2+} level. Early investigations with human and porcine muscle in vitro demonstrated that susceptible muscle was more sensitive to caffeine-induced contractures.[14] Caffeine and other methylxanthines are known to increase the release and to decrease the reuptake of Ca^{2+} from the SR in normal muscle preparations, and to cause contractures if present in a sufficiently high concentration. Muscle strips from MH-susceptible humans and pigs usually develop contractures at much lower concentrations of caffeine. This increased sensitivity to caffeine forms the basis for the in vitro diagnosis of MH.[15] It also suggests that perhaps the defect in MH muscle is the SR handling of Ca^{2+}, since similar contractures can be induced in normal muscle with higher doses of caffeine.

Using calcium-specific microelectrodes, Lopez et al. have shown that intracellular Ca^{2+} levels are abnormally high in MH susceptible muscle biopsies without triggering agents or caffeine.[16] This high resting level is antagonized by dantrolene. Other experiments on porcine tissues have shown an enhancement of calcium-induced calcium release in isolated SR vesicles.[17] The size of the calcium channel appears to be normal, however, its function appears abnormal.[18]

An abnormality of mitochondrial function has been suggested as the muscle defect in MH because a breakdown of oxidative metabolism occurs early in an MH episode and because at high levels of intracellular Ca^{2+} the mitochondria actively sequester Ca^{2+}. Microscopically, the mitochondrial morphology and number in MH muscle are normal. Isolated mitochondrial preparations from MH-susceptible muscles also appear to function normally, even in the presence of halothane, thus making the mitochondrion an unlikely location for the defect in MH.

A probable component of the defect in MH is the excitation-contraction (EC) coupling mechanism, which alters the handling of Ca^{2+} by the SR. Halothane is known to augment the increase in intracellular Ca^{2+} by affecting EC coupling, as well as having effects on the SR.[19] Caffeine also affects the EC coupling mechanism as well as the release and uptake of Ca^{2+} by the SR. Caffeine augments intracellular Ca^{2+} levels by this mechanism. The increased sensitivity of MH-susceptible muscles to caffeine is abolished by disrupting the T-tubule system, which underlies EC coupling.[20] Furthermore, drugs that decrease the effectiveness of EC coupling, such as dantrolene or procainamide, cause weakness in normal muscle and prevent contractures in MH-susceptible muscles. The fact that depolarizing agents can precipitate MH also lends support to this possible mechanism, since their effects should be primarily extracellular and on the EC coupling mechanism.

Recent experimental data have suggested that perhaps a generalized membrane defect, in lipid composition or function, is responsible for the variety of transport protein and channel function differences seen in MH-susceptible muscle. Inhibition of phospholipase A_2 diminishes the succinylcholine- and halothane-induced contractures in MH-susceptible human muscle biopsies. Treatment of normal fibers with lipolytic agents made them sensitive to halothane-induced contractures.[21] A defect in erythrocyte ATPase in MH-susceptible pigs supports a membrane defect and may lead to a simpler diagnostic and screening test for human MH.[22]

In summary, MH muscle experiences abnormal flux in sarcoplasmic Ca^{2+} concentration, probably due to defects in SR release and reuptake of Ca^{2+} in conjunction with EC coupling. This genetically determined abnormality may be in all cellular membranes and may be due to lipid composition or function. A further elevation of Ca^{2+} is triggered by anesthetic agents by their direct effect on the SR release and uptake of Ca^{2+}. In an attempt to reduce the sarcoplasmic Ca^{2+} concentration, active sequestration occurs, huge amounts ATP are consumed, and lactate is formed.

Muscle metabolism increases greatly, and contracture may occur. The mitochondrial Ca^{2+} levels rise, due to active sequestration, and oxidative phosphorylation is inhibited. Inefficient energy pathways are utilized to satisfy the metabolic demands of the muscle cell. As listed in Table 15-2, the sources of heat generation in MH are from these active processes in muscle. Gluconeogenesis and lactate metabolism in the liver also contribute to heat production. A generalized stress reaction ensues, with elevation of the levels of stress-related hormones. Heat-dissipating mechanisms (vasodilation and sweating) are abolished and temperature may rise further.

Cardiac dysrhythmias are a common early feature of MH. The cardiac dysrhythmias probably result from abnormal Ca^{2+} regulation in the myocardium, and are augmented by the hypermetabolic state. A primary functional abnormality of cardiac muscle is also possible. The metabolic demands during an MH crisis should be easily met by a normal cardiac system (as in athletes during periods of exercise), but with MH this does not occur. Whether this is due to a

Table 15-2. Sources of Heat Production and Failure of Cooling Mechanisms in Malignant Hyperthermia

Process	Location
Heat production	
Muscle contraction	Muscle
Muscle relaxation	Muscle
Lactate metabolism	Liver
Gluconeogenesis	Liver
Heat loss	
Vasodilation	Circulation
Sweating	Skin

cardiovascular abnormality or the effects of the anesthetic trigger agent is not known.

As energy sources are depleted, skeletal muscle cells leak their contents, causing increased CPK and myoglobin concentrations in the blood. This can result in renal failure. Cardiac arrest and cardiovascular collapse are the most dreaded events in an MH crisis. The ultimate outcome is related to the degree of hyperthermia and the severity of secondary complications.

That multiple biochemical abnormalities have been found in different MH-susceptible tissues and patients raises the interesting possibility that MH is a multifactorial disease. Some classic clinical episodes have had convincingly negative biopsy studies, lending support to this idea. There may be more than one genetic defect that may lead to the same common final pathway. This theory is supported by the varying inheritance patterns in pigs (and humans) as well. MH probably should be thought of as a syndrome of altered muscle calcium regulation rather than a specific disease. There are probably several different defects that can produce this frightening clinical picture. An implication of this hypothesis is that no specific test would ever be able to rule out the presence of susceptibility with certainty.

CLINICAL PRESENTATION OF MALIGNANT HYPERTHERMIA

Malignant hyperthermia may present as a fulminant, rapidly fatal crisis in which temperature elevation occurs as quickly as 1°C every 5 minutes, or as a more insidious increase in metabolic rate heralded by a gradual increase in the heart rate, PCO_2, and lactate. The usual signs are listed in Table 15-3. Successful treatment requires early detection, diagnosis, and prompt therapy. With the availability of intravenous dantrolene, which appears to be a specific treatment for MH, the mortality rate should be greatly reduced.

As shown in Table 15-3, the early signs of MH are nonspecific indicators of increased metabolism. Tachycardia with or without other dysrhythmias is present and occurs first in almost all episodes of MH. Tachypnea or, if the patient is paralyzed, a rise in the PCO_2 is also very common. When a patient makes an effort to breathe despite what is believed to be an adequate dosage of muscle relaxant, an arterial or venous blood gas measurement should be obtained to identify the cause of the stimulus to breathe and to monitor for the development of MH.

An effective alternative to blood gas analysis at this juncture is capnography.[23,24] With capnography an elevated end-tidal PCO_2 can be detected and machine-induced causes (such as rebreathing) can be diagnosed. For confirmation of the development of an MH crisis arterial (or venous) blood gas sampling is necessary. Mixed acidosis (respiratory and metabolic) is an early finding on blood sampling and should imply the occurrence of MH. A high PCO_2 and a low bicarbonate or large base deficit will be seen. Arterial hypoxemia is unusual but may be observed.

Table 15-3. Clinical Signs, Laboratory Findings, and Time Course in a Malignant Hyperthermic Crisis

Early clinical
    Tachycardia
    Tachypnea
    Muscle rigidity

Middle (established)
    Cardiac dysrhythmias
        Supraventricular tachycardias
        Ventricular dysrhythmias
    $\uparrow$ PCO_2
    $\downarrow$ HCO_3, $\uparrow$ base deficit
    $\downarrow$ PO_2
    Dark blood
    Mottled skin
    Hypertension
    $\uparrow$ Lactate

Late (undiagnosed)
    Fever
    Warm CO_2 absorber
    $\uparrow$ K^+
    $\uparrow$ CPK
    Myoglobinuria
    $\uparrow$ Ca^{2+}
    $\downarrow$ Mg^{2+}
    Seizures
    Renal failure
    Cadiovascular collapse
    Disseminated intravascular coagulopathy

Late signs of the hypermetabolic state include dark blood in the operating field, caused by venous desaturation and hypercarbia; skin mottling (hypercarbia); and a color change and warming of the CO_2-absorbent material as a by-product of processing the huge amount of CO_2 generated during an MH episode.

Localized (masseter spasm) or generalized muscle rigidity is often present. Careful studies in the porcine stress syndrome have shown that lactate production develops very early in the MH episode; increased CO_2 production follows rapidly, and somewhat later in the course, tachycardia and rigidity occur. Blood gas monitoring for the development of metabolic and respiratory acidosis is the best and earliest means of identification of developing MH, although capnography may help by indicating a developing problem with CO_2 removal.

The last and most grave sign of MH is a rise in body temperature. If this is undetected and untreated, the prognosis becomes poor. The relationship between temperature elevation and mortality is shown in Table 15-4, summarizing an analysis of 94 MH episodes by Britt and Kalow.[25] Although the worsening outcome with increased temperature may be related to delay in appropriate treatment, severe temperature elevation causes significant mortality itself.

The late consequences of MH include muscle necrosis, resulting in hyper-

Table 15-4. Relationship of Maximum Temperature During a Malignant Hyperthermic Crisis and Mortality

Maximum Temperature (°F)	Died	Survived	Total	Percent Survived
99.0–102.9	0	6	6	100
103.0–106.9	9	14	23	61
107.0–110.9	37	8	45	18
>111.0	5	1	6	17
Not specified	6	8	14	57
Total	57	37	94	36

Chi-square for significance of regression of survival on maximum temperature = 21.37.
$P < 0.000004$.
(From Britt et al.,[25] with permission.)

kalemia, and myoglobin release, which may cause renal failure. If the syndrome progresses to this degree CPK and aldolase levels are invariably massively elevated as well. The acidosis and hyperkalemia may lead to cardiac failure and worsening dysrhythmias. Clotting abnormalities, including disseminated intravascular coagulopathy, are often present in severe episodes.

Other clinical conditions that may mimic the hypermetabolic state of MH are thyroid storm and systemic sepsis; however, the metabolic abnormalities and their progression in MH are generally more severe than in either of these other two entities. The finding of an extremely elevated CPK may help differentiate these causes of hypermetabolism from MH, but this information will not be available during a critical episode.

For the successful treatment of MH, early detection of the syndrome is essential. Since the early signs are subtle and nonspecific, a high degree of suspicion and an aggressive, rapid interoperative workup are mandatory. The earliest diagnostic changes are seen in acid-base balance, therefore, blood gas analysis must be immediately (within 15 minutes) available in any setting in which general or major regional anesthesia is to be given. Once the diagnosis of MH is entertained, a prearranged treatment plan must be started immediately.

Occasionally, patients will develop rigidity after being given succinylcholine. This is an adverse reaction to the drug and may be a heralding sign for MH. The rigidity may be generalized or confined to the masseter muscles. Inability to open the mouth is common. This rigidity usually lasts for about 10 minutes, after which relaxation occurs. It may be more common if a potent agent is also being administered. Some experts believe that about 50 percent of patients who develop masseter muscle rigidity or spasm after being given succinylcholine will be MH susceptible.[26] How to proceed should masseter muscle rigidity occur is a matter of controversy, and is discussed in further detail in a later section of this chapter.

INTRAOPERATIVE DIAGNOSIS OF MALIGNANT HYPERTHERMIA CRISIS

Figure 15-2 outlines an intraoperative diagnostic protocol for working up a possible case of MH. If the usual causes of tachycardia (such as light levels of anesthesia and increased surgical stimulus) are ruled out, an arterial or venous

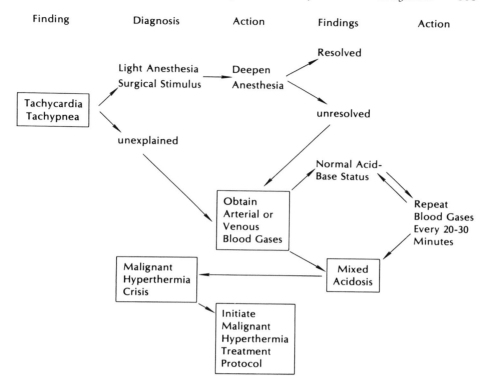

| Finding | Diagnosis | Action | Findings | Action |

Fig. 15-2. The intraoperative diagnosis of an MH crisis can be made by following this algorithm to evaluate a patient with the nonspecific findings of tachycardia and/or tachypnea.

blood gas analysis should be obtained. Since the arteriovenous difference in acid-base status is small, the pH, PCO_2, and base excess of either blood source can be appropriately interpreted. If capnography is used, a rise in end-tidal PCO_2 may indicate increased CO_2 production if alveolar ventilation is kept constant. This suspicion should lead to obtaining a blood sample for pH and metabolic evaluation. If a significant metabolic acidosis (base deficit greater than -8 mEq/L) is present or if a mixed acidosis is present despite confirmed adequate ventilation, MH is presumed to exist and therapy must be started.

If the arterial blood gas results are not abnormal but tachycardia or the dysrhythmia persists, end-tidal PCO_2 monitoring or frequent arterial blood gas measurements should be continued to watch for the development of MH. MH may develop at any point in the anesthetic course or even in the recovery room.

Since there is no reliable way to screen for the risk for the development of MH prior to administering an anesthetic, any anesthetizing area where agents known to precipitate MH are to be used must provide for rapid arterial blood gas analysis and the necessary drugs and equipment for treating MH. The requirements for an MH crisis are no different from those of a cardiac arrest: resuscitative equipment, a preformulated treatment plan, and people trained to respond must be readily available. Should MH occur in an anesthetizing location not associated with a hospital (e.g., an outpatient surgical center or dental office), a prior agreement with a hospital for expeditious transfer of the patient must be formalized and a transfer policy established. Treatment of MH must be initiated prior to transfer and continued uninterrupted during transport.

TREATMENT OF A MALIGNANT HYPERTHERMIA CRISIS

Once the intraoperative diagnosis of MH is entertained, a prearranged and practiced treatment protocol must be initiated. A suggested protocol is shown in Table 15-5. Of primary importance is discontinuing the precipitating agents and terminating the surgical procedure. This primarily means stopping the potent agents and succinylcholine. Hyperventilation with 100 percent O_2 and the use of an open system or changing any rubber parts in the breathing circuit along with high gas flow will help remove residual potent vapors. Changing the anesthetic machine to one that has not recently carried a potent agent has been suggested, however, this is costly, cumbersome, requires extra personnel, and should not be allowed to interrupt resuscitation or delay definitive pharmacologic treatment with dantrolene. Having a machine on "stand-by" for this purpose is not necessary.

Intravenous dantrolene is lifesaving and must be rapidly available to the op-

Table 15-5. Suggested Malignant Hyperthermia Treatment Protocol

Discontinue potent agents
    Change hoses
    High-flow oxygen (15 to 20 L/min)
Discontinue depolarizing agents
Hyperventilate
Get help
Mix dantrolene solution

Monitor core and peripheral temperature
Prepare to actively cool patient
Give dantrolene 2.4 mg/kg IV
Increase IV rate to increase urine output (2 to 3 ml/kg/hr); use iced lactated Ringer's solution if possible
Repeat dantrolene 1 mg/kg every 5 min until tachycardia, tachypnea resolve
If temperature is >39.5°C place ice packs on axillae and groins
If temperature is >41.5°C immerse patient in ice water, lavage stomach, body cavities, and rectum with iced saline
If temperature is >43°C consider cardiopulmonary bypass cooling
If ventricular ectopy persists, give lidocaine 1 mg/kg

Monitor central venous pressure, arterial blood gases (A-line), urinary output, and twitch tension
Send blood samples for clotting studies, platelet count, and fibrin split products, CPK, lactate, K^+, Mg^{2+}, Ca^{2+}, and PO_4^{-2}, and urine sample for myoglobin analysis
If K^+ >5.5, give 50% dextrose 1 ml/kg with regular insulin 0.1 U/kg
Induce diuresis with fluids, mannitol, or furosemide

Table 15-6. Relationship of Dantrolene Dose and Survival of Malignant Hyperthermia Episode

Dose of Dantrolene (mg/kg)	Number of Patients[a]	
	Died	Survived
<1.0	1	9
1.0–1.99	2	19
2.0–2.99	1	15
3.0–5.99	2	5
6.0–8.99	0	4
≥9.0	0	8

[a] Data include only patients receiving official formulation prior to cardiac arrest.

(From Britt,[27] with permission.)

erating room suite in a large enough quantity to start therapy (2.4 mg/kg). Once this is used, as much as 15 mg/kg (30 vials of lyophilized drug) must be easily accessible. Owing to solubility difficulties, dantrolene comes as a powder with mannitol and buffer, and must be mixed with sterile water immediately prior to use. As soon as the diagnosis is made, someone should start dissolving the dantrolene, since it may take 5 to 10 minutes to achieve solution. Rapid mixing devices may aid in this process.

Dantrolene given intravenously has been shown to completely reverse human MH if given in sufficient amounts and early enough in the course of the crisis.[27] In Tables 15-6 and 15-7 the relationship of mortality to dantrolene dose and maximum temperature are depicted. No patient receiving more than 6 mg/kg dantrolene died in the period of this study (1975 through 1981).

In this study population the maximum temperature (indirectly related to time in delay of treatment) decreased with the administration of dantrolene; and mortality at any specific peak temperature was less if dantrolene had been administered. If dantrolene is administered more than 12 hours after the development of MH or after a peak temperature of 43 degrees centigrade is reached, there is no improvement in the survival rate or quality of survival. Without dantrolene, the mortality in MH is high; with early detection and treatment with

Table 15-7. Relationship of Dantrolene Therapy, Maximum Temperature, and Survival of a Malignant Hyperthermia Episode

Dantrolene (mg/kg)	Number of Patients			
	Died		Survived	
	Yes	No	Yes	No
Max temp. (°C)				
≤37.9	1	0	53	7
38.0–39.9	10	2	104	3
40.0–41.9	19	4	72	17
42.0–43.9	29	1	26	6
≥44	4	0	0	0

(From Britt,[27] with permission.)

dantrolene, the mortality should be extremely low.[28] It must be remembered that in human studies of mortality, results may not be entirely reliable since the diagnosis of MH can only be made with reasonable certainty in survivors. Patients dying may do so due to causes other than MH.

In studies with pigs, no pig expired from MH, despite continuation of the precipitating agent, when dantrolene was given prior to the rise in temperature.[29] The metabolic changes abated in minutes, and the temperature increase was prevented. Thus, in pigs, dantrolene is completely protective even in the face of continuing precipitating agents. Although not tested in humans for ethical reasons, this is probably also true.

The initial treatment dose of intravenous dantrolene should be 2.4 mg/kg.[30] The muscular relaxant (and therapeutic) effects of dantrolene last 8 to 12 hours. Five to 10 minutes after the initial dose of dantrolene, incremental doses of 1 mg/kg should be given until the signs of hypermetabolism resolve. This usually will occur after the initial loading dose. Tachycardia and tachypnea should regress. Up to 16 mg/kg have been used clinically, however, if there is no improvement after 10 mg/kg a condition other than MH is probably present. Monitoring and dantrolene treatment should be continued for 24 to 72 hours, depending on the severity of the episode, since the recrudescence of MH has been reported as long as 24 hours after the initial episode.[31]

Dantrolene causes a decrease in muscle strength. A maximum 75 percent twitch-tension depression may occur in human peripheral muscle. By its effect on EC coupling,[32,33] dantrolene decreases the release of Ca^{2+} from the SR and increases Ca^{2+} reuptake. Patients receiving other nondepolarizing neuromuscular relaxants during anesthesia often require prolonged mechanical ventilation due to the synergistic effects of dantrolene.

Of equal importance with giving dantrolene is treating or preventing a lethal rise in body temperature, especially if diagnosis has been delayed. Provisions and a protocol for rapidly cooling a hyperthermic patient must be available in the operating suite. Cooling mattresses are not very efficient in a full-blown episode. Placing the patient in a plastic sheet filled with ice water is more efficient, and placing ice on the axillae and groin areas helps in cooling. Cold intravenous fluids may be given. Cardiopulmonary bypass has been used for rapid cooling,[34] but is available only in unusual circumstances. Care must be exercised to avoid hypothermia and its inherent complications.

Other measures are supportive and related to the secondary complications of the crisis. If the PCO_2 is elevated, vigorous hyperventilation should be established and maintained. Metabolic acidosis should be treated with sodium bicarbonate only if the arterial pH is less than 7.2. Invasive monitoring of urine output, central venous pressure, and arterial pressure (for repeated arterial blood gas determination) is indicated. If hyperkalemia occurs, treatment with insulin and glucose is indicated (1 ml/kg of 50 percent glucose solution with 0.1 unit regular insulin/kg over 10 to 30 minutes is a convenient and effective dosage). A fluid diuresis should be induced to prevent renal failure from myoglobinuria. This will also help treat any hyperkalemia that may be present. Alkalinization of the urine with a bicarbonate infusion will help clear myoglobin if this substance is identified in the urine.

The dantrolene preparation used in treating MH contains a significant amount of mannitol, and large amounts of a crystalloid solution may be needed to maintain intravascular volume and urine flow after the diuretic effects are manifested. Glucose-containing solutions should be avoided (except when treating hyperkalemia with insulin), as these have been shown to impair neurologic recovery after cerebral ischemia.[35]

Cardiac dysrhythmias usually clear with dantrolene, but if necessary, lidocaine can be used to treat them. Some suggest using procainamide, since it may decrease intracellular Ca^{2+} concentrations. A dosage of 10 mg/kg every 5 minutes up to a total of 0.1 g/kg and followed by 100 to 400 μg/kg/min can be used in the pediatric patient. Hypotension and widening of the QRS complex may occur with procainamide.

The use of lidocaine in MH has been controversial in the past but is now believed to be safe and effective for local anesthesia and treatment of cardiac dysrhythmias. Cardiac function may need to be supported with inotropic agents. Calcium administration probably should be avoided, as should digitalis preparations. Clotting abnormalities should be corrected with appropriate component replacement. Steroids probably have no effect on the syndrome and may increase infectious complications.[36]

Calcium channel-blocking agents have no specific role in the treatment of MH, since their sites of action are calcium channels in the extracellular membrane. Recent work suggests that dantrolene may also block these so-called slow channels.[37] The combination of dantrolene and the calcium channel blocker verapamil causes a synergistic depression of cardiac contractility.[38] Dantrolene has been shown to occasionally cause asystole when given as a bolus to hyperthermic swine.[39] Calcium channel blockers, therefore, should not be used to treat MH.

Once the syndrome is effectively controlled, continued monitoring for its recurrence is indicated.[31] Dantrolene should be continued for 24 to 72 hours, depending on the severity of the episode. A dose of 1 mg/kg IV should be given every 8 hours if the symptoms are controlled. With evidence of continuing dysfunction (tachycardia, tachypnea) this dose should be increased until symptoms are abolished.

With the availability of dantrolene and a low threshold for its use, patients known to be MH susceptible should be at low risk of death in the operating suite. The preoperative identification of unsuspected susceptible persons remains problematic.

DIAGNOSTIC WORKUP FOR SUSCEPTIBILITY TO MALIGNANT HYPERTHERMIA

With increased education, safe and versatile anesthetic agents, intravenous dantrolene, and availability of treatment carts for acute episodes, the risk to patients susceptible to MH is decreasing. For scientific study, social reasons, and

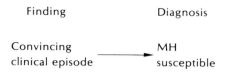

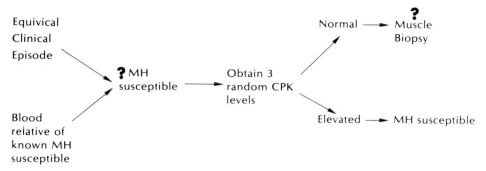

Fig. 15-3. MH susceptibility may be determined preoperatively, as illustrated in the above chart.

patient psychological needs, diagnostic studies, including muscle biopsy, may be indicated.

There are several ways in which patients may be diagnosed as being MH susceptible. These are illustrated in Figure 15-3. Patients who survive a convincing clinical episode are considered susceptible and require no further workup. If the episode is equivocal but the patient has been found to have an abnormally high CPK and no evidence of any other myopathy, he or she should be considered MH susceptible. Patients who have had an equivocal episode and normal CPKs on several determinations should be considered for referral to a diagnostic center for possible muscle biopsy studies. With rare exception, the results of invasive tests will not alter anesthetic management even if the results are considered negative. Biopsy results may help increase understanding of the disease of malignant hyperthermia, and a negative result may help alleviate some of the patient's fears. At this point a negative result cannot be interpreted to completely rule out the possibility of anesthetic difficulty.

Families of MH-susceptible patients report a higher than expected incidence of several medical conditions. MH-susceptible patients also report several findings more frequently than their unaffected relatives. The findings in Tables 15-8 and 15-9 should be sought when evaluating a person or family for MH susceptibility.[40]

The current standard diagnostic test for malignant hyperthermia is an in vitro halothane, caffeine, or halothane and caffeine contracture study.[41] This test must be performed on a properly obtained, rapidly tested leg muscle biopsy sample

Table 15-8. Abnormalities and Medical Illnesses Seen in Malignant Hyperthermia-Susceptible Patients

Personal History	Family History
Squint	Squint
Ptosis	Ptosis
Hernia	Hernia
Kyphoscoliosis	Kyphoscoliosis
Dislocated joints	Dislocated joints
Slipped disc	Slipped disc
Feet abnormalities	Feet abnormalities
Muscle, bone, and joint disease	Muscle, bone, and joint disease
Undescended testicle	Heart disease
Heart disease	Bleeding
Diabetes	Sudden death
Cramps	Congenital abnormalities
Muscle weakness	Sudden Infant Death Syndrome
Blackouts	
Temperature changes	
Anxiety	
Sports injury	

(From Smith,[40] with permission.)

Table 15-9. Factors Distinguishing a Malignant Hyperthermia-Positive Group of Patients From Other Patient Groups

Previous postoperative problems
    Fever
    Muscle swelling
    Muscle weakness

Personal history
    Squint
    Backache
    Heart disease
    Muscle cramps
    Muscle weakness
    Blackouts
    High fevers
    Febrile convulsions
    Anxiety
    Road accidents

Family history
    Squint
    Foot abnormality
    Muscle, bone, and joint disease
    Diabetes
    Bleeding
    Sudden Infant Death Syndrome
    Congenital abnormality

(From Smith,[40] with permission.)

using a standard testing protocol. A standardized protocol has recently been adopted by centers in North America.[42] The European Malignant Hyperthermia Group established a testing protocol in 1983 that includes a dynamic contracture study as well.[43] Other noninvasive tests, including CPK determinations,[44] a tourniquet test,[45] motor-unit counting,[46] and the ATP depletion test[47] have not proven reliable. Studies of white cells and platelets have shown conflicting results.[48] The results of diagnostic tests based on calcium uptake by the SR in frozen specimens have not correlated well with caffeine contracture studies and are no longer considered reliable.[49] Recent work with red cells has shown a defect in the plasma membrane of MH-susceptible patients.[50] Magnetic resonance imaging studies on the intact arm have shown promising results in diagnosing susceptibility as well.[51] As yet none of these tests can replace the caffeine-stimulated in vitro muscle biopsy study.

The difficulty with the caffeine contracture study is that it must be performed immediately on the biopsy specimen in a laboratory with considerable experience in the identification of normal and abnormal muscles. The differentiation between normal and MH-susceptible muscle is based on a quantitative difference in susceptibility to caffeine- or halothane- (or a combination of halothane and caffeine) induced contracture. The patient must travel to a center where this test is performed. An up-to-date list of active centers and patient referral is available through the Malignant Hyperthermia Association of the United States (MHAUS), Box 3231, Darien, CT 06820.

MHAUS functions as a professional and lay support group and information clearinghouse. In addition to the 24-hour hotline, they sponsor an annual patient-oriented conference. Patients should be referred to MHAUS for eduction through a newsletter (the Communicator), information and referral telephone service ((203) 655-3007), and 24-hour emergency medical information service (MH Hotline: (209) 634-4917). Membership is free, as are the periodic mailings of the newsletter.

Because of the uncertainty of inheritance patterns, all blood relatives of a person with a clinical history of MH or biopsy-proven MH should be considered susceptible unless biopsy has proven them normal. This is true even if they have had one or more uneventful episodes of anesthesia with known MH triggering agents.[52] Any relative with an elevated CPK is considered susceptible, and no further testing is required. Those with normal CPKs on three or more separate occasions require a biopsy to lower the possibility of susceptibility.

Another concern is in interpretation of the contracture test. At least four fascicles must be tested as often in susceptible patients several fascicles will test negative. Each laboratory establishes its own standards and determines positive and negative results. A contracture to 2 percent halothane alone is considered the most positive response. Unfortunately, only 20 percent of susceptible patients will have this result. The other positive response is a shift in sensitivity to caffeine or halothane and caffeine. With invasive testing false-negative results may occur in as many as 2 to 5 percent of the tests.[53]

Relatives of known MH-susceptible persons should be informed of their potential for anesthetic-related problems and should wear or carry a Medic Alert identification. They should be encouraged to join the Malignant Hyperthermia Association of the United States to increase their understanding of the disorder. Several excellent publications are available from MHAUS at a small charge. Patient information about MH is also available through the Muscular Dystrophy Association.

ANESTHESIA FOR PATIENTS SUSCEPTIBLE TO MALIGNANT HYPERTHERMIA

When a patient is identified as being MH susceptible, a careful approach to anesthesia should prevent MH from developing. While it is impossible to guarantee that an episode of MH will not develop, with the availability of intravenous dantrolene and a high degree of vigilance a good outcome should be anticipated.

The need for prophylactic pretreatment has been brought into question. In a large group of patients (956 patients), 93.7 percent of whom had general anesthesia for muscle biopsy without dantrolene pretreatment, there were no cases of intraoperative MH (643 positive biopsies).[54] In the recovery room four patients exhibited mild signs of MH, only two of whom required treatment with dantrolene. None of these patients was significantly affected.

With careful monitoring, dantrolene readily at hand, and nontriggering anesthetic agents, pretreatment of MH-susceptible surgical patients is unnecessary. This approach may be modified if the patient has had a previous aggressive MH course or is exhibiting signs of MH prior to induction, or the surgery is emergent or very stressful.

Precipitating agents of MH, especially the potent anesthetic vapors, must be avoided. Previously unused breathing hoses should be used. Preferably, MH-susceptible patients should be treated as the first cases of the day in the operating room so that no residual vapors remain from prior anesthetics. The gas machine should be flushed for 15 minutes with oxygen to remove any traces of vapors.[55]

When appropriate for the surgical procedure, regional anesthesia is probably the technique of choice for MH-susceptible patients. Local anesthetics of either type are acceptable. Lidocaine (an amide), once contraindicated, has been used in MH-susceptible patients without complication, and is now considered safe.

Patients should be relaxed and comfortable on arriving in the operating room. This can be achieved with premedication and a confident, reassuring approach by the anesthesiologist. Preoperative anticholinergics (e.g., atropine and glycopyrrolate) should be avoided, since they may cause tachycardia (thus masking the early signs of an MH episode) and reduce heat loss.

A list of safe agents for MH-susceptible patients is presented in Table 15-10. Nitrous oxide is safe or at least of very low triggering potential. Nondepolarizing muscle relaxants, especially pancuronium, have a good record. Pancuronium in vitro prevents caffeine-induced contractures in MH-susceptible muscles, but it may cause tachycardia and mask the development of clinical MH. The newer nondepolarizers, atracurium and vecuronium, are safe. Vecuronium may have

Table 15-10. Anesthetic Agents That Have Been Used Safely in Malignant Hyperthermia Susceptible Patients

Althesin	Muscle relaxants (nondepolarizing)
Anticholinergics	Pancuronium
Atropine	Metocurine
Ipratropium	Curare
Glycopyrrolate	Vecuronium
Barbiturates	Atracurium
Thiopental	Narcotics
Thiamylal	Morphine
Phenobarbital	Meperidine
Pentobarbital	Codeine
Methohexital	Fentanyl
Benzodiazepines	Sufentanil
Diazepam	Alfentanil
Lorazepam	Pentazocine
Midazolam	Nalbuphine
Dropiderol	Hydromorphone
Etomidate	Butorphanol
Ketamine	Nitrous oxide
Local anesthetics	Propofol
Lidocaine	Reversal agents
Procaine	Naltrexone
Tetracaine	Naloxone
Bupivacaine	Anticholinergics–anticholinesterases
Etidocaine	
Cocaine	

a slight advantage due to its similarity to pancuronium. Neither drug causes tachycardia sufficient to interfere with MH diagnosis.

Narcotics, including morphine, fentanyl, sufentanil, and alfentanil, are without triggering effects. Barbiturates (e.g., thiopental, methohexital) are safe, and may be used for premedication and induction. Etomidate is safe for induction but due to its depression of adrenal hormone release, it may be best avoided. Diazepam, midazolam, lorazepam, and droperidol are safe. Propofol does not cause MH in susceptible swine, and is probably safe in humans.

Ketamine is not a triggering agent but may cause tachycardia and rigidity, making the diagnosis of MH more difficult.[56] Anticholinesterase agents (e.g., neostigmine, edrophonium, and physostigmine) may be used safely to reverse neuromuscular blockade, and anticholinergic agents must be used carefully with them to prevent bradycardia. The dose should be adjusted downward.

The known MH-triggering drugs are listed in Table 15-11. All of the potent vapors have been associated with the triggering of MH, as has cyclopropane and diethyl ether. Depolarizing muscle relaxants are contraindicated, as they release Ca^{2+} from the SR. Chlorpromazine (Thorazine) should be avoided, as it may cause the uncoupling of oxidation phosphorylation and heat production.[57]

The anesthesia machine should not have been used with a potent agent just prior to use on an MH-susceptible patient. Using fresh hoses and flowing oxygen

Table 15-11. Anesthetic Agents Known to Precipitate a Malignant Hyperthermia Crisis

Potent vapors
    Halothane
    Enflurane
    Isoflurane
    Ether
    Methoxyflurane
    Trichloroethylene
    Sevoflurane
Cyclopropane
Depolarizing muscle relaxants
    Succinylcholine
    Decamethonium
Chlorpromazine

through the machine for 10 to 15 minutes is adequate to remove most of the potent agents. Triggering is really a dose-dependent issue rather than all-or-nothing situation. An open circuit bypasses the need to replace the CO_2 absorber canister.

With attention to preoperative preparation, a safe and acceptable anesthetic can be administered. A high index of suspicion and a low threshold for giving intravenous dantrolene will allow the anesthesiologist to confidently assure the patient of a safe anesthetic experience.

Psychological support of the patient and any potentially affected relatives is important. All blood relatives should be counseled to inform their anesthesiologists that they may be susceptible to MH. Medic Alert or other identifying information should be carried.

The counseling anesthesiologist must take time to explain that MH is not a "disease" but a condition that is usually only a problem in an anesthetic procedure. It is, however, potentially lethal. Education about the disease and open discussion with anesthesia caregivers are the best guarantee of a safe surgical experience in the future. All potentially MH-susceptible persons should be encouraged to become members of MHAUS.

Most of the fear of MH has come from practicing physicians and hospitals that have experienced fatalities from it. As information has become more widespread, safer anesthetic agents have been developed, and intravenous dantrolene has become available, this fear has become unfounded. If an anesthesiologist suspects MH susceptibility, it is possible to administer a nontriggering anesthetic, and likely that the early signs of MH will be correctly identified. Caring for known MH-susceptible patients should not evoke great fear if proper precautions are taken.

The possibility of MH occurring in a patient not known to be susceptible is real. Early suspicion, confirmation by blood gas measurement, and a rapid response are essential for patient survival in such a case.

CONTROVERSIAL ASPECTS
Masseter Muscle Rigidity

Occasionally, after the administration of succinylcholine to facilitate endotracheal intubation, difficulty in opening the mouth is encountered. This clinically significant but poorly defined occurrence has been termed *masseter muscle rigidity*, *masseter spasm*, or *trismus*. It may be due to anatomic abnormalities of the temporomandibular joint that were unrecognized prior to induction of anesthesia, the presence of a myopathy such as myotonic dystrophy, an adverse reaction to succinylcholine, or an extreme response of the normal effects of succinylcholine on masseter tone, or it may herald the development of MH. Considerable controversy exists regarding cause and appropriate response should this condition occur.

The first issue in dealing with MMR is definition. A mobile jaw that becomes "stiff" after succinylcholine must be observed. Often, difficulty in opening the mouth is encountered in patients with temporomandibular inflammation or arthritis or other intra- or extraoral pathology. This may not be apparent on casual examination and a history and examination of the upper airway should be carried out prior to anesthetic induction. Since this may be difficult to do in children, pre-existing conditions may be easily unrecognized in these patients.

In "true" MMR, relaxation occurs after 6 to 10 minutes and intubation is usually easily accomplished at that time. Maintenance of airway patency is usually adequate during MMR, and difficulty with the airway should not be confused with MMR. If adequate ventilation cannot be provided and light anesthesia has been administered, generalized increased muscle tone and struggling may occur as the short-acting relaxant wears off. This is not MMR. An inadequate dose of succinylcholine could produce the same effect.

In children receiving halothane and succinylcholine, Schwartz et al. reported an incidence of MMR of 1 percent.[58] If 50 percent of those with MMR are MH susceptible the incidence of MH in children would be 1 in 200. This is clearly not so. Children in this study may have had inadequate doses of succinylcholine, which, along with the effects of succinylcholine on jaw tone described below, may account for the high incidence of MMR. It has been demonstrated that children may require as much as 2 mg/kg and neonates as much as 3 mg/kg of succinylcholine to completely block neuromuscular transmission.[59] Probably the most common cause of MMR after succinylcholine is inadequate drug dose.

The effects of succinylcholine on jaw tone in normal subjects has recently been investigated. Van Der Spek et al. showed in a cat model that the amount of mouth opening produced by a standard force was reduced after a dose of succinylcholine adequate to provide complete twitch abolition in the limbs.[60] This effect compared to vecuronium persisted for 30 minutes. Applying the same method in two other studies in children, Van Der Spek et al. demonstrated the same findings in humans.[61,62] This reduced mouth opening was so profound in several cases as to pose difficulties with intubation. Increased tension (and hence reduced mouth opening) occurred in 87 percent of children, was profound in about 1 percent, and lasted for up to 10 minutes. This 1 percent incidence of

MMR is consistent with the findings of Schwartz et al. Potent anesthetic agents were continued in all these children and no evidence of MH was seen.

Smith et al. studied baseline tension and twitch tension during increasing blockade by incremental succinylcholine administration in masseter muscles and adductor pollicis muscles in 10 adult humans administered light isofluorane anesthesia.[63] They found that sensitivity was identical for both muscle groups. However, six patients developed significant increases in baseline masseter tone despite abolition of twitch. This effect was abolished at higher doses of succinylcholine.

MMR in children is commonly the result of succinylcholine on masseter muscle tone. Since children are relatively less sensitive to the relaxant effects of this drug, they exhibit an increased tone at the routine dosages. Treatment of this condition is to use a larger dose of succinylcholine.

In rare instances MMR may herald MH. To continue surgery, anesthetic techniques that do not precipitate MH should be used. These agents were described earlier in this chapter. The early signs of MH (tachycardia and tachypnea) should be watched for and periodic arterial blood gas analysis (every 10 to 30 minutes) must be obtained or capnographic monitoring initiated. If metabolic acidosis occurs, dantrolene should be given and the patient presumed to be MH susceptible.

If the anesthetic proceeds uneventfully, CPK and urine myoglobin levels should be obtained intraoperatively and postoperatively for at least 24 hours. A very high CPK level (greater than 20,000 IU/L) correlates with the presence of MH susceptibility.[64] If the CPK level is less than 20,000 IU/L, a muscle biopsy should be considered at a future time to ascertain MH susceptibility or the presence of other myopathy, such as muscular dystrophy or myotonia. The patient must be treated as susceptible in future anesthetic exposures unless the biopsy result is negative. In any event succinylcholine should be omitted from future anesthetic plans as rhabdomyolysis may occur and renal failure ensue.[65]

Outpatient Surgery for Malignant Hyperthermia-Susceptible Patients

Some have said that a patient susceptible to MH should not have surgical procedures performed in an outpatient facility. This is too rigid a standard. With proper monitoring and observation, a prearranged treatment protocol, adequate assistance, appropriate procedures and patient selection, adequate dantrolene, and blood gas measurement availability, a safe and cost-effective experience is probable. Although many centers will not wish to provide this degree of investment, outpatient surgery is not contraindicated in patients with MH susceptibility. Prophylactic treatment with dantrolene should not be used if the patient is to be sent home after the procedure. The patient should be monitored for several hours in the recovery area or admitted overnight to the hospital if any suspicion of an MH episode occurs.

Patients should remain close to the hospital for at least 24 hours and be told to contact the anesthesiologist immediately should any evidence of MH occur after leaving the facility. An agreement should be prearranged with an acute care hospital and appropriate personnel contacted when such a patient is to be treated. The patient should know whether to go to the emergency room or the outpatient facility if a concern arises.

Implications of Malignant Hyperthermia Susceptibility Outside the Operating Room

Because pigs with PSS develop MH to a variety of normal life stresses and often die without exposure to anesthetic agents, concern has been raised that patients may have a similar response. Some have suggested that MH-susceptible patients reduce physical activity and stress in their lives. They suggest no military service, no contact sports, no heat exposure, and reduction in exposure to stress situations. Although there are a few suggestive cases of unexpected death in families of MH-susceptible persons, it is unwarranted at this time to insist that MH-susceptible persons observe such activity restrictions.

Because caffeine and other methylxanthines are used to induce in vitro contracture in MH-susceptible muscles, some believe that patients known to be susceptible should avoid dietary caffeine for fear of triggering an MH episode. The use of aminophylline and theophylline for wheezing in these patients has also been questioned. In a theoretical analysis of therapeutic levels of caffeine and theophylline, Flewellen and Nelson concluded that dietary and therapeutic levels are safe.[66]

Some patients with MH experience skeletal muscle cramps, aches, pains, and spasms. Oral treatment with dantrolene has helped some but not all of these patients. If tried, a low dose (1 to 2 mg/kg PO) once daily should be used, but should be discontinued after several days to avoid complications.

Intraoperative Fever

Often the first time the anesthesiologist becomes concerned about the possibility of MH is when the patient's temperature begins to rise. The hypermetabolism of MH is only one (and the least common) cause of this finding. A differential diagnosis of fever is given in Table 15-12. Environmental warming (especially in children) is the most common cause of a rising temperature in the operating room when aggressive warming measures are taken. Infection, drug reactions, and febrile blood reactions are also common. Less common are hyperthyroid crisis and pheochromocytoma. Malignancy often is associated with fever. Pulmonary aspiration and atelectasis may be the cause of fever.

Fever is a late sign of MH. In the absence of other signs of hypermetabolism, fever is *never* the presenting finding in MH. Appropriate workup (described in detail earlier) includes blood gas analysis. Without increased CO_2 production and a base deficit fever is not due to MH. Other causes must be sought.

Table 15-12. Interoperative Causes of Temperature Elevation

Overzealous warming
Infection
Localized
Generalized sepsis
Drug reaction
Hyperthyroid storm
Pheochromocytoma
Blood transfusion reaction
Pulmonary aspiration
Atelectasis
MH

Other Uses of Dantrolene

There are several clinical syndromes in which dantrolene may be of some value. The first is a syndrome of hyperthermia that is induced with chronic antipsychotic medication. It occurs in a small group of psychiatric patients and is called the neuroleptic malignant syndrome (NMS). This syndrome has some similarities to MH in that it involves uncontrolled metabolism, muscle rigidity, elevated CPK, and hyperthermia, and often leads to death. It usually develops after long-term antipsychotic treatment, and may persist for days to weeks before the patient recovers or dies. There are several reports of dantrolene ameliorating this condition.[67] Whether the condition is a variant of MH is not known, however, in one study muscle biopsies in patients recovering from NMS had a high percentage of positive caffeine-induced contractures.[68] The most commonly held belief is that NMS is caused by central nervous system dopamine elevation. Bromocryptine has been more effective than dantrolene in this condition.[69]

Patients with heat stroke have been given dantrolene, with a variable response. It may be that MH-susceptible persons are also at an increased risk for heat stroke, and that those who respond to dantrolene are MH susceptible. This has not been proven.

Dantrolene has antiarrhythmic properties. This is probably due to calcium channel-blocking effects in the myocardium. These effects have not been investigated clinically, but may be useful in control of ischemia-induced ventricular dysrhythmias. The risk of myocardial depression discussed earlier must be kept in mind if dantrolene is used in conjunction with other calcium channel-blocking drugs.

REFERENCES

1. Denborough MA, Lovell RRH: Anaesthetic deaths in a family. Lancet 2:45, 1960
2. Gronert GA: Malignant hyperthermia. Anesthesiology 53:395, 1980
3. Britt BA, Locher WG, Kalow W: Hereditary aspects of malignant hyperthermia. Can Anaesth Soc J 16:89, 1969
4. Kelstrup J, Reske-Nielsen E, Haase J, et al: Malignant hyperthermia in a family: A

clinical and serological investigation of 139 members. Acta Anaesthesiol Scand 18:58, 1974

5. McPherson E, Taylor CA: The genetics of malignant hyperthermia: Evidence for heterogeneity. Am J Med Genet 11:273, 1982

6. Brownell AKW: Malignant hyperthermia: Relationship to other diseases. Br J Anaesth 60:303, 1988

7. Britt BA: Malignant hyperthermia: A pharmacogenetic disease of skeletal and cardiac muscle. N Engl J Med 290:1140, 1974

8. Brownell AKW, Paasuke RT, Elash A, et al: Malignant hyperthermia in Duchenne muscular dystrophy. Anesthesiology 58:180, 1983

9. Larsen UT, Juhl B, Hein-Sorensen O, de Fine Olivarius B: Complications during anaesthesia in patients with Duchenne's muscular dystrophy. Can J Anaesth 36:418, 1989

10. King JO, Denborough MA: Anesthetic-induced malignant hyperpyrexia in children. J Pediatr 83:37, 1973

11. Isaacs H: High serum creatine phosphokinase levels in asymptomatic members of the families of patients developing malignant hyperpyrexia—A genetic study. In Gordon RA, Britt BA, Kalow W (eds): International Symposium on Malignant Hyperthermia. Charles C Thomas, Springfield, IL, 1973

12. Schaib A, Paasuke RT, Brownell KW: Central core disease, clinical features in 13 patients. Medicine 66:389, 1987

13. Frank JP, Harati Y, Butler FJ, et al: Central core disease and malignant hyperthermia syndrome. Ann Neurol 7:11, 1980

14. Moulds RFW, Denborough MA: Biochemical basis of malignant hyperpyrexia. Br Med J 2:241, 1974

15. Nelson TE, Austin KL, Denborough MA: Screening for malignant hyperthermia. Br J Anaesth 29:169, 1977

16. Lopez JR, Alamo L, Caputo C, et al: Intracellular ionized calcium concentration in muscles from humans with malignant hyperthermia. Muscle Nerve 8:355, 1985

17. Mickelson JR, Ross JA, Reed BK, Louis CF: Enhanced Ca^{2+}-induced release by isolated sarcoplasmic reticulum vesicles from malignant hyperthermia susceptible pig muscle. Biochem Biophys Acta 862:318, 1986

18. Mikelson JR, Gallant EM, Litterer LA, et al: Abnormal sarcoplasmic reticulum ryanodine receptor in malignant hyperthermia. J Biol Chem 263:9310, 1988

19. Rosenberg H: Sites and mechanisms of action of halothane on skeletal muscle function in vitro. Anesthesiology 51:331, 1979

20. Rosenberg H, Hilf M: The importance of T-tubular function in the pathophysiology of malignant hyperthermia. Anesthesiology 59:A229, 1983

21. Fletcher JE, Rosenberg H: In vitro muscle contractures induced by halothane and suxamethonium. Br J Anaesth 58:1433, 1986

22. Thatte HS, Mickelson JR, Addis PB, Louis C: Erythrocyte membrane Atpase and calcium pumping activities in porcine malignant hyperthermia. Biochem Med Metabol Biol 38:355, 1987

23. Triner L, Sherman J: Potential value of expiratory carbon dioxide measurement in patients considered to be susceptible to malignant hyperthermia. Anesthesiology 55:482, 1981

24. Verburg, MP, Oerlemans FTJJ, van Bennekom CA,et al: In vitro induced changes in pigs. Physiological and biochemical changes and the influence of dantrolene sodium. Acta Anaesthesiol Scand 28:1, 1984

25. Britt BA, Locher WG, Kalow W: Malignant hyperthermia: A statistical review. Can Anaesth Soc J 17:301, 1970

26. Flewellen EH, Nelson TE: Halothane-succinylcholine induced masseter spasm: Indicative of malignant hyperthermia susceptibility? Anesth Analg 63:693, 1984
27. Britt BA: Dantrolene. Can Anaesth Soc J 31:61, 1984
28. Kolb ME, Horne ML, Martz R: Dantrolene in malignant hyperthermia. A multicenter study. Anesthesiology 56:254, 1982
29. Gronert GA, Milde JH, Theye RA: Dantrolene in porcine malignant hyperthermia. Anesthesiology 44:488, 1976
30. Flewellen EH, Nelson TE, Jones WP, et al: Dantrolene dose response in awake man: Implications for management of malignant hyperthermia. Anesthesiology 59:275, 1983
31. Matthew A: Recrudescence after survival of an initial episode of malignant hyperthermia. Anesthesiology 50:454, 1979
32. Cambell KP, Shamoo AE: Chloride-induced release of actively loaded calcium from light and heavy sarcoplasmic reticulum vesicles. J Membrane Biol 54:73, 1980
33. Morgan KG, Bryant SH: The mechanism of action of dantrolene sodium. J Pharmacol Exp Ther 201:138, 1977
34. Ryan JF, Donlon JV, Malt RA, et al: Cardio-pulmonary bypass in the treatment of malignant hyperthermia. N Engl J Med 290:1121, 1974
35. Lockwood AH, Bogue L, Yap E, et al: Increased glucose metabolism causes cerebral acidosis during hypoxia. Ann Neurol 20:155, 1986
36. Jasttemski M, Sutton-Tyrell K, Vaagenes P, et al: Glucocorticoid treatment does not improve neurological recovery following cardiac arrest. JAMA 262:3427, 1989
37. Salata J, Jalife J: Effects of dantrolene on the electrophysiological properties of canine Purkinje fibers. J Pharmacol Exp Ther 220:157, 1982
38. Lynch C III, Durbin GC, Fisher NA, et al: Effects of dantrolene and verapamil on atrioventricular conduction and cardiovascular performance in dogs. Anesth Analg 65:252, 1986
39. Rubin AS, Zablocki AD: Hyperkalemia, verapamil, and dantrolene. Anesthesiology 66:246, 1987
40. Smith RJ: Preoperative assessment of risk factors. Br J Anaesth 60:317, 1989
41. Rosenberg H, Reed S: In vitro contracture tests for susceptibility to malignant hyperthermia. Anesth Analg 62:415, 1983
42. Larch MG, for the North American Malignant Hyperthermia Group: Standardization of the caffeine halothane muscle contracture test. Anesth Analg 69:511, 1989
43. Ellis FR, Fletcher R, Halsall PM, et al: A protocol for the investigation of malignant hyperpyrexia (MH) susceptibility. Br J Anaesth 56:1267, 1984
44. Ellis FR: Evaluation of creatine phosphokinase in screening patients for malignant hyperthermia. Br Med J 3:511, 1975
45. Roberts JR, Ali HH, Ryan JF: A tourniquet test for malignant hyperthermia (abst). p. 67. In Proceedings of the International Anesthesia Research Society Annual Meeting, Hollywood, FL, 1979
46. Britt BA, McComas AJ, Endrenyi L, et al: Motor unit counting and the caffeine contracture test in malignant hyperthermia. Anesthesiology 47:490, 1977
47. Britt BA, Endrenyi L, Kalow W, et al: The adenosine triphosphate (ATP) depletion test: Comparison with the caffeine contracture test as a method of diagnosing malignant hyperthermia susceptibility. Can Anaesth Soc J 26:117, 1979
48. Rosenberg H, Fisher CA, Reed SB, et al: Platelet aggregation in patients susceptible to malignant hyperthermia. Anesthesiology 55:621, 1981
49. Nagarajan K, Fishbein WN, Muldoon SM, et al: Calcium uptake in frozen muscle biopsy sections compared with other predictors of malignant hyperthermia susceptibility. Anesthesiology 67:680, 1987

50. Ohnishi ST, Katagi H, Ohnishi T, et al: Detection of malignant hyperthermia susceptibility using a spin label technique on red blood cells. Br J Anaesth 61:565, 1988
51. Olgin J, Argov Z, Rosenberg H, et al: Non-invasive evaluation of malignant hyperthermia susceptibility with phosphorus nuclear magnetic resonance spectroscopy. Anesthesiology 68:507, 1988
52. Halsell PJ, Cain PA, Ellis FR: Retrospective analysis of anaesthetics received by patients before susceptibility to malignant hyperpyrexia was recognized. Br J Anaesth 51:949, 1979
53. Gallant EM, Rempel WE: Porcine malignant hyperthermia: False negatives in the halothane test. Am J Vet Res 48:488, 1987
54. Cunliffe M, Lerman J, Britt BA: Is prophylactic dantrolene indicated for patients undergoing elective surgery? Anesth Analg 66:s35, 1987
55. Beebe JJ, Sessler DI: Preparation of anesthesia machines for patients susceptible to malignant hyperthermia. Anesthesiology 69:395, 1988
56. Dershwithz M, Sreter FA, Ryan JF: Ketamine does not trigger malignant hyperthermia in susceptible swine. Anesth Analg 69:501, 1989
57. Rosenberg H: Malignant hyperthermia syndrome. Anesth Analg 56:466, 1977
58. Schwartz L, Rockoff MA, Koka BN: Masseter spasm with anesthesia: Incidence and implications. Anesthesiology 61:772, 1984
59. Meakin G, McKiernan EP, Morris P, Baker RD: Dose-response curves for suxamethonium in neonates, infants and children. Br J Anaesth 62:655, 1989
60. Van Der Spek AFL, Reynolds PI, Aston-Miller JA, et al: Differing effect of agonist and antagonist muscle relaxants on cat jaw muscles. Anesth Analg 69:76, 1989
61. Van Der Spek AFL, Fang WB, Ashton-Miller JA, et al: Increased masticatory muscle stiffness during limb muscle flaccidity associated with succinylcholine administration. Anesthesiology 69:11, 1988
62. Van Der Spek AFL, Fang WB, Ashton-Miller JA, et al: The effects of succinylcholine on mouth opening. Anesthesiology 67:459, 1987
63. Smith CE, Donati F, Bevan DR: Effects of succinylcholine at the masseter and adductor pollicis muscles in adults. Anesth Analg 69:158, 1989
64. Rosenberg H, Fletcher JE: Masseter muscle rigidity and malignant hyperthermia susceptibility. Anesth Analg 65:161, 1986
65. Miller ED, Sanders DB, Rowlingson JC, et al: Anesthesia-induced rhabdomyolysis in a patient with Duchenne's muscular dystrophy. Anesthesiology 48:146, 1978
66. Flewellen EH, Nelson TE: Is theophylline, aminophylline or caffeine (methylxanthines) contraindicated in malignant hyperthermia susceptible patients? Anesth Analg 62:115, 1983
67. Weinberg S, Twersky RS: Neuroleptic malignant syndrome. Anesth Analg 62:878, 1983
68. Caroff SN, Rosenberg H, Fletcher JE, et al: Malignant hyperthermia susceptibility in neuroleptic malignant syndrome. Anesthesiology 67:20, 1987
69. Levenson JL: Neuroleptic malignant syndrome. Am J Psychiatry 142:1137, 985

16

MISCELLANEOUS POTHOLES

Frederic A. Berry

There are many miscellaneous potholes that confront the anesthesiologist on a daily basis. Many of these occur in the postanesthesia care unit and in the ambulatory surgery unit. Therefore, this chapter primarily focuses on a discussion of these two areas.

THE POSTANESTHESIA CARE UNIT

The postanesthesia care unit (PACU) has several functions. It serves as (1) a general recovery room for patients undergoing routine surgery, (2) a short-term intensive care unit for postoperative patients with serious and, one would hope, transient problems (e.g., those with a spinal fusion who need airway and circulatory stabilization in the immediate postoperative period, before being discharged to the ward), and (3) an intensive care unit for the postoperative patient awaiting transfer to the regular intensive care unit. Many patients may need intensive care for several days postoperatively. Their postoperative response to anesthesia and surgery will determine whether they may return to the routine ward after short periods of observation or will require a longer period of intensive care nursing. An example of a patient who requires a longer period of intensive care is the child with velopharyngeal incompetence who has undergone the construction of pharyngeal flaps designed to improve speech. The airway problems of these children are anatomic narrowing and obstructive sleep apnea.[1,2] The genioglossal muscles normally pull the tongue forward, out of the oropharynx. The airway obstruction is thought to occur when there is a depression of genioglossal muscle tone due to sleep. This allows the negative pressure created by the child's inspiratory efforts to pull the tongue back into the pharyngeal airway, resulting in obstruction. In one reported case, a child with Treacher Collins syndrome who had velopharyngeal incompetence underwent a tympanoplasty and developed obstructive sleep apnea in the immediate postoperative period.[3] This precipitated the development of postobstructive pulmonary edema 40 minutes after the surgery. Obstructive sleep apnea is potentially fatal, and children at risk for it have to be monitored very carefully. It should always be kept in mind that the recovery room is an extension of the operating room.

Problems in the Postanesthesia Care Unit

The end of surgery does not mean the end of problems. For the purposes of discussion, problems in the PACU may be divided into three categories: (1) those of a pre-existing disease unrelated to surgery, (2) those of the disease or surgical condition necessitating the surgery, and (3) complications of anesthesia, surgery, or both.

A patient may present with pre-existing disease unrelated to surgery but which necessitates special awareness through the entire surgical period. An example of this is the premature nursery graduate with residual lung disease, apneic and bradycardic episodes, or both.

The second group comprises those in whom a disease or surgical condition necessitates surgery. This category consists mainly of trauma victims, who may present with contused lungs, pneumothoraces, head injuries, and so forth. Sometimes the extent of the lesion is not well known at the time of surgery, and the patient requires a period of observation in the recovery room before being triaged to the appropriate nursing unit. Other types of patients who fit into this category include those who need anesthesia and bronchoscopy for the removal of a foreign body or those with airway disease who require surgery on the airway. An example of such a disease is juvenile papillomatosis.

It is evident from this list of potential postanesthesia problems that the anesthesiologist must keep some basic concepts in mind when forming the anesthetic plan. The anesthetic plan includes the intraoperative management of the patient as well as the potential postoperative complications and the methods that can be used to minimize or avoid them.

At times there will be expected or unexpected complications, such as aspiration or obstruction with postobstructive pulmonary edema or traumatic croup. When this occurs the anesthesiologist should remain with the patient in the recovery room until the patient is stable and the recovery room team understands the problem and has a plan to manage it. This may necessitate a delay in starting the next case.

The remainder of this section discusses the problems with which the anesthesiologist is usually presented when summoned to the PACU. Each problem must be sorted out in a systematic, stepwise fashion. The first step is to examine the patient while listening to the history. Sometimes the cause of the problem will be evident from the history, and sometimes not. The condition of the patient can often be determined as the anesthesiologist approaches the bedside. A glance at the patient's appearance, the oximeter, the electrocardiogram, and the overall situation will often indicate to the anesthesiologist whether the problem is a severe one that requires cardiopulmonary resuscitation, or whether there is time for a more systematic evaluation. Most problems in the postoperative period are associated with the adequacy of the airway and with ventilation. The use of the oximeter in the PACU has led to an earlier appreciation of airway and ventilation problems as well as the effectiveness of therapeutic measures to treat them. The next step is to determine the patency of the airway as well as the degree of respiratory effort and ventilation. A history should be obtained from the PACU nurse to determine if there is an increasing or decreasing level of consciousness, a change in the respiratory pattern, or any other change. A review of the vital signs may provide information about whether or not the child has slowly been developing hypercarbia. If the diagnosis is not evident, various laboratory and radiographic information, such as a chest x-ray, arterial blood gases, hematocrit, and blood chemistries, should be obtained. The surgeon should be notified immediately if there is any significant problem with the patient.

The Obstructed Airway

The most frequent and earliest postanesthesia problem is that of the obstructed airway. The presenting signs include desaturation, stridor, retraction, lethargy, and unconsciousness. The problem may begin in the operating room, with laryngospasm, breathholding, and apnea, and continue into the immediate postoperative period. The reasons for upper airway obstruction include (1) traumatic edema, (2) a foreign body such as a sponge lodged in the airway, (3) secretions and blood, and (4) anesthetic depression of the airway and protective airway reflexes. If the problem is determined to be anesthetic depression of the airway and protective airway reflexes, the use of an oral or nasal airway along with proper positioning of the head will unobstruct the airway until the patient can awaken and recover the protective reflexes. The timing of extubation requires a great deal of clinical judgment, and even then endotracheal tubes may be left in too long, with a resulting coughing and traumatic croup, or may be removed too early, with resulting airway obstruction. At times a child will initially tolerate extubation well, but will experience airway obstruction after the stimulus of the surgery and the immediate postoperative period are diminished. At times the protective airway reflexes are incompletely recovered, resulting in episodes of apnea, laryngospasm, and coughing. This may or may not be associated with desaturation, depending on the degree of laryngospasm. The airway with incompletely recovered protective reflexes is a very difficult type of airway to manage, because as long as the airway is partially obstructed, the patient's ventilation will be impaired, which means that there will be delayed awakening and a prolonged period of marginal protection of the airway. The use of an oral airway in an attempt to remove the airway obstruction may precipitate more laryngospasm, apnea, and coughing. If the patient is identified as being in this transitional state of anesthesia, with incompletely recovered protective reflexes and the resultant laryngospasm, apnea, and inadequate ventilation, the administration of lidocaine 1.5 mg/kg IV, which will temporarily depress the protective reflexes, will allow the child to ventilate more effectively, thereby reducing the anesthetic level of inhalational agents and permitting control of the airway to be regained. There is a temporary deepening of the general anesthesia by the lidocaine, but after 5 to 10 minutes, the lidocaine will have only a minimal residual effect.

At times, however, the laryngospasm will persist, and may result in bradycardia and severe desaturation. At this point more active measures must be taken, such as ventilation with a bag and mask and the administration of succinylcholine 2 mg/kg IV. This will allow ventilation, reoxygenation, and evaluation of the patient. If a foreign body or blood and secretions are irritating the airway, the child should be laryngoscoped so that an appropriate diagnosis can be made. If the airway obstruction has been an ongoing problem, producing several episodes of hypoxia, the most conservative approach, after suctioning of the airway, would be to reintubate and leave the patient intubated until more awake and able to maintain the airway reflexes. This is a judgment call. The dose of lidocaine can be repeated twice in 5 minutes, but no more than 6 mg/kg of lidocaine (without epinephrine) should be administered in any 1-hour period.

Respiratory Distress

The main presentation of patients with respiratory distress is dyspnea, tachypnea, wheezing, or use of the accessory muscles of ventilation. They may have a persistent cough. The cough may be irritative or it may produce frothy or blood-tinged secretions. The major causes of the respiratory distress in such cases are pneumonia, aspiration pneumonitis, postobstructive pulmonary edema, pneumothorax, residual paralysis, or asthma. The evaluation of the patient depends on the history, physical examination, and appropriate laboratory and radiographic studies. If the patient is in severe respiratory distress, the initial priority is to support ventilation by increasing the FiO_2, ventilating with a bag and mask, and finally, establishing an endotracheal airway if indicated. If the child is stable, increasing the FiO_2 may provide sufficient supportive care while the evaluation is performed. The history may be positive for asthma, heart failure, or a previous respiratory infection. A rapid evaluation of the heart and lungs provides information about breath sounds, rales, wheezes, and other signs. A quick test of muscle strength will provide information about the possibility of neuromuscular blockade and whether or not adequate reversal of the effects of muscle relaxants has been accomplished. If the child is cooperative and awake, the head-lift test is a good method for determining residual weakness. Uncooperative children must be evaluated on the basis of their ability to sustain muscle movement. Jerky muscle movements indicate residual paralysis. The ability of an infant to sustain a knee lift is an indication that the infant has had a sufficient reversal of the effects of muscle relaxants. A nerve stimulator can be used in the unconscious or uncooperative patient. If residual weakness is present, it can be managed by further reversal, or if attempts at reversal are unsuccessful, by ventilatory support. Arterial blood gas and serum electrolyte measurements may reveal the causative factor or factors. Temperature monitoring will rapidly determine whether hypothermia is a factor. The child who is chronically ill with end-stage renal disease or any other severe systemic illness may need to be monitored intensively for several hours after having apparently returned to a normal state of neuromuscular activity.

If no obvious, rapidly treatable reason is found for the respiratory distress, a chest x-ray should be obtained to determine if the child has pneumonia, pulmonary edema, pneumothorax, or asthma. Arterial blood gas measurement will assist in determining the presence and degree of any respiratory failure and the child's metabolic status. Correlation of the history, fluid management, and cardiac evaluation will assist in the differentiation between the four major causes of pulmonary edema: aspiration, cardiac failure, obstruction, and fluid overload. The therapy depends on the cause. If an endotracheal tube is inserted, all of the conditions listed above will benefit from positive end-expiratory pressure (PEEP). Attempting to clear the secretions in this situation by suctioning will only make them worse. Diuretics and morphine are effective in reducing the preload of cardiac pulmonary edema, as well as that in fluid overload. Additionally, morphine will provide sedation during therapy in all cases of pulmonary edema. If the problem is cardiac, or the reason for the problem is not clear, intensified monitoring is indicated. If fluid balance is a problem, a Foley catheter should be inserted. If repeated blood gas measurements are required for management, an arterial line is quite helpful. A central venous pressure (CVP) line can help in estimating vascular volume and right heart performance when used in conjunction with other findings. Finally, if the cardiac output or left ventricular function is in question, a pulmonary artery catheter may be useful. In summary, respiratory distress must be aggressively diagnosed and treated in a stepwise manner in order to make an early diagnosis and thereby improve the outcome.

Postoperative Analgesia

A problem that infants and children often have when they come into the recovery room is postoperative pain (see Ch. 11). In very young children this can sometimes be very difficult to evaluate, but chronic irritability, crying, tachycardia, sweating, and other signs and symptoms are indicative of either pain or hypoxia. Use of the pulse oximeter and examination of the patient will usually reveal which of the two is the problem. If the problem is pain, I usually administer morphine 0.05 mg/kg for infants over 6 months of age and morphine 0.02 mg/kg if the patient is under 6 months of age. I prefer morphine over fentanyl because most of the pain that infants and children have is going to last for several hours, and morphine is a longer-acting narcotic. The argument is often given that outpatients should only be given fentanyl because it is short acting. My feeling is that the child doesn't know that he's an outpatient, nor does he care. The child's major concern is that he is in pain and needs relief. My major concern and obligation is to provide that relief. If the pain persists despite the first dose of narcotic, the same dose of morphine is repeated. It requires approximately 5 to 10 minutes for morphine to have a peak effect, therefore this much time must be allowed to pass between doses. If the child is particularly upset and the problem does not seem to be entirely that of pain, a small dose of valium (0.05 mg/kg) will often calm the child. The next step is to send the child back to the parents so that they may comfort the child, or have the parents come to the recovery room to be with their child. The latter is by far the best option, and is the routine in our ambulatory as well as inpatient recovery rooms. Our policy is that the parents are allowed to be with their child as soon as the child is awake and calling for them. Parents in the recovery room can greatly ease the burden on the PACU nurses as well as provide a much more satisfactory recovery from anesthesia for the child and a much more satisfying medical experience for the parents. In addition, it may allow the anesthesiologist to meet with the parents if they are present when the anesthesiologist comes to the recovery room between cases. This is particularly important in ambulatory surgery, where the anesthesiologist may not get to see the parents again on the day of surgery.

Delayed Awakening

There are a variety of reasons for delayed awakening after surgical anesthesia. The patient may have received an overdose of a central nervous system depressant such as a narcotic or barbiturate. Other causes of delayed awakening include ventilation-perfusion abnormalities, which slow the removal of volatile anesthetics from the pulmonary system and therefore from the CNS. Anything that interferes with ventilation, perfusion, or both has the potential for delaying the patient's awakening. Any of the causes of pulmonary edema can cause delayed awakening, owing to either hypoxia or the slow removal of volatile anesthetics. At times, although the dose of intraoperative narcotics may have been calculated to be appropriate for the child's age, the patient may be sensitive to the dose because the child is on the far end of the normal bell-shaped dose-response curve or because of an underlying medical illness. Children with renal disease have an increased sensitivity to narcotics. It is also important to recheck the nurse's notes to make sure that the dosage and type of premedication that was ordered was that which was administered. A careful physical examination will reveal any pulmonary problems. Blood gas measurements should be obtained to determine whether hypercarbia is initiating or compounding the depression caused by drugs. Monitoring the patient's temperature is important to ensure that hypothermia does not initiate or compound the problem, since a low temperature will depress ventilation and circulation. It is important to establish the cause for the delayed awakening in order to treat it appropriately. It is also important to decide if there is a problem before treatment is initiated. Delayed awakening is no problem if its cause is benign and the child is not in danger from an obstructed airway or other complication. It is better to allow the child to awaken slowly and steadily from a mild narcotic overdose than to administer a dose of naloxone and create a hyperactive, upset child who is in pain. On the other hand, if the child has delayed awakening and also has recurrent upper airway obstruction with desaturation, and the cause is believed to be a narcotic overdose, a small dose of naloxone (0.01 mg/kg IV) may reduce the airway obstruction, and with the resulting improved ventilation, recovery may occur more rapidly. If there is a response to naloxone but not an adequate reversal of the narcotic effect, the dose should be repeated and titrated to achieve the desired effect. Because of the relatively short action of intravenous naloxone compared to the long action of narcotics, the naloxone must also be given intramuscularly for sustained reversal of the narcotic effect. The intramuscular dose is the same as the total intravenous dose.

Nausea and Vomiting

The most frequent postoperative problem with general anesthesia is nausea and vomiting. Some patients never have it, some patients always have it, and many have it only occasionally. There are two main techniques to treat—or prevent—nausea and vomiting. The first is to administer a small dose of an antiemetic agent such as droperidol intraoperatively, for surgical procedures that are associated with a high incidence of nausea and vomiting (i.e., eye muscle surgery, middle ear surgery, and abdominal surgery). The dose that proved effective in one report of reduced vomiting after strabismus surgery in children is 75 μg/kg.[4,5] The children were divided into two groups, one receiving droperidol and the other a placebo. The incidence of vomiting was 43 percent in the droperidol-treated group and 85 percent in the placebo group. The children who received the droperidol did not have a delayed recovery from anesthesia.

The other technique for reducing the incidence and severity of nausea and vomiting is to keep patients NPO until they are ready to take oral fluids. This is the method I prefer. Patients are usually able to tolerate oral fluids when they are hungry. Hunger, in most patients, indicates a functioning intestinal system. Thirst is not a good indicator of the ability to tolerate fluids. It is difficult to tell whether infants and children up to the age of 2 to 3 are hungry or thirsty. In older children, however, hunger becomes a valuable indicator. Even after what is considered minor surgery, it may take 4 to 6 hours for children to become hungry after anesthesia. It is our procedure to start almost every patient on intravenous fluids and to administer sufficient fluids to supply the patient's replacement and maintenance needs. If the patient has recovered sufficiently from surgery to be able to protect the airway and meet all of the other criteria for discharge, I do not insist on his being able to take fluids before he can go home; the patient can go home and take small amounts of fluids only when hungry. My recommendation is to allow the child to have 1 to 2 ounces of fluid, wait approximately 15 to 20 minutes to see what happens, and then repeat that same amount of fluid if there is no difficulty. The fluid should be either a soft drink or clear fruit juice. The fluid intake is then increased as tolerated, and food is added as the fluid is tolerated. Giving fluids prematurely will often induce vomiting in a patient who would not otherwise have had it. Certain institutions require patients be able to take oral fluids before discharge. I do not agree with this philosophy. It should also be remembered that ice chips are fluids. Motion has been demonstrated to be a cause of nausea and vomiting. For this reason, we discourage early ambulation of patients following anesthesia and surgery. They should be kept as quiet as possible until they have recovered almost completely from the effects of anesthesia. There are institutions that require their ambulatory surgery patients to be able to ambulate before discharge. This may account for the high incidence of admission from certain ambulatory units because of nausea and vomiting.

Fluid Management

One of the frequent questions in the recovery room is what to do about the child who accidentally pulls out the IV and what to do if the child needs to have medications given on a regular basis or will be NPO. There is no question that in these situations the IV has to be restarted. If the child has had a long NPO period and very little fluid was administered, the IV may need to be restarted. In order to minimize the chance of this occurring, I administer generous amounts of fluid during surgery. (The guidelines for fluid maintenance are outlined in Chapter 4). I also administer generous amounts of fluids (15 to 25 ml/kg/hr) in the recovery room for the first hour or two, so that if the patient's IV does come out, sufficient fluid will have been given to tide the patient over until fluids can be taken orally.

Hypertension and Hypotension

The two major causes of hypotension in the recovery room are hypoxia and unrecognized fluid and blood loss. The initial supportive care for patients with hypotension consists of immediate assessment of ventilation while increasing the FiO_2 and ventilating the patient and immediate assessment of the circulation while increasing the vascular volume with a bolus of lactated Ringer's solution or saline (15 ml/kg in 20 minutes). The operative site or bandages must be quickly checked to see whether there has been excessive or unrecognized blood loss. If there is a question of volume loss, a hematocrit should be done.

The evaluation of hypertension is a bit more difficult. At times it is difficult to determine whether the hypertension is a recent development or a long-term problem. There are many causes of postoperative hypertension, and it is important for the clinician to have a list of the differential diagnoses for this condition so that the appropriate diagnostic and therapeutic steps can be taken. There have been no studies in children such as those in adults to evaluate the factors that could contribute to the development of postoperative hypertension. Gal and Cooperman reported a series of 60 patients among 1,844 consecutive recovery room admissions who were determined to have significant postoperative arterial hypertension.[6] Hypertension was defined as two consecutive arterial pressure readings with a systolic pressure in excess of 190 mmHg and a diastolic pressure of 100 mmHg. Sixty percent of these patients had a history of hypertension, and those who had complications attributable to hypertension came mainly from this group. Table 16-1 lists the factors that were believed possible to contribute to postoperative hypertension. When the patients with a history of hypertension were eliminated, the largest group by far had hypertension on the basis of pain. A surprising finding was that 17 percent of the patients had hypertension for which no cause could be found. It is obvious from the causes listed that a careful clinical evaluation of the patient is necessary. If the reason for the hypertension is not obvious, a blood gas analysis should be done

Table 16-1. Factors Possibly Contributing to Postoperative Hypertension in Adults

Factor	Present in Patients (%)
Pain	36
Emergence excitement	17
Reaction to endotracheal tube	15
Hypercarbia	15
Excess fluid administration	7
Hypothermia	7
Hypoxia	2
Hypertension by history	58
Uncertain	17

(From Gal and Cooperman,[6] with permission.)

to determine if hypercarbia is the cause for the hypertension. If the cause is still not found, a reevaluation must be performed at frequent intervals until either the hypertension disappears or the cause is found. I have not addressed the definition of hypertension in children. There are no studies to suggest what the guidelines for it should be. However, to pick an arbitrary number, any persistent systolic blood pressure that is 30 percent greater than the average blood pressure for the patient's age indicates the need for evaluation.

Disorientation and Agitation

A decrease in the use of scopolamine and a reduction in the dose of ketamine have markedly decreased the number of patients who are disoriented and agitated in the recovery room. However, the problem still exists. Scopolamine premedication was formerly responsible for disorientation in a significant number of patients. However, many institutions, including ours, have reduced the incidence of disorientation by virtually eliminating this drug as a premedication. Initially, ketamine was recommended in a dose of 7 to 10 mg/kg IM. Most clinicians have greatly modified this dose downward. At present, I use 3 mg/kg IM, and if further ketamine is to be used, I start an IV and administer the drug intravenously. Most patients who receive ketamine will also receive small doses of intravenous barbiturates or lidocaine. They will often have some mild postoperative nystagmus, but hallucinations and prolonged disorientation are unusual. There are still a small but significant number of children who do go through a period of disorientation and agitation as they are awakening from the effects of general anesthesia. The pulse oximeter will rule out hypoxia. If they have received no narcotic and appear agitated or disoriented, I administer morphine 0.05 mg/kg IV. At times, barbiturates, atropine, scopolamine, ketamine, valium, and midazolam have been reported to cause disorientation, agitation, or both. These are reports that physostigmine can reverse these effects. The dose is 0.5 mg, and can be repeated once. Parents are allowed to be with their child in the recovery room as soon as the child is sufficiently awake. Often the agitation will disappear when the parents arrive.

Postintubation or Traumatic Croup

The most frequently occurring type of croup familiar to anesthesiologists is postintubation croup. Postintubation croup in years gone by was a relatively frequent occurrence in the recovery room, but for unknown reasons in the past several years there has been an apparent decrease in the incidence of croup. However, some children do have a short episode of croup in the initial 30 to 60 minutes after extubation. Children who are most susceptible to developing croup are those between 1 and 4 years. For reasons that are not entirely clear, infants under 1 year[7] of age appear to be relatively resistant to the development of postintubation croup. Perhaps one of the reasons for the reduction in the incidence of postintubation croup has been the recommendation that there be an air leak of between 15 and 25 cmH$_2$O after intubation.[8] This test is performed by putting repressure on the rebreathing bag while listening with a stethoscope over the larynx to determine when the leak occurs. Table 16-2 gives the endotracheal tube dimensions for infants up to age 1 year. One formula for determining the tube size for children age 1 year and older is (16 + age)/4. If there is no leak, the endotracheal tube is removed and the next smaller size tube is introduced. Coughing with the endotracheal tube in place has been associated with postintubation croup. It is most difficult for the anesthesiologist to prevent coughing completely, since an attempt is made to have children very lightly anesthetized at the termination of surgery so that they can rapidly recover their protective airway reflexes. There is a fine line between the stimulation provided by the endotracheal tube and the resulting cough, and the ability to determine at which moment the tube should be removed so as to avoid such a problem while still accomplishing the objective of control of airway reflexes. The old concept of extubating patients while they were deeply anesthetized has largely become a minority view. Intravenous lidocaine has been used at the end of surgery to tide the patient over the irritable period after the anesthetic is discontinued and before it is time for extubation. The dose is 1.5 mg/kg, which can be repeated once within 5 minutes. Lidocaine is a general anesthetic, and depresses the protective reflexes while anesthetic gases are being eliminated and the protective reflexes regained. If the patient is extubated too early and coughs or has laryngospasm, the anesthesiologist is faced with a very difficult situation.

Table 16-2. Dimensions of Endotracheal Tubes[a]

Patient Age	Internal Diameter (ID) (mm)	Total Length (Oral) (cm)[b]	Distance to Mid-trachea (cm)
Premature (2 kg)	2.5	10–11	8
Full-term	3.0	11–12	9–10
6 months	3.5	14	10–11
12 months	4.0	14	11–12

[a] Average size for age. Occasionally one size 0.5-mm ID smaller or larger will be required in normal children.

[b] For nasal tubes, add 2 to 3 cm length.

Please refer to the discussion of the obstructed airway earlier in the chapter for the further management of these patients.

Clinical Course of Traumatic Croup

Traumatic croup usually appears within 30 to 60 minutes of the time of extubation. It takes a reasonable tidal ventilation to elicit the signs and symptoms that will occur with edema and the subsequent obstruction of the subglottic region. The current therapy for traumatic croup includes oxygen, steroids, racemic epinephrine, and sedation. The use of oxygen can cause an undesired response in some infants or children, depending on their state of cooperation. A child who is in no pain, is comfortable, and is not frightened will often accept a face mask with oxygen. However, if the child is in pain, is not fully awake, is upset, or is having other difficulty, attempts at placing a face mask with oxygen may make matters much worse. At this time, the judicious use of intravenous sedation or analgesia may well calm the child and decrease the severity of the croup as well as allowing oxygen to be administered. The child who is having pain should be given a small dose of morphine (0.05 mg/kg IV). In addition to the analgesia, the morphine will also sedate the child, and this may well accomplish the desired objectives. If, on the other hand, the child is moderately depressed from a narcotic, reversing the narcotic will sometimes awaken the child and the croup may disappear. Narcotics are the drugs that can be reversed most successfully, and a small intravenous dose of naloxone should be given if it is thought that narcotics are the cause of the problem. The initial dose is 0.01 mg/kg IV. Unfortunately, the age at which traumatic croup develops is also the age at which cooperation is at its low point. The presence of the parents can often calm a child like nothing else. When possible, it would seem wise to allow the parents to be with their child during this period.

Steroids have proven to be of considerable value in the treatment of infectious croup, but there are no studies of their value in traumatic croup.[9] Most clinicians have had occasional success with steroids in traumatic croup. Since there is little harm with a few doses, I administer steroids if the croup symptoms are increasing or if the croup persists for longer than 30 minutes with the child at rest. The important point to remember is that the dosage must be adequate. The dose of dexamethasone is 0.5 to 1 mg/kg. If improvement is going to occur, it will do so within 30 to 60 minutes. If necessary, the dosage can be repeated within 4 to 6 hours.

The most rapid mode of therapy is administration of racemic epinephrine.[10] This is a mixture of levo- and dextro-epinephrine. The levo form is the active component. The drug is diluted with water or saline in an 8:1 ratio and administered by any method that will nebulize the mixture. The mechanism of action of the racemic epinephrine is vasoconstriction of the edematous tissue. Racemic epinephrine will last for approximately 1 hour, after which the effects will dissipate. In cases of subglottic edema, there is a concern for rebound. Racemic epinephrine can be repeated every 1 to 2 hours as needed. It is rare for a child with traumatic croup to need reintubation. However, the patient's basic disease may be some form of tracheal stenosis or subglottic stenosis, which, when coupled with the trauma of intubation or instrumentation, may cause edema and resultant further narrowing of the subglottic area, making the conservative methods of therapy listed above ineffective and possibly necessitating reintubation and sometimes tracheotomy.

Criteria for Discharge After Croup

After the development of traumatic croup, the question that arises is when can the child be released from the recovery room or ambulatory care unit, or, if the symptoms continue, when should the child be admitted to a hospital. A child that is symptomatic at rest (i.e., has retractions, tachypnea, and stridor) should either remain in the recovery room or be admitted to an intensive care unit for further care. If, on the other hand, the child is asymptomatic while at rest and develops symptoms only when crying or agitated, he can be returned to the hospital ward or can be discharged home from the ambulatory care unit. However, there must be a period of observation of at least 2 hours after the last dose of racemic epinephrine. If there is doubt, the child should be admitted.

THE AMBULATORY SURGERY UNIT

There is an enormous movement toward ambulatory surgery, which is being led by the insurance companies. This is somewhat of a paradox, since 20 years ago these very same insurance companies would not cover surgery done on an ambulatory basis. How times change!

There are many advantages as well as disadvantages to ambulatory surgery. The advantages are well documented, and have been emphasized and publicized. The disadvantages receive scant attention. There are four major disadvantages: (1) insufficient time to develop rapport with the patient; (2) insufficient time for patient evaluation; (3) potentially uncontrolled and unknown access to food; and (4) a reliance on the family or friends to identify postoperative complications and seek medical help. Most parents and older children are aware of the implications of being NPO. This is usually not a problem with the infant under 1 to 2 years unless the siblings are tired of hearing their brother or sister cry and give them food. It may become a problem as children get older. They understand that they are to have nothing to eat or drink, but still do not understand the reasons. Therefore, the occasional child will sneak food. In addition, they may be afraid to tell anyone when questioned, for fear of punishment. There is no foolproof way to prevent this problem, but it must be discussed with the patient and family. The insufficient time to develop rapport refers not only to the establishment of rapport with the child, but also with the family. This rapport is extremely important in securing the confidence of the family unit, which results in a much smoother induction and in better perioperative care of the child. The other aspect of the establishment of rapport with the family is that it is well known to increase trust in the physician, which decreases the interest of the family in litigation should there be a complication.

Another disadvantage of ambulatory surgery is the insufficient time to obtain further laboratory work or consultation. There is no question that if the clinician feels very strongly that additional laboratory work or consultation is required, it should be obtained. However, there are situations in which the additional information may be useful or helpful but is not mandatory. Since obtaining the additional information or consultation would result in either an inordinate delay in surgery or perhaps cancellation of the surgery until another time, this additional information should not be obtained.

The last disadvantage of ambulatory surgery is that the family must be able to identify postoperative complications and then seek medical assistance. We give all ambulatory patients and their families a list of possible postoperative anesthetic complications as well as a phone number that they may call if they think there is a problem. The responsibility to do so, however, lies with the parents or friends, and not with a nurse on a ward or a physician making postoperative rounds.

There appears to be no limit as to the type or length of surgery that can be performed in an ambulatory surgery unit. However, there are some guidelines that are helpful in determining which patients are best served in this facility.

Patient selection has undergone a great change since the early days of ambulatory surgery, when only ASA I or II patients were treated in an ambulatory setting. Now ASA III patients are routinely treated and, in some centers, ASA IV patients are treated, with the expectation that a certain percentage of these patients will be admitted following surgery. The issue of whether or not to treat emergency patients certainly depends on the type of emergency. Superficial lacerations, fractures, and other less serious problems certainly can be treated on an ambulatory basis, whereas life-threatening or more severe types of injuries need to be treated in an inpatient setting.

The issue of what is required for preoperative evaluation—in terms of both physical and laboratory examinations—has elicited a certain amount of controversy. One of these is the question of time interval: when was the physical examination done and what time interval can elapse before the examination is no longer acceptable? Much of this is determined by local hospital guidelines. Another issue is whether or not the staff physician has to do the preoperative physical examination and what routine laboratory work needs to be done. The Joint Commission on Accreditation of Hospitals is quite clear on the issue of routine laboratory work: there is no such thing as routine laboratory work. The only laboratory evaluations that should be done are those that are indicated.

The surgical procedure may be the final indicator of whether or not the surgery can be performed in an ambulatory setting. Surgical procedures that are very painful, long, or may engender large amounts of blood loss are better done in an inpatient hospital setting.

Patient Selection

The Child With a Runny Nose

The child with a runny nose (see Ch. 9) presents a special problem because so many children present with both allergic disease and respiratory tract infection. It is most difficult to sort out these two diseases—particularly in the time period that is allowed for the preoperative evaluation. Often the patient, having been well 2 or 3 weeks prior to the surgical date when the preoperative physical was done, shows up on the day of surgery with a runny nose. The problem is to determine whether this is a benign or an infectious runny nose. There are those that believe that if the patient has a mild respiratory tract infection it is permissible to do minor surgical procedures such as insertion of middle-ear ventilation tubes. There are others who disagree with this position, believing that the intraoperative and postoperative problems that may occur in children with respiratory tract infections may result in either a bad outcome or the potential for postoperative difficulties. At any rate, the child with a runny nose is one of the more difficult issues for the anesthesiologist. The guideline I use is whether this runny nose is typical for that child. If the mother says this runny nose is different from the usual, serious consideration should be given to postponing surgery. A severe cough or a temperature of 38°C in conjunction with a runny nose would strongly suggest that an infectious process may either be present or be incubating and that elective surgery would best be postponed until there has been an appropriate period for the respiratory tract infection to clear. If the procedure is a short one, such as the insertion of middle-ear ventilation tubes, it may be acceptable to do the surgery. However, it should be remembered that the presence of these children in the preoperative, operative, and postoperative areas exposes other patients and the medical team to the viral infection.

The Child With Heart Disease or a Heart Murmur

Children who have known heart disease or a heart murmur usually have had a consultation with a cardiologist or a pediatrician, and their condition is well known before surgery. It is desirable have a written medical evaluation with a description of the lesion and its hemodynamic consequences. One requirement for the ambulatory patient is that the clinical condition be stable, and if there is any question, the cardiologist or pediatrician should be contacted to make sure that the child is ready for surgery. Antibiotic prophylaxis needs to be considered in all of these patients who have known heart disease or a heart murmur. It is my routine either to administer the prophylaxis orally 1 to 2 hours before surgery or to wait until after the induction of anesthesia, begin an IV, and then administer the antibiotics intravenously.

The child who presents with a new murmur that has not been evaluated is an area of controversy. It is my opinion that if the child is stable, growing well, and has no symptomatology, ambulatory surgery can be performed with a follow-up evaluation of the murmur. Others believe that all murmurs need evaluation before ambulatory surgery.

The Child With Mitral Valve Prolapse

The most common cardiac diagnosis of childhood is mitral valve prolapse, which has been reported in as many as 11 percent in a study of healthy students.[11] Mitral valve prolapse occurs in approximately 5 percent of the adult population.

The primordium of the mitral valve develops during the seventh week of fetal life as the thoracic cage and vertebra are beginning chondrification and ossification. The result is that there may be associated anomalies with mitral valve prolapse, such as pectus excavatum, straight-back syndrome, or connective tissue disorders. The pathophysiology of mitral valve prolapse is a progressive myxomatous degeneration. In addition there are abnormal cardiovascular regulatory mechanisms secondary to an imbalance of the sympathetic nervous system.

The diagnosis of mitral valve prolapse in children is very difficult because there has not been complete agreement as to the diagnostic criteria. In one study in which superior systolic motion of the mitral valve was used as a diagnostic criteria, approximately 35 percent of children in the 10- to 18-year age group were found to have superior systolic motion.[11] Therefore, it has been suggested that more restrictive diagnostic criteria be developed that consider several factors, including the degree of leaflet displacement and the presence of superior systolic motion in more than one echocardiographic view.

The electrocardiogram in these patients is usually normal. The most frequent cardiac dysrhythmia is that of premature ventricular complexes (PVCs). In one study of 103 children with mitral valve prolapse, 16 patients had PVCs with treadmill exercise and 39 had PVCs on ambulatory electrocardiograms.[12] Four patients developed what were considered as serious ventricular ectopia (i.e., multifocal PVCs, ventricular tachycardia, or couplets).

The patient with mitral valve prolapse may present several different clinical problems depending on age and whether or not the patient has a known diagnosis of mitral valve prolapse. Mitral valve prolapse has been reported as a cause of dysrhythmias during anesthesia.[13] Therefore, one of the differential diagnoses of dysrhythmias during anesthesia is mitral valve prolapse. There is an age- and sex-related incidence of the development of mitral valve regurgitation in patients with mitral valve prolapse. After the age of 50, there is a sharp increase in the incidence of the development of severe mitral regurgitation. The incidence in men is approximately double that of women.[14]

Therefore, with patients with a known diagnosis of mitral valve prolapse, certain pathophysiologic concerns need to be kept in mind as the anesthetic management is planned. It is known that emotional upset may precipitate dysrhythmias, therefore it is important to have a preoperative discussion with the patient and the family in order to allay their apprehension and at the same time explain what some of the problems may be. Some patients may benefit from sedative premedication, and this should be discussed with the child and parents. As part of the anesthetic management, it would be important to avoid drugs that are known to produce a tachycardia, since tachycardia will decrease ventricular volume and worsen the prolapse of the mitral leaflets. It is important to maintain a normal intravascular volume for the same reason. If tachycardia or ventricular ectopia develops, it is important to use intravenous β-blockers to control the heart rate. The question of whether to administer antibiotic prophylaxis has not been fully answered because there is a risk of developing anaphylaxis with antibiotics just as there is a risk of developing bacterial endocarditis. However, it should also be remembered that in one study of subacute bacterial endocarditis, mitral valve prolapse accounted for one-third of the cases. The endocarditis has been reported to develop with either regurgitation or merely with a systolic click. Therefore, it would seem prudent to use antibiotic prophylaxis for patients with mitral valve prolapse who are to undergo dental, gastrointestinal, or genitourinary surgery or nasotracheal intubation.

Children who develop persistent unexpected or unexplainable ventricular dysrhythmias during surgery should be referred to a cardiologist for evaluation. Recent innovations in the development of noninvasive cardiac diagnosis may well provide an answer. It would also be helpful to the family to be aware that their child has such a problem, since sudden death has been reported to occur in patients with mitral valve prolapse.

The Child With Down Syndrome

Down syndrome (trisomy 21) is one of the most frequent genetic disorders, occurring in approximately 1 in 800 live births. Infants with Down syndrome are often small for gestational age, with approximately 20 percent weighing less than 2.5 kg at birth. In one series of anesthetic procedures in patients with Down syndrome, 71 percent of patients were below the tenth percentile for weight. Of these patients 44 percent presented for cardiac surgery, so this fact is partially responsible for the large percentage in this low-weight group.[15]

The most frequently associated congenital defect is a congenital heart defect (CHD).[16] The overall incidence of CHD in infants with Down syndrome is approximately 25 percent, and in some series has been reported as high as 50 percent. The most frequently occurring group of lesions in Down syndrome are endocardial cushion defects. Other congenital heart defects, such as tetralogy of Fallot and ventricular septal defects, occur less frequently. With the exception of tetralogy of Fallot, which has reduced pulmonary blood flow due to a right to left shunt, all of these other lesions are associated with an increase in pulmonary blood flow secondary to a left to right shunt. There has been concern that infants with Down syndrome, even those without a cardiovascular defect, have an increase in hypertensive pulmonary vascular disease. This clinical impression has not been substantiated by autopsy findings.

Children with Down syndrome appear to have either an absolute or a relative increase in pulmonary infections. It is not clear whether it is related to the frequent occurrence of congenital heart disease, an immune deficiency, or the hypotonia. At any rate, individual examination of these patients should determine whether they have increased secretions and/or a sensitive airway and what measures should be taken. Children with a sensitive airway and secretions tend to obstruct during the induction of anesthesia, often terrorizing the anesthesiologist with episodes of laryngospasm, apnea, cyanosis, and, occasionally, bradycardia. These children should be evaluated to see if they would benefit from the administration of an anticholinergic before anesthesia. There has been concern that children with Down syndrome have an increased sensitivity to atropine, particularly with an increased response of heart rate. However, these concerns have not been documented, and several studies have shown no unexpected problems with the usual doses of atropine in these children. Therefore appropriate doses of an anticholinergic can be used as in any other patient. Glycopyrrolate is the preferred anticholinergic, since it is a better drying agent and does not appear to have the same degree of tachycardia.

Children with Down syndrome do have the potential for perioperative airway problems.[15] The increased propensity for respiratory tract infections can result in a child with a sensitive airway. In addition, however, the child with Down syndrome has a relatively large tongue, a flat small nose, and hypotonia. All of these factors make airway management more difficult both during induction and at the time of extubation. Anesthetic technique needs to be tailored toward having the child's airway reflexes as intact as possible at the end of surgery. For this reason, heavy intraoperative narcotic analgesia should be used only if the patient is going to remain intubated for a period of time. If extubation is anticipated at the end of surgery, administration of small doses of narcotic along with regional anesthesia would be the method of choice for postoperative analgesia, followed by small doses of additional narcotic titrated in the postoperative period as indicated. In the study by Kobel et al., 23 percent of the endotracheal tubes inserted were smaller than those that would have been predicted for age.[15] Therefore, one needs to be prepared to use a smaller size endotracheal tube than expected for age, carefully checking to make sure that there is a leak with positive-pressure ventilation (15 to 25 cmH$_2$O). If intubation is difficult even with a smaller tube, consideration should be given to cancelling the surgery and/or calling in a pediatric endoscopist to diagnose the reason for the airway difficulty. The clinician needs to have a high degree of suspicion for subglottic stenosis, particularly if the endotracheal tube does not pass easily and there is no air leak. A history of what happens to the child's breathing pattern with a respiratory infection may increase suspicion about subglottic stenosis. Another clue is if the child has a history of asthma, which may actually be subglottic stenosis.

Another major problem is the fact that 10 to 15 percent of all patients with Down syndrome have a tendency for atlantoaxial instability. Approximately 10 percent of patients with this instability will end up with an overt subluxation. Two recent cases have been reported in the anesthesia literature in which the patient developed subluxation at some time in the perioperative period.[17,18] Both of these children had undergone major cardiovascular surgery and the exact time that the subluxation occurred was not clear. In both cases, the child was symptomatic at discharge. The cord compression was discovered on a follow-up visit and surgical repair resulted in a good outcome. The conclusion of these investigators was that these children need aggressive evaluation to determine if there are symptoms or signs of atlantoaxial instability. There are differences of opinion as to what type of medical workup is indicated. One consideration for the anesthesiologist is whether an orthopaedic or neurologic evaluation before surgery would be useful. The other issue is whether cervical spine films are indicated. Most pediatricians would obtain a cervical spine series as part of the usual evaluation of a child with Down syndrome. The radiographs would be obtained at age 3 years or older. One recent study of neurologic complications in patients with Down syndrome strongly suggested that in the cases of symptomatic subluxation that have been reported, the patients had neurologic symptoms for a period of 1 month before the actual subluxation was determined.[19] Davidson believed that radiographs were not necessary, and that if a neurologic examination was performed, it would be more effective. Therefore, the major issue for the anesthesiologist at the time of surgery is whether there are any neurologic changes in the period preceding surgery and what types of neurologic changes that are suggestive of cord compression to look for after surgery. The major physical findings are those of weakness, a positive Babinski sign, increased deep tendon reflexes, and incontinence. Another very important sign and symptom is pain in the neck and torticollis. The parent should be aware of these symptoms and should be looking for them in the postoperative period. These parents need continual emotional support in the raising of these children.

The Premature Nursery Graduate

Another major thrash for the anesthesiologist is that of the premature nursery graduate. Advances in medical technology have resulted in the survival of a large percentage of premature infants who have undergone intensive care therapy after birth, and these infants may present to surgery with a whole host of neurologic and respiratory problems. The three major concerns in premature nursery graduates are residual lung disease, subglottic stenosis, and apnea. The most frequent surgical procedures are examination under anesthesia, retinopathy of prematurity therapy, and herniorrhaphy. There is no question that the hernias found in the first year of life are different from those found after 1 year of life, as those of the first year of life have a much higher incidence of incarceration (31 percent).[20] Therefore, it is inappropriate to delay repair of hernias until the child is 1 year of age. For that reason, it is important to learn how to evaluate the premature infant and to determine at what conceptual age surgery can be performed on an ambulatory basis. Infants who have been intubated and ventilated are at risk for developing residual lung disease,[21] the most severe form of which is bronchopulmonary dysplasia. It is hoped that information about the child is available at the time he is evaluated for any type of surgery. If in doubt, surgical procedures on premature nursery graduates with bronchopulmonary dysplasia should be on an inpatient basis because they can then be more appropriately evaluated and treated.

Conceptual Age and Ambulatory Surgery

There has been an enormous debate over what postconceptual age is appropriate for ambulatory surgery in the premature nursery graduate.[22-24] The postconceptual age is the gestational age plus the postnatal age. There is great variability in the opinions; they range from allowing ambulatory surgery in the premature nursery graduate at 44 to 46 weeks postconceptual age in some centers to allowing ambulatory surgery only when the infant has reached 60 weeks of postconceptual age in other centers. Unfortunately, the studies that have looked at these various age groups have not studied similar types of patients and the surgical techniques employed. However, at the present time it would appear that the premature nursery graduate with no other high-risk condition may undergo ambulatory surgery somewhere between 48 and 50 weeks of postconceptual age. If there are special problems, such as bronchopulmonary dysplasia, or any other concern on the part of the physician, consideration should be given to admitting these patients overnight.

Postoperative Apnea in Former Premature Infants

There is an extensive literature that documents that premature infants undergoing general anesthesia at various postconceptual ages are prone to develop apnea and/or bradycardia in the perioperative period. The problem is thought to be due to an immature respiratory center, and the incidence of these episodes is inversely correlated with gestational age and weight. Furthermore, it is thought that the immature respiratory center of the preterm infant is more easily depressed by anesthetics, endorphins, and other drugs. The following definition of apnea came from the clinical studies of Welborn et al.[25] Brief apnea is defined as a respiratory pause of less than 15 seconds not associated with bradycardia. Prolonged or potentially life-threatening apnea is defined as a respiratory pause of 15 seconds or longer or less than 15 seconds if accompanied by bradycardia. The key factor here is the bradycardia, which is defined as a heart rate of less than 100 bpm for at least 5 seconds. Periodic breathing is defined as three or more periods of apnea lasting from 3 to 15 seconds separated by less than 20 seconds of normal respiration. The usual way to report periodic breathing is as a percentage of time in the normal respiratory pattern that periodic breathing occurs. To determine this, the total time in minutes of periodic breathing is divided by the total sleep time in minutes to determine the percentage of periodic breathing. Less than 1 percent periodic breathing is considered normal. Neonatologists for a long time have used methylxanthines in the treatment of the apnea of prematurity. Caffeine has the distinct advantage over theophylline of being a more potent central nervous system and respiratory stimulant and having fewer side effects.[26] There is a significant reduction in the elimination rate of drugs in infants; neonates will have an elimination half-life of caffeine that varies from 37 to 231 hours.

The major problem with general anesthesia in the premature infant under 46 weeks of postconceptual age is the development of apnea and bradycardia. Welborn and her colleagues have demonstrated quite conclusively that caffeine can greatly minimize and in some age groups eliminate the problem of postoperative apnea.[25] They recommend that caffeine 10 mg/kg IV be administered at the beginning of surgery. The type of caffeine used is a caffeine base, which needs to be made up in the hospital pharmacy. However, the numbers are small yet, and we have to wait for further studies to be absolutely sure of its preventive effects in these patients. This group of patients (under 48 to 50 weeks postconceptual age) still need to be admitted and monitored overnight.

Anesthetic Techniques

A great deal has been made about the various anesthetic techniques for ambulatory surgery, but it is my opinion that the anesthetic technique should be tailored to the needs of the patient and that it makes no difference if the patient is an inpatient or an outpatient. This means that if the patient needs rectal methohexital for induction, it should be used even though it may prolong the recovery period. For the child between 1 and 5 years of age, I prefer to use rectal methohexital as an induction technique. For the child aged 5 to 12 years, we allow the parents to be present for an inhalational induction, and if the child will accept it, we start an IV and do an intravenous induction. The techniques used for induction and maintenance depend on the skill of the anesthesiologist and the needs of the patient.

Postoperative Analgesia

There has been a great deal of controversy about appropriate postoperative analgesia for outpatients. The issue is patient comfort. If morphine is needed, it should be given for postoperative pain. We use a combination of narcotics and local and regional anesthesia whenever possible (see Ch. 11). We do not require that the patient be able to ambulate before discharge, as this would mean that caudal anesthesia would have a limited application in the ambulatory surgery setting and that the patient would have to remain in the ambulatory surgery unit for a long period of time.

Discharge Criteria

Discharge criteria is also an area of controversy. It is my opinion that a patient should be discharged when comfortable and essentially recovered from the anesthesia, and when the parents feel comfortable about taking the child home. We give ample intravenous fluids so that we do *not* require patients be able to take oral fluids before discharge. It is my opinion that premature forcing of oral fluids will either cause or increase postoperative vomiting. Many patients vomit on the trip home, therefore our instructions are that oral fluids should be started only when the patient is hungry, not thirsty. There is no need to require that a patient ambulate before being discharged. Having the patient get up and walk around is another cause of postoperative vomiting. The patient should be kept as quiet as possible and allowed to be transported home according to the criteria listed above.

Admission Criteria

The first tenet of ambulatory surgery admission is, if there is any question about discharging the patient, the patient should be admitted. The parents should be carefully questioned about their feelings, and if they have any hesitation about taking the child home, the child should be admitted. Other indications for postoperative admission include uncontrolled pain, pernicious vomiting, croup that is not improving or is getting worse, and aspiration pneumonia or postobstructive pulmonary edema.

REFERENCES

1. Brouillette RT, Fernbach SK, Hunt CE: Obstructive sleep apnea in infants and children. J Pediatr 100:31, 1982
2. Kravath RE, Pollak CP, Borowiecki B, et al: Obstructive sleep apnea and death associated with surgical correction of velopharyngeal incompetence. J Pediatr 96:645, 1980
3. Roa NL, Moss KS: Treacher Collins syndrome with sleep apnea: Anesthetic considerations. Anesthesiology 60:71, 1984
4. Lerman J, Eustis S, Smith DR: Effect of droperidol pretreatment on postanesthetic vomiting in children undergoing strabismus surgery. Anesthesiology 65:322, 1986
5. Christensen, S, Farrow-Gillespie A, Lerman J: Incidence of emesis and postanesthetic recovery after strabismus surgery in children: A comparison of droperidol and lidocaine. Anesthesiology 70:251, 1989
6. Gal TJ, Cooperman LH: Hypertension in the immediate postoperative period. Br J Anaesth 47:70, 1975
7. Koka BV, Jeon IS, Andre JM, et al: Postintubation croup in children. Anesth Analg 56:501, 1977
8. Finholt DA, Henry DB, Raphaely RC: The "leak" test—A standard method for assessing tracheal tube fit in pediatric patients. Anesthesiology 61:A450, 1984
9. Kairys SW, Olmstead EM, O'Connor GT: Steroid treatment of laryngotracheitis: A meta-analysis of the evidence from randomized trials. Pediatrics 83:5683, 1989
10. Westley CR, Cotton EK, Brooks JG, et al: Nebulized racemic epinephrine by IPPB for the treatment of croup. Am J Dis Child 132:484, 1978
11. Warth DC, King ME, Cohen JM, et al: Prevalence of mitral valve prolapse in normal children. J Am Coll Cardiol 5:1173, 1985
12. Kavey R-EW, Blackman MS, Sondheimer HM, Byrum CJ: Ventricular arrhythmias and mitral valve prolapse in childhood. J Pediatr 105:885, 1984
13. Berry FA, Lake CL, Johns RA, Rogers BM: Mitral valve prolapse—Another cause of intraoperative dysrhythmias in the pediatric patient. Anesthesiology 62:662, 1985
14. Wilcken DEL, Hickey AJ: Lifetime risk for patients with mitral valve prolapse of developing severe valve regurgitation requiring surgery. Circulation 78:10, 1988
15. Kobel M, Creighton RE, Steward DJ: Anaesthetic considerations in Down's syndrome: Experience with 100 patients and a review of the literature. Can Anaesth Soc J 29(6):593, 1982
16. Greenwood RD, Nadas AS: The clinical course of cardiac disease in Down's syndrome. Pediatrics 58:893, 1976
17. Moore RA, McNicholas KW, Warran SP: Atlantoaxial subluxation with symptomatic spinal cord compression in a child with Down's syndrome. Anesth Analg 66:89, 1987
18. Williams JP, Somerville GM, Miner ME, Reilly D: Atlanto-axial subluxation and trisomy-21: Another perioperative complication. Anesthesiology 67:253, 1987
19. Davidson RG: Atlantoaxial instability in individuals with Down syndrome: A fresh look at the evidence. Pediatrics 81:857, 1988

20. Rescorla FJ, Grosfeld JL: Inguinal hernia repair in the perinatal period and early infancy: Clinical considerations. J Pediatr Surg 19:832, 1984

21. Kraybill EN, Runyan DK, Bose CL, Khan JH: Risk factors for chronic lung disease in infants with birth weights of 751 to 1000 grams. J Pediatr 115:115, 1989

22. Liu LMP, Cote CJ, Goudsouzian NG, et al: Life-threatening apnea in infants recovering from anesthesia. Anesthesiology 59:506, 1983

23. Kurth CD, Spitzer AR, Broennle AM, Downes JJ: Postoperative apnea in preterm infants. Anesthesiology 66:483, 1987

24. Welborn LG, Ramirez N, Oh TH, et al: Postanesthetic apnea and periodic breathing in infants. Anesthesiology 65:658, 1986

25. Welborn LG, Hannallah RS, Rink R, et al: High-dose caffeine suppresses postoperative apnea in former preterm infants. Anesthesiology 71:347, 1989

26. Murat I, Moriette G, Blin MC, et al: The efficacy of caffeine in the treatment of recurrent idiopathic apnea in premature infants. J Pediatr 99(6):984, 1981

INDEX

Page numbers followed by f denote figures; those followed by t denote tables.

in children, 28
with difficult airway, 29–30
dosage, by route of administration, 26t, 135t
indications for, 26, 135–136
during laryngoscopy, 30
in older infants, 28
oral, pharmacokinetics of, 30
preceding bronchoscopy, 210–211
routine administration of, controversy over, 26
safe, for MH-susceptible patients, 402t
with sensitive airway, 29
in treatment of asthma, 303
Antidiuretic hormone
appropriate secretion of, 97–98
differentiated from inappropriate secretion of antidiuretic hormone, 100
hyponatremia caused by, 117
inappropriate secretion of. *See* Inappropriate secretion of antidiuretic hormone
inhibition of, 96
release of, 96
Antiemetics, as premedications, 30–33
Antifog solution, 205
Apgar, Virginia, 11
Apgar score, in congenital diaphragmatic hernia, 142
Apnea
physiology of, 175
postoperative
ambulatory surgery and, 429–430
anesthetic technique and, 161–162
Arnold-Chiari malformation
anesthetic management in surgery for, 357
defined, 357
Arteriovenous malformations, anesthetic management in treatment of, 352
Artificial airways
supportive care of, in acute epiglottitis, 254–255
in treatment of laryngotracheobronchitis, 262–263
Aspiration
as cause of death, 33
in child with sensitive airway or secretions, 275
foreign body. *See* Foreign body aspiration
indicators of risk, 33
Aspiration pneumonitis, in differential diagnosis of pulmonary edema, 369
Asthma, 285–322
α-adrenergic drugs in treatment of, 300, 301t, 302t, 303

allergic, immunopathologic agents potentially operative in, 291, 291t
anesthesia in child with, 309–315
anesthesia maintenance in patient with, 313–314
anticholinergic drugs in treatment of, 303
atopic or allergic, 286
classification of, 286t, 286–288
clinical evaluation of, 295–298
confused with epiglottitis, 246
corticosteroids in treatment of, 305–306
cromolyn sodium in treatment of, 303, 305
dual-phase response in, 294
effects on pulmonary physiology, 294–295
emotional factors in, 287
exercise-induced, 286
extrinsic, 286
glucocorticoid action in, 305t, 305–306
impaired α-adrenergic responses in, 293t
incidence of, 285, 309
induction in patient with, 312–313
intraoperative bronchospasm in patient with, treatment of, 314–315
intrinsic, 286, 287–288
laboratory findings in, 296–297
morbidity and mortality from, 285
muscle relaxants in patient with, 313
pathogenesis of, 289–295
autonomic regulation disorders in, 293
disordered immune function in, 293
epithelial damage in, 293
smooth muscle alterations in, 292
theories of, 292–293
pathology of, 288–289
macroscopic findings, 288
microscopic findings, 288–289
patient history in, 295
premedication in patient with, 311–312
preoperative evaluation in, 310–311
pulmonary function testing in, 298
pulmonary function values in children with, 297t
radiography in diagnosis of, 296
and respiratory tract infection, 286–287
signs and symptoms in, 296
theophylline in treatment of, 298, 300
treatment of, 298–307
immunotherapy, 306
pharmacologic agents, 298–306
physical therapy, 307
psychotherapy, 307
Atelectasis
as complication of respiratory tract infection, 281f, 281–283, 282f
in infant, 130